Aspects of Human Nutrition

World Review of Nutrition and Dietetics

Vol. 57

Series Editor
Geoffrey H. Bourne, Grenada, West Indies

KARGER

Basel · München · Paris · London · New York · New Delhi · Singapore · Tokyo · Sydney

Aspects of Human Nutrition

Volume Editor
Geoffrey H. Bourne
St. Georges University School of Medicine, Grenada, West Indies

26 figures and 36 tables, 1988

KARGER

Basel · München · Paris · London · New York · New Delhi · Singapore · Tokyo · Sydney

World Review of Nutrition and Dietetics

Library of Congress Cataloging-in-Publication Data
Aspects of human nutrition.
(World review of nutrition and dietetics; vol. 57)
Includes bibliographies and index.
1. Nutrition. I. Bourne, Geoffrey H. (Geoffrey Howard), 1909-. II. Series.
[DNLM: 1. Nutrition.
W1 W0898 v. 57 / QU 145 A8379]
QP141.A1W59 vol. 57 612.3 s [612.3] 88-9155
ISBN 3-8055-4810-9

Bibliographic Indices
This publication is listed in bibliographic services, including Current Contents® and Index Medicus.

Drug Dosage

The authors and the publisher have exerted every effort to ensure that drug selection and dosage set forth in this text are in accord with current recommendations and practice at the time of publication. However, in view of ongoing research, changes in government regulations, and the constant flow of information relating to drug therapy and drug reactions, the reader is urged to check the package insert for each drug for any change in indications and dosage and for added warnings and precautions. This is particularly important when the recommended agent is a new and/or infrequently employed drug.

Printed in Switzerland by Thür AG, Offsetdruck, Pratteln
ISBN 3-8055-4810-9

Advisory Board

Contents

Wld Rev. Nutr. Diet., vol. 57, pp. 1–23 (Karger, Basel 1988)

The Knowledge of Human Nutrition and the Peoples of the World[1]

Debabar Banerji

Centre of Social Medicine and Community Health, School of Social Sciences, Jawaharlal Nehru University, New Delhi, India

Contents

Social Origins of the Science of Human Nutrition

By projecting the current knowledge concerning nutritional requirements back in history, it can safely be asserted that when human beings have been able to acquire adequate resources to satisfy their hunger and appetite, it is very unlikely that they would have suffered from deficiency of one or more nutritional elements to such an extent as to manifest specific forms of malnutrition or undernutrition on a large scale. Develop-

[1] Draft of a paper for publication in the *International Review of Nutrition and Dietetics.*

ment of a superior nervous system, which enables the humans to learn, to retain learning and to transmit the learnt knowledge to the fellow humans, has given them an overwhelming advantage over other living beings in the struggle for existence. It has also enabled them to have enormous power to exploit and 'conquer' nature. Because of population growth and migration, human beings have colonised different parts of the globe. They have adapted themselves to widely different ecological conditions and in this process developed different food habits. Despite the very different physical conditions of living, the incidence or prevalence of nutritional disorders was negligible, as long as they were able to eat well.

However, different types of nutritional disorders emerged as public health problems as man started to exploit man. This led to institution of slavery and employment of serfs and class and/or caste differentiation and exploitation. Wars, feudal relations of production and industrialisation and the resulting urbanisation precipitated famines and various degrees and forms of malnutrition and undernutrition. Thus, the root causes of nutritional disorders are social, economic and political. When these factors generate conditions where people are not able to eat well and/or are forced to live under bad environmental conditions, they lead to various deficiency disorders. Significantly, under such social conditions this fundamental basis of nutritional status of a population is also not expected to receive adequate attention. Instead, very active efforts are made to generate an enormous body of knowledge exploring the minutiae of specific nutritional disorders. The symptoms are emphasised and so the root cause gets obscured. As would be pointed out later, sometimes active efforts are made to develop nutritional ideas which subserve commercial and political interests.

The classical case of high incidence of scurvy among seamen undertaking long voyages in sailing ships and of the discovery of antiscorbutic properties of citrus fruits and some other green vegetables was the forerunner of use of citrus fruit juice in the diet to prevent deficiency of vitamin C. The citrus food industry generated such an intensive motivation among people to consume the vitamin that a glass of citrus fruit juice has become a standard cultural fixture of the breakfast table of most people in Western countries. It is noteworthy that in the excitement of the discovery of antiscorbutic properties of citrus fruits and because of the zeal to expand the market for citrus fruits and synthetic vitamin C, it was overlooked that scurvy occurred on a large scale mostly under very exceptional conditions, e.g. during long voyages in sailing ships, during long sieges and when mothers had to go for work, and substitute mother's milk with improperly prepared milk powders. Compulsions of the market ordained that knowledge concerning vitamin C and scurvy in the practice of human nutrition should favour the industries which produce them; scientific knowledge was so manipulated and twisted that consumers became a mere means for expansion of the industries.

Expectedly, the desperate conditions of living which resulted from the exploitative social relations during the Industrial Revolution in the West brought into sharper focus some other ecology-related nutritional disorders – rickets, osteomalacia, night blindness, keratomalacia and, as pointed out above, infantile scurvy. These disorders were mere symptoms of the wider malady of the conditions which compelled large masses of people to live under most degrading ecological settings. It is, therefore, logical that these disorders became virtually unknown when the living conditions of the masses were improved in Western countries. Similarly, large outbreaks of beriberi occurred only under extreme conditions of famines and wars. In fact, while conclusive evidence of pathological outcome of eating polished rice was established in birds, very few cases of clinical beriberi were observed among the millions of humans who had been eating polished rice for generations.

It may also be noted that people did manifest deficiency symptoms when they colonised some special regions – iodine deficiency areas and areas having high fluoride content in drinking water are classical examples. However, even in these special cases little work has been done to explain why the poor suffer more than the rich; nor has much effort been made to study the process of formation of entirely new goitrous zones. Is it possible to isolate iodine-deficiency simple goitre from other environmental conditions where the disease is endemic?

Thus, outbreaks of some of the classical cases of nutritional disorders are rooted in the special ecological, social and economic conditions. They can be traced back to widespread disruption of ecological balance which is associated with exploitative relations of production. Social and economic forces which create such conditions also ensured that such issues are kept out of the body of knowledge of nutrition sciences. Instead, market forces were allowed free play to actively generate nutritional knowledge which helps in increasing the sale of the food and drugs industry.

A noteworthy feature of forming the body of knowledge of the science of human nutrition is that in the course of time, because of pressure from market forces, knowledge concerning these nutritional disorders (along many others) got uprooted from their ecological and cultural moor-ıgs and became isolated entities, with their specific curative agents which are derived mostly from the products of the pharmaceutical industry. Nutritional education made rapid strides to 'sell' such ideas concerning nutritional disorders and their cures.

Overlap with Biochemistry and Other Medical Sciences

Tracing the history of nutrition science leads to another geneological line. Apparently to gain respectability as a 'science', it has claimed its pedigree from chemistry, biochemistry, physiology and the clinical medical sciences. It has adopted aspects of knowledge generated in these fields as its own. Therefore, it also shares some aspects of social origins of these sciences. Joseph Priestley, Antoine Lavoisier, Carl Voit and Louis Pasteur form a part of the pantheon of nutrition science, side by side with Eijkman, Atwater, McCarrison, Hopkins, McCollum, Rose, Williams and King. This cross-fertilization triggered a series of scientific breakthroughs: identification of the nutritional elements, balanced diets, digestion of food and working out the complex pathways in the metabolism of the different elements. Various forms of primary nutritional disorders were identified as outcomes of specific nutritional deficiencies. Reciprocally, nutritional science was utilised in understanding different aspects of etiology, pathogenesis and clinical management of a wide variety of general diseases. Nutrition education, food processing, food safety and animal nutrition became additional components of nutrition science.

Undoubtedly, these advancements made major contributions to the body of knowledge of nutrition science and of biochemistry, physiology and the clinical sciences. However, they also had adverse consequences that are of far-reaching significance. With the increasing 'scientific' content in the body of knowledge of nutrition, the focus of studies moved farther and farther away from the study of problems of nutrition in humans in their ecological settings. Biochemical laboratories and animal houses became the major places for study of human nutrition. Some of these spilled into clinical wards of hospitals. Gussow [38] has called it 'scientification of food'.

This was not unintentional. Researches in laboratories and animal houses were actively promoted by the market interests because nutrition became a very happy hunting ground for rapid growth and proliferation of the food and drugs industry in affluent Western countries. Nutrition scientists had talked of a high incidence of protein deficiency among people and they advocated use of animal (first-class) proteins as against 'second-class' vegetable proteins. This created a large market for the protein food industry. Later, it was conceded that the 'class' concept of proteins is not tenable and that estimates of incidence of protein deficiency was highly exaggerated: most often a negative protein balance occurred because, in the absence of adequate carbohydrates to meet the calorie requirements, body proteins had to be burnt. The sale of 'essential' amino acids was boosted by exploiting the experiments of Rose on rats. Later, it turned out that very few cases of specific amino acid deficiency were observed in humans, even after they were exposed to prolonged conditions of food deprivations – for example, during a stay in a concentration camp, during hunger strikes or famines. The sale of vitamins, minerals, including so-called trace elements, and various forms of tonics skyrocketed. Bottles of specially 'developed' combinations of vitamins and minerals became common fixtures of dining tables of affluent people. Later, epidemiological analyses revealed that less than one in a hundred of the consumers would have suffered any form of avitaminosis or other deficiency conditions had they not taken the pills prescribed by physicians and nutritionists (at the insistance of the food and drug industry). The industry also rapidly expanded the market for baby food by extolling their virtues, but it was only discovered later that in many poverty-stricken countries, its high-pressure sales promotion actually led to the deaths of large numbers of children [68].

Professionalisation of the Practice of Nutrition

The forces which have shaped the body of knowledge of human nutrition also influenced the formation of the profession of nutritionists. Assessment of the nutritional status of people, determination of nutritional requirements, nutritional analysis of different diets and making recommendations for balanced diets, diagnosis and management of primary nutritional disorders, meeting dietary requirements in certain other clinical conditions, cooking and processing of foods and food toxicology are some of the major areas which came within the purview of this profession. In addition, there are the well-known areas of interests which it shares with the medical sciences, including biochemistry. Obviously, these areas do not carry enough weight, either in the form of research or as action programmes, to place nutritionists very high in the prestige hierarchy of professions. Because of this, the profession has not been able to attract adequate numbers of talented persons. This has formed a vicious cycle. Nutritionists have become inward looking and insular and, therefore, more vulnerable to exploitation by market forces.

In fact, so pervasive has been the influence of the market forces in research and practice of human nutrition that a new subprofession has come into existence. This is the profession of nutrition education. Unwittingly or otherwise, there have been several occasions when nutritionists and nutrition educators had become covert sales agents of the food and drugs industry – selling 'first-class' proteins, 'essential' amino acids, vitamins and minerals, for instance. Because of their preoccupation with findings from researches conducted in laboratories, animal houses or clinical wards, the ecological, epidemiological, sociological, economic and political factors which influence the nutritional status of an individual or a group did not receive adequate attention. Pleading to look at 'food through a macroscope', Gussow [38] observed: 'Fearing... that we would not be taken seriously as scientists... we have attended to the ever smaller and smaller; breaking down food, food handling, food processing, food functions, into manageable, microscopic pieces; looking at the isolated effects of the isolated behaviors on isolated food substances in isolated biological systems. I believe it is time now for some of us in the field of food and nutrition to take up our macroscopes rather than our microscopes, to begin the task of looking at connections not merely between nutrients and cells; or between food handling, food textures and food toxins; but of looking at the connections between farmers and producers; between food policies and environmental policies; between toxic wastes and the opportunity to produce safe, affordable food; between tax policies, development policies, and landuse policies and our ability to retain farmland; between the cost of energy and the cost of food.'

Going still further in subservience to vested interests, sometimes nutritionists have also ended up in offering active support to the dominant political power centres by blaming the victims for their unsatisfactory nutritional conditions. Health educators are examples of another professional group which is often used by a political system to blame the victims for their poor state of health [13]. The profession of home economists also took over some of the functions of nutritionists by making a science of home making [38]. Social workers also belong to this group. It is important that the social and political contexts of origin of such professionals are properly analysed.

Nyswander [48], who had been one of the founders of the profession of health education, had deeply regretted such approaches which divert people's energy from changing the social context of behaviour to changing of individual behaviour. Looking back at her work at the end of her career, she observed: 'My efforts were expanded in working out symptoms of closed societies, the basic conditions giving rise to symptoms were untouched... Have I actually helped maintain the status quo in these situations? Have I not taught people to accept those gifts approved by the establishment which would make life more bearable but which would not threaten the power of the establishment?' In market-dominated countries, no profession can escape the influence of the market forces. However, in the cases of nutrition, nutrition education, home economics, social work and health education, the influence is much more pervasive and dominant. In fact, they can be called the more favoured proginies of the market forces.

Illich [40] has given an account of the awe some distortion of the practice even of so 'strong' a discipline as medicine – through generation of various types of iatrogenesis, professionalisation, centralisation and commercialisation. Professionals simply cannot claim political or social neutrality. In fact, they are products of these forces and they have to make an active effort to dissociate themselves from that legacy.

Social and political analysis of the generation of knowledge of science of human nutrition and its practice and professionalisation should thus form a part of the wider analysis generation of knowledge of the science as a whole. This should be a prelude to formation of plans of social, political and scientific and technological action to correct the distortions. As pointed out in the following paragraphs, the distortions are much more serious in countries of the third world and their implications are of much more far-reaching significance. Actions to correct the distortions are therefore far more urgent in these countries.

Discussion of the implications of using the conventional knowledge of human nutrition in third world countries and identification of the issue in the formulation of alternative approaches requires covering of a wide area. As many of the issues discussed are overlapping in nature (e.g. primacy of calorie requirements and the question of poverty and its measurement), it becomes impossible to totally avoid repetition of certain arguments.

Implications for Third World Countries

In the first place, these countries are much poorer than those of the West. There are large numbers of people who are hungry and who live under degrading environmental conditions. There has been economic exploitation of third world countries by the industrialised countries during the colonial period. After the third world countries attained political independence, grossly unfair terms of trade have been imposed on them. Within individual countries, there is acute polarisation of the population between the rich and the poor and there is very pronounced social and economic injustice. These are the major causes of poverty and hunger. Food habits are different as the people in third world countries have very different ecological and cultural backgrounds.

Secondly, as in any other field of science and technology, the flow of knowledge in the field of human nutrition is also almost a one-way process, with the third world being at the receiving end. There is little endogenous generation of knowledge. There is abject dependence on the West in all aspects – in developing the body of knowledge, in obtaining equipment, in developing research ideas and in the education and training of personnel.

There is thus a strong streak in the research and practice of human nutrition which is culturally alien to peoples of these countries. Undoubtedly, scientific knowledge has universal relevance. However, it is often overlooked that decisions to generate aspects of scientific knowledge have strong social, economic and political overtones. Further, around the central core of scientific knowledge, technology has acquired a thick envelope of sociocultural accretions of Western countries [45]. Nutritionists in third world countries have not been very successful in performing the difficult task of separating the thick sociocultural overcoatings from the central scientific core and then placing the latter within a new envelope which blends properly with the local sociocultural situation.

They preferred the softer option of remaining dependent on Western scholars. They got ready made models and modules for teaching, practice and research. Delving into intricacies of working out metabolic pathways of different dietary elements with the mediation of enzymes, vitamins and hormones and involvement in various forms of experiments on animals tended to impart a scientific aura to the profession. This also helped promotion of international exchange of ideas among nutritionists which, in turn, tended to provide justification for the dependence of scholars in the third world on those from the West. Under such conditions they became easy victims for manipulation by the food and drugs industry. Development of an above-down approach of nutrition education was the next logical step. Nutrition educators were employed to exhort people to give up many of their 'traditional' views on nutrition and adopt 'scientific' approaches suggested by the professionals. Bottle-feeding, high-protein diets and vitamins, tonics and trace element supplements are examples of such 'scientific' approaches.

Lately, a still more ominous trend has appeared in the field of human nutrition. This comes perilously close to misuse or distortion of science to subserve the dominant political ideology. It was declared, on the basis of laboratory and field studies, that severe malnutrition during late pregnancy and early infancy causes permanent brain damage [25, 47, 52]. This assertion implies that the body of a child sacrifices the vital brain cells during nutritional deprivations well before other less vital cells (e.g. muscles and connective tissues) and that there are tools available to measure permanent mental damage caused by destruction of brain cells and that these tools are equally reliable and valid cross-culturally. This contention received widespread acceptance, so much so that the then Secretary General of the United Nations [67] issued a special message, expressing deep concern over the danger of hundreds of millions of children becoming permanent mental cripples and urging immediate action to bridge what he called the global 'protein gap'. Exponents of this view felt so confident or they were in so much hurry that they did not care to collect epidemiological data on the present stage of mental health of persons who formed the infant cohorts when they were exposed to severe deprivation during the Russian Revolution, during the Bengal Famine or during their incarceration in concentration camps during World War II [5]. Nor did they appear to be concerned over the political implications of their contentions: that in a totalitarian society a dictator may invoke the 'scientific' findings of these eminent nutritionists to declare that a large proportion of the population of that country as mentally retarded because they suffered from severe nutritional deprivations during the very early phases of their lives [5]. They could then be condemned to work as 'hewers of wood' and 'drawers of water' in the service of the ruling class.

Not learning lessons from the case of nutrition and mental health, the cry of permanent mental retardation has once again been raised – this time in relation to endemic goitre [41, 42]. Indeed, there might be some cases of cretinism among those who suffer from endemic goitre and this might cause some mental damage. But what does that mean against the background of ecological conditions which lead to an infant mortality of anything between 200 and 300 per 1,000 live births and maternal mortality of more than 10 per 1,000 child births and high mortality and morbidity rates due to a host of infectious diseases and due to severe undernutrition? Concern for the mental damage of the cretins ought to have been balanced with the far more extensive deaths and debilities due to other unfavourable ecological conditions. Even within the narrow confines of the problem of endemic goitre, the focus ought to have been on political and administrative factors which had hampered iodisation of the salt in the goitrous regions over the past 30 years or more [28, 29].

Again, ignoring widespread prevalance of hunger, degrading conditions of the environment, high unemployment, landlessness and drought, some nutrition statistitions have developed arguments to claim that the actual estimates of prevalence of malnutrition in India and other third world countries have been grossly overestimated; they have gone further to claim that smaller size of people is an adaptive phenomenon and that they are nutritionally 'normal' for their size: small is beautiful [57, 64].

Major Nutritional Issues in the Third World

The Primacy of Calorie Requirements

It is interesting that it took nutritionists so much of time to 'discover' that calorie deficiency is by far the most common nutritional disorder in the third world [30, 59]. It is also worth noting that this important finding was made by nutrition research workers from the third world. Had this issue been looked at from the other end, it could have been seen that in the very process of food consumption to meet the calorie requirement, over a period of time, it becomes very 'difficult' for a subject to 'avoid' consuming proteins, fats, vitamins and minerals to degrees which meet the 'normal' body requirements for these components. This forms the basis of the contention that if a person is able to consume food which meet the calorie requirements, most often the requirements of the other components are also met. Prevalence of protein deficiency symptoms are not common among these people. Prevalence of symptoms of deficiency of a specific amino acid is still rarer, if not absent altogether. Prevalence of protein deficiency may be higher in some African countries where the staple food has higher starch content. It will also not be common to get cases of iron or calcium deficiency

among individuals who are able to have enough food to satisfy their hunger. Similarly, it would be rare to find cases of beriberi, pellagra, scurvy, rickets, osteomalacia, night-blindness and kerotomalacia in this group. Indeed, such conditions of avitaminosis are rare even among those who barely manage to satisfy their hunger for 6 or 9 months in a year.

It can thus be concluded that if people get opportunities to get enough food to satisfy their hunger and meet their calorie needs, the need for intervention from nutritionists will be limited only to a few special conditions. For dealing with the rest of the problems, they will have to get involved in the social, economic and political issues that come in the way of satiation of hunger and meeting the calorie needs. This opens up large new areas of interests in the field of human nutrition. One can go further and assert that it would be decidedly counter-productive, if nutritionists allow themselves to be manipulated by the food and drugs industry in exaggerating the extent of prevalence or incidence of nutritional disorders which need intervention in the form of vitamins, minerals or tonics.

There have been numerous instances of prescription of vitamin C by physicians to desperately poor people even when there is no evidence whatsoever of deficiency of that vitamin. Sometimes the prescriptions are in the form of the brand name of a multinational company. This is over a hundred times more expensive than the locally produced ascorbic acid pill. And, if at all there is any scientific justification for taking the vitamin, why not ask the villager to take some vitamin-C-rich locally available fruits (e.g. *amla*) which can be obtained virtually free of cost? Similarly, numerous families in third world countries have been financially ruined in the process of procuring the protein or amino acid concentrates or high-class protein food (e.g. milk, chicken, fish, eggs, etc.) prescribed by physicians or nutritionists for their patients.

There is also the need of cultural adaptation and formation of inexpensive nutritional alternatives for undertaking dietetic treatment of certain general diseases (e.g. diabetes mellitus and peptic ulcers). Similar reassessments and readjustments are also needed for the other areas, e.g. nutritional assessment, food processing and food technology. When such alternatives are developed through endogenous research efforts, it will be possible to give up dependence on the Western models. This is a major challenge for nutrition scientists of the third world.

Thus, while the issue of people having access to food which satisfies hunger and meets the calorie requirements opens up some very critical areas in the field of human nutrition in the third world, it also sets in motion a process which challenges some of the well-established concepts in education, practice and the research in nutrition. It calls for correction of the imbalances that have crept in because of overemphasis on nutritional research that are conducted in animal houses, in biochemical laboratories and in clinical wards. The alternative would be to start from the people. Problems for laboratory or clinical research should emerge from study of the nutritional problems as they exist among people and what these problems mean to the people, socially, culturally as well as economically. Development of nutrition science and technology ought to be subordinated to the needs of the people, rather than people becoming victims of exploitation by market forces [6]. There ought to be social control over education, training, practice and research in human nutrition.

This would require adoption of an epidemiological approach [7], which includes taking into account the social and economic dimensions of problems. This will provide an entirely different perspective for generation of a new body of knowledge in human nutrition. For instance, even among those who suffer from long spells of hunger every year, only a few might manifest symptoms due to specific deficiency conditions. For the rest, who form by far the great majority, mere administration of vitamins or amino acids is of little consequence. Providing food that meets the calorie needs is the prime consideration.

Nutrition and Poverty

Hundreds of millions of people in the third world are unable to get the minimum calorie requirements because they do not have enough resources to buy food – they are poor. Because of poverty, they live under miserable environmental conditions. The environment is bad in terms of access to protected drinking water supply, facilities for disposal of wastes, infestations with parasites and pests, housing, clothing, and so on. They have high rates of mortality and morbidity. Illiteracy is also very high.

Over the past several years, many countries of Africa, particularly those of the sub-Sahara (Sahel), have been experiencing extreme conditions of deprivation – famines, leading to deaths of hundreds of thousands of people, particularly children. This invoked emergency responses from the more affluent countries, several international agencies and groups of individuals like the pop singer Bob Geldoff and his colleagues from different parts of the world.

While the 'generous' response received worldwide publicity and acclaim, including the spectacular communicational extravaganza in the form of World Aid, it went virtually unnoticed that a major cause of the predicament of the countries of the Sahel region and elsewhere in the third world lies in the grossly unfair terms of trade between them and the affluent industrialized countries of the West. On the basis of a scholarly analysis of the severe drought of 1972 in the Sahel region of Africa, using an interdisciplinary approach, Garcia and his colleagues [23, 24] have asserted that many of the assumptions underlying the responses of the more developed countries have been faulty. The authors claim that at stake is the whole development process and the role of science and technology transfer in development. Nothing short of the total structural change in the underlying practices that are considered as 'normal' for today's society will reduce the third world's vulnerability to climate adversity as a trigger of socioeconomic instability and frequent catastrophe. These forecasts, made in 1978–1981, have proved prophetic. The authors go on to describe the Sahel case as a textbook example of what are called social dimensions of drought. Pre-colonial ethics have response mechanisms ingrained in the structure of social relations, which were at the basis of production systems. An analysis of the historical evolution of the system of social relations and the disruption of the response mechanism is presented as a solid foundation for the diagnosis of the Sahelian catastrophe in the early 1970s.

In addition to such catastrophic famines, hundreds of millions of people in the third world are victims of chronic starvation. The problem is social, economic and political, rather than nutritional in the conventional sense. Here too, disruption of the production systems due to deterioration in social relations remains the main cause. Behar [12] is one of the earlier exponents of this line of thinking. According to him, 'malnutrition is one of the consequences of social injustice, and at the same time one of the mechanisms for maintaining it'. There was a growing awareness of the need of meeting the new challenges of the profession in the XIII International Congress of Nutrition [66].Discussing this in a paper, Gussow and Eide [39] have pleaded for a reconsideration of 'prevailing assumptions about ignorance of ordinary eaters and pay more attention to the ignorance – or need for education – of the power brokers and policy makers whose decisions in the variety of settings affect the quality, distribution, comprehensibility, safety and sustainability of the food supply'. They visualise formation of a second generation of nutritionists who are exposed to knowledge based on understanding of the real political, social, economic and other sources of people's food problems and the ways to resolve these problems within the constraints imposed by a globe of finite resources.

In a Workshop he had organized at the same International Congress of Nutrition, Schuftan [56] has emphasised that nutritionists simply cannot steer clear of economic, political or ideological issues. To decline to take a stance on fundamental political issues, according to him, was itself a vote for the status quo and contribution to the perpetuation of maldevelopment. Nutritionists should take the roles of advocates and change agents.

Cultural and Biological Dimensions of Hunger

Involvement of nutritionists in the issues associated with the question of poverty, hunger and degrading conditions of living opens up the important area of study of the cultural and biological consequences of hunger. For instance, there is substantial evidence to assert that the levels of living of the lower 60–70% of the population of India had not improved at least during the three decades of 1941–1970 [8]. As late as in 1977, the Union Ministry of Health and Family Welfare [32] admitted that as much as four fifths of the rural population had no access to health services, government or private. But then, there is sound evidence, based on a reasonably reliable census data, that the expectation of life at birth in the country has shot up from 31.8 in 1941 to 45.6 years in 1971 [11, p. 159]. There had also been a marked decline in infant mortality. It is not possible to explain this paradoxical situation fully. However, there is some evidence [1, 21, 36] to indicate possibilities of some sort of biological adjustment over a period of time in the metabolic system of the people affected by chronic hunger and ill health, so that they are able to survive even at lower levels of subsistence. Though this expanding lowest category of the poor and destitute come nearer, in social and political terms, to a vegetative existence, they cannot be biologically labelled as dead. Whatever the possible mechanism, acquisition of ability by man to further lower the survival threshold, both in immunological and nutritional terms, has profound social and political implications. In the 1940s, the weak died in large numbers when they went below the threshold of the minimum conditions of survival. But in the ecological conditions of the 1970s and the 1980s, a significant proportion of the weak, who would otherwise have died away, somehow manage to survive in a state of weakness which is even more pronounced than what was the case in the 1940s. This group thus becomes a still easier prey to the machinations of the power elites. This adds a new and a very disturbing dimension to the power struggle of the havenots to wrest their rights from the haves [7].

The above considerations also provide an interesting angle for understanding the implications of the sharp fall in birth and death rates in the Kerala State of India [49] and in Sri Lanka [37]. In the haste to attribute this phenomenon to high rates of literacy, land reforms, food distribution system and greater access to health services, the exponents of this line of explanation have overlooked the stark fact that a large number of the people are hungry, they live under most degrading environmental conditions and there are high levels of unemployment or underemployment. Are they healthy? Are they nutritionally 'normal' [11, pp. 349–357]?

Measurement of Undernutrition

Diet surveys have been used as a tool for measuring the prevalence of undernutrition and malnutrition in a country. However, considering the extensive prevalence of undernutrition in a country like India and use of undernutrition as a measure of poverty, several attempts have been made to determine how far consumption data obtained through nationwide sample surveys (NSS) [19] can be used as a substitute for elaborate nutrition surveys. The idea was to convert the quantum of consumption of an individual into intake of calories in food.

This has stimulated prolonged and intensive debates among economists [15–18, 20, 43, 44, 54, 55], statisticians [60–65], nutritionists [14, 22, 26, 27, 53, 57], epidemiologists and anthropologists [7, 50] in India. The issues of the debates are inter- and intra-individual variations, the question of adaptation leading to the slogan 'small is beautiful' and to biological, cultural and political implications of hunger.

It may, however, be noted that apart from the various statistical and non-statistical errors that can creep in due to defects in conceptualisation of the survey, or in collection of data, the findings of a survey provide a snapshot view of a flux at any given point of time or, within a given period, if the survey covers a given period. Undoubtedly, it is desirable to have systematic, quantitative data on consumption of calories among individuals in a community and to process such data with the help of different statistical and mathematical methods. However, at the same time, the limitations of such survey data should be clearly recognised and these should be highlighted against conceptualisation of the entire dynamics of the biological, social, cultural and economic consequences of hunger and deprivation among human beings in the country.

Unfortunately, in the debate among statisticians and economists on aspects of measurement of undernutrition in India, the symbols that have been used to describe the reality have been derived on the basis of assumptions which suffer from serious limitations. The temptation to play mathematical games with these symbols was so strong that the symbols have been used to signify far more than what they were meant to symbolise. They have often taken the place of the reality.

The most outstanding flaw in the debate on poverty and hunger is that the scholars have not adequately realised that there is an enormously wide range of categories between those who just somehow manage to satisfy their physiological need and those who die of starvation or of starvation-related diseases [9, p. 220]. When a human being is unable to satisfy his hunger, apart from this being a problem having considerable social, cultural, economic and political implications, it also becomes a stark biological problem of survival. When he finds himself worsted in the struggle for existence, the human biological being 'fights' back to survive in an effort to stop the downward slide and also to regain the lost ground. Therefore, in terms of biological survival, apart from the two categories consisting of those who are able to regain the lost ground and those who continue to slide down right to the point of death due to hunger, there are numerous individuals in other categories of the hungry who continue to slide down or climb up or remain for varying periods in a steady state while remaining within the very wide range provided by the two extremes. The position of an individual in this wide spectrum is determined by the number of days in a year he/she has to suffer from varying degrees of hunger. Therefore, the number of days in a year an individual suffers from varying degrees of hunger is a point of central concern for those who want to have a sensitive tool for measuring the degree of undernutrition in a population [7]. The question of the degree to which a human body economises on whatever it is able to eat, by lowering its basal metabolic rate or by otherwise increasing the efficiency of utilisation of the calories in performing work, is of secondary importance and this should not be allowed to cloud the central fact – that the individual is hungry.

Thus, apart from measuring undernutrition with the help of survey data, it is necessary to obtain data on a more fundamental human feeling – the feeling of hunger. How many people are hungry? How many months in a year do they have to go hungry? What effort do these people make to stave off hunger? What are the cultural implications of hunger? Cultural anthropologists can make important contributions by finding answers to such questions in the study of undernutrition in a community.

Political Economy and Sociology of Knowledge of Human Nutrition

As pointed out earlier, as a result of interplay of social and political forces, very deliberate efforts have been made to project human nutrition merely as body of almost 'aseptic' scientific knowledge: it is considered as ahistorical and apolitical in character and it has little to do with social and cultural forces. Social, cultural and psychological considerations are taken into account when it comes to 'motivating' people to give up their 'traditional' nutritional practices and accept whatever is handed down to them by nutrition educations or projected through various media of mass communication. These forces have also shaped the profession of nutritionists – researchers, teachers, trainers and practitioners.

However, the foregoing discussion has drawn attention to a number of dimensions to the conventional knowledge of human nutrition. It has identified the cultural and biological dimensions and the social and political issues in the measurement of undernutrition. 'Launching' of the concept that severe malnutrition during infancy causes permanent brain damage provides an instance of active involvement of 'scientists' in politically motivated activities.

Indeed, nutrition scientists are particularly vulnerable to manipulation by political forces and the market forces which control the political forces. Unlike physical scientists, it is often difficult for them to be very precise about issues concerning human nutrition. This limitation is exploited by the market forces which use nutrition 'science' to promote their products. Why did it take such a long time for the eminent nutritionists in India to realise that rather than protein deficiency, it is calorie deficiency which is of central concern? Why did they hitch the individual minimum protein requirements so high on earlier occasions? Why were they so vociferous about superior attributes of animal proteins – the so-called first-class proteins? Why did they overplay the importance of essential amino acids and vitamins? Why is it that such a huge market has been created for many 'tonics' which obviously have no nutritional value? What about the high-pressure salesmanship of baby food? Why did the nutrition scientists not pay enough attention to basing their research on people as they exist in the community? Instead, why did they attach undue importance to nutrition research in the animal house or in the laboratory? Such issues come within the purview of study of sociology of knowledge [58] and political economy [46]. It is important, particularly for scholars in the third world, to develop these areas of study so as to rectify the distortions in the knowledge of human nutrition. From the issues raised earlier in this presentation, one can make a strong case for inclusion of ecological, epidemiological, sociocultural, historical, economical and political considerations within the body of knowledge of human nutrition. It is claimed here that such broad-based interdisciplinary contributions are necessary to make the science of nutrition more relevant to the needs of the peoples of the world.

Practice of Public Health Nutrition: An Epidemiological Approach

While a different type of action is needed to rectify the root causes of chronic undernutrition, some efforts have been made to deal with the effect through the launching of large-scale supplementary nutrition programmes to provide protection to the particularly vulnerable groups in a community. In India, for instance, this is done by providing food to the mothers and children in particularly deprived populations of the country through programmes, such as the Applied Nutrition Programme [34], Supplementary Nutrition Programme [3], Integrated Child Development Scheme (ICDS) [11, pp. 328–329; 33] and Mid-day Meals Scheme [31] for school-going children. The ICDS is of particular interest because, apart from extensive coverage involving more than five million children and 500,000 mothers [35], who constitute a very substantial proportion of the deprived sections of both rural and urban populations of the country, it seeks to integrate supplementary feeding programmes for expectant mothers and children with programmes of health and nutrition education, adult literacy, non-formal education of children and a package of maternal and child health services. There have also been nationwide community nutrition drives against specific nutritional disorders: administration of iron and folic acid against pregnancy anaemias [11, p. 286] and of vitamin A [51] to children against nutritional blindness.

Interestingly, the practice of public health nutrition has shifted the focus of nutrition research from the laboratory or clinical ward to the people – to the community. Epidemiological analysis becomes the starting point, because it is necessary to determine the size, distribution, time trends and the detriments (including cultural, social and economic detriments) of nutritional problems in a community and their linkages with other community health problems. This provides a framework for identification of problems which need further study in research institutions. Defining of the different epidemiological dimensions of the problem also provides the base for identification of different packages of technology and delivery systems for solution of the problem, choice of the 'optimal' package with or without the use of mathematical models, testing them under real-life field conditions (test run) and, finally, their implementation on a nationwide scale. This is called an approach of operational research [2, 4]. This approach of optimising an organised complexity (involving, for example, social, cultural, economic and ecological background of the people, their nutritional problems, the possible technological interventions, the delivery systems and the overall political framework) has also a built-in system for evaluation of the programme and its implementation.

Summary

Historically, despite very different physical conditions of living, the incidence or prevalence of nutritional disorders was negligible, as long as people were able to eat well. Different types of nutritional disorders emerged as public health problems as man started to exploit man – slavery, feudal and capitalistic production relations, unequal terms of international trade, and so on. The root cause of nutritional disorders are social, economic and political. Apparently, to gain respectability as a science, human nutrition has also claimed its origin from chemistry, biochemistry, physicology and the clinical medical sciences. This has led to what Gussow has termed as 'scientification of food'. Because of this, the focus of studies has moved farther and farther away from studies of problems of nutrition in humans in their ecological settings. Biochemical laboratories and animal houses became the major places of study. This was not unintentional. This was actively promoted by the food and drug industry because it helped to expand its markets. These market forces also influenced the formation of the profession of nutritionists and nutrition educators. These professionals are mostly inward looking and insular. This has made them particularly vulnerable to exploitation by the market forces. Unwittingly or otherwise, there have been several occasions when they became covert sales agents of the food and drugs industry.

They promoted the sale of items which are proven to have no scientific rationale. Sometimes they have offered active support to the dominant political power centres by obscuring the basic social, economic and political cause of undernutrition and blaming the victims for their plight. Even more disturbing has been the trend of branding people as permanent mental cripples without producing convincing evidence.

The distortions are much more serious in third world countries and their implications are of much more far-reaching significance. Actions to correct the distortions are therefore far more urgent in these countries. The task before scholars in the third world is to give up their abject dependency on those from the Western countries and formulate, mostly endogenously, an alternative body of knowledge which is in tune with the specific conditions prevailing in these countries. For this they will have to restore the focus on the people rather than on laboratories. The approach has to be an epidemiological one, with biochemical research problems being identified to elaborate the conditions which are directly observed among people with the help of epidemiological studies. In the alternative approach suggested, meeting the calorie requirements will be of prime importance for action programmes. As the question of meeting the calorie needs is linked with the question of poverty, biological, cultural, social, political and economic dimensions of poverty will form important components of research, practice and education and trainig in human nutrition in third world countries.

References

1 Anand, B.K.; et al.: Studies on Shri Ramanand Yogi during his stay in an air-tight box. Indian J. med. Res. *49:* 82–89 (1961).

2 Andersen, S.: Operations research in public health. Publ. Hlth Rep. *79:* April (1964).

3 Bagchi, K.: Public Health Nutrition in Developing Countries (Academic Publishers, Calcutta 1986).

4 Banerji, D.: Operational research in the field of community health. Opsearch *9:* 135–142 (1972).

5 Banerji, D.: Political issues in health, population and nutrition. Social Sci. *7:* 159–168 (1978).

6 Banerji, D.: Epidemiological issues in nutrition. Indian J. Nutr. Diet. *16:* 89–194 (1978).

7 Banerji, D.: Measurement of poverty and undernutrition. Econom. polit. Weekly *XVI:* No. 39 (1981).

8 Banerji, D.: Impact of draught on nutrition and health status of the population of India; in Garcia, Escudero, Draught and man: the 1972 case history report of an IFIAS Research Project, vol. 2, pp. 104–112 (Pergamon Press, Oxford 1982).

9 Banerji, D.: Poverty, class and health culture in India, vol. 1 (Prachi Prakashan, New Delhi 1982).

10 Banerji, D.: Cultural and biological consequences of hunger; in Basu, Malhotra, Proc. Indian Statistical Institute Golden Jubilee Int. Conf. on Human Genetics and Adaptation; pp 309–325 (Indian Statistical Insitute, Calcutta 1983).

11 Banerji, D.: Health and family planning services in India: an epidemiological, socio-cultural and political analysis and a perspective (Lok Paksh, New Delhi 1985).
12 Behar, M.: Nutrition and the future of mankind. Proc. 13th Pacific Science Congr., Vancouver 1975).
13 Brown, E.R.; Margo, G.E.: Health education: can the reformers be reformed? Int. J. Hlth Serv. *8:* 3–16 (1978).
14 Chafkin, S.: Bashing nutritionists: the small but healthy? Hypothesis. Econ. polit. Weekly *20:* 896 (1985).
15 Dandekar, V.M.: Below the poverty line. Econ. polit. Weekly *14:* 233–236 (1979).
16 Dandekar, V.M.: On measurement of poverty. Econ. polit. Weekly *16:* 1241–1250 (1981).
17 Dandekar, V.M.: On measurement of undernutrition. Econ. polit. Weekly *17:* 203–212 (1982).
18 Dandekar, V.M.: Measurement of undernutrition. Proc. Nutr. Society of India, No. 27, pp. 1–35 (1982).
19 Dandekar, V.M.; Rath, N.: Poverty in India (Indian School of Political Economy, Poona 1971).
20 Dasgupta, R: Undernutrition and poverty: measurement problems. Margin *14:* 83–88 (1981).
21 Dubos, R.; Dubos, J.: The white plague (Little, Brown, Boston 1952).
22 Garby, L.: Undernourishment, energy requirements and adaptation: a physiologists point of view. Econ. polit. Weekly *18:* 2035–2036 (1983).
23 Garcia. R.V.: Drought and man: the 1972 case history. Report on an IFIAS Project. Nature Pleads not Guilty, vol. 1. (Pergamon Press, Oxford 1981).
24 Garcia, R.V.; Escudero, J.C.: Drought and man: the constant catastrophe: malnutrition, famines and drought, vol. 2 (Pergamon Press, Oxford 1982).
25 Glaxo Symposium on Nutrition Growth and Development: Session IV, Nutrition and Mental Development. Indian J. med. Res. *59:* suppl., pp. 177–220 (1971).
26 Gopalan, C.: Small is healthy? For the poor, not for the rich. NFI Bull. *October:* 1–5 (1983).
27 Gopalan, C.: Development and deprivation: the Indian experience. Econ. polit. Weekly *18:* 2163–2168 (1983).
28 Gopalan, C.: The National Goitre Control Programme: a sad story; in Nutrition Foundation of India: The National Goitre Control Programme – a blue-print for its intensification, pp. 55–57 (NFI, New Delhi 1983).
29 Gopalan, C.: Prevention and control of endemic goitre. NFI Bull. *7:* No. 4 (1986).
30 Gopalan, C.; Narsingarao, B.S.: Nutritional constraints on growth and development in current Indian dietaries. Indian J. med. Res. *59:* suppl., p. 111 (1971).
31 Government of India: Report of the Committee on Pre-School Children Feeding Programmes (Planning Commission, New Delhi 1972).
32 Government of India: Health care services in rural areas: draft plan (Ministry of Health & Family Welfare, New Delhi 1977).
33 Government of India: Integrated child development services scheme, pp. 1–31 (Ministry of Education & Social Welfare, New Delhi 1978).
34 Government of India: Report of 2nd Regional Workshop on Special Nutrition Programme – Conclusions and Recommendations, Calcutta (NIPCCD, New Delhi 1980).

35 Government of India: Sixth Five-Year Plan 1980–1985 (Planning Commission, New Delhi 1981).
36 Grigg, E.R.N.: Arcana of tuberculosis. Am. Rev. resp. Dis. *78:* 151–172; 426–453, 583–603 (1958).
37 Gunatilleke, G. (ed.): Intersectoral linkages and health development: case studies in India (Kerala State), Jamaica, Norway, Sri Lanka, and Thailand, publ. No. 83 (WHO, Genève 1984).
38 Gussow, J.D.: Growth, truth and responsibility: food is the bottom line. Occasional Paper Series, vol. 11, No. 6 (University of North Carolina, Greensboro 1981).
39 Gussow, J.D.; Eide, W.B.: The challenge to the profession: How do we transfer what we want to teach? In Taylor, Jenkins, Proc. 12th Int. Congr. of Nutrition, pp. 929–932 (Libbey, London 1985).
40 Illich, I.: Limits to medicine – medical nemesis: the expropriation of health (Penguin Harmondsworth 1977).
41 Kochupillai, N. et al.: Present status of endemic goitre as a problem of public health: South East Asia; in Stanbury, Hetzel, Endemic goitre and endemic cretinism, p. 101 (Wiley, New York 1980).
42 Kochupillai, N.; Godbole, M.M.: Iodised oil injections in goitre prophylaxis: possible impact on the new-born. NFI Bull. *7:* No. 4 (1986).
43 Krishnaji, N.: On measuring incidence of undernutrition: What is a consumer unit? Econ. polit. Weekly *16:* 1509–1511 (1981).
44 Krishnaji N.: On measuring incidence of undernutrition: a note of Sukhatme's procedure. Econom. polit. Weekly *16:* 989–992 (1981).
45 Leavell, H.R.: Health administrators in the making. NIHAE Bull. *1:* 15–19 (1968).
46 McKinlay, J.B.: Issues in the political economy of health care (Tavistock, London 1984).
47 National Academy of Sciences (USA): Relationship of nutrition to brain development and behaviour (National Academy of Sciences, Washington 1973).
48 Nyswander, D.B.: The open society: its implications for health educators. Hlth Educ. Monogr. *22:* 3–15 (1967).
49 Panikar, P.G.K.; Soman, C.R.: Health status of Kerala: paradox of economic backwardness and health development (Centre for Development Studies, Trivandrum 1984).
50 Payne, P., Cutler, P.: Measuring malnutrition: technical problems and ideological perspectives. Econ. polit. Weekly *19:* 1485–1496 (1984).
51 Ramalingaswami, V.: Knowledge and action in the control of vitamin A deficiency. Ann. N.Y. Acad. Sci. *300:* 210–220 (1977).
52 Ramamurthi, D.: Malnutrition and mental retardation in developing countries. Baroda J. Nutr. *8:* 5–13 (1981).
53 Rand, W.M.; Scrimashaw, N.S.: Protein and energy requirements – insights from long-term studies. NFI Bull. *5:* 1–2 (1984).
54 Rao, V.K.R.V.: Some nutritional puzzles: a note. Econ. polit. Weekly *16:* 1205–1208 (1981).
55 Rao, V.K.R.V.: Measurement of poverty: a note. Econ. polit. Weekly *16:* 1433–1436 (1981).
56 Schuftan, C.: Ethics and ideology in the battle against malnutrition; in Taylor, Jenkins, Proc. 13th Int. Congr. Nutrition, London, pp. 89–91 (Libbey, 1985).

57 Seckler, D.: Newer concepts in nutrition and their implications for policy; in Sukhatme, Malnutrition and poverty: newer concepts in nutrition and their implications for policy, p. 127 (MACS Research Institute, Pune 1982).
58 Straus, R.: The nature and status of medical sociology. Am. sociol. Rev. *22:* 200–204 (1957).
59 Sukhatme, P.V.: Assessment of adequacy of diets at different income levels. Econ. polit. Weekly *12:* special No., pp. 1373–1384 (1978).
60 Sukhatme, P.V.: Nutrition policy: need for reorientation. Econ. polit. Weekly *15:* 1101–1105 (1980).
61 Sukhatme, P.V.: Measuring the incidence of undernutrition: a comment. Econ. polit. Weekly *16:* 1034–1036 (1981).
62 Sukhatme, P.V.: On measurement of poverty. Econ. polit. Weekly *16:* 1318–1324 (1981).
63 Sukhatme, P.V.: Malnutrition and poverty: newer concepts in nutrition and their implications for policy (MACS Research Institute, Pune 1982).
64 Sukhatme, P.V.: Measurement of undernutrition, Econ. polit. Weekly *17:* 2000–2016 (1982).
65 Sukhatme, P.V.: Protein and energy requirements: a reply to Rand and Scrinshaw. Econ. polit. Weekly *20:* 1892–1894 (1985).
66 Taylor, T.G.; Jenkins, N.K. (ed.): Proc. 13th Int. Congr. Nutrition (Libbey, London 1985).
67 United Nations: International action to avert the impending protein crisis (United Nations, WHO, New York 1968).
68 World Health Organization: Breast feeding (Genève 1979).

Debabar Banerji, MD, Centre of Social Medicine and Community Health,
School of Social Sciences, Jawaharlal Nehru University, New Mehrauli Road,
New Delhi 110067 (India)

Wld Rev. Nutr. Diet., vol. 57, pp. 24–74 (Karger, Basel 1988)

Studies of the Dietary Habits, Food Consumption and Nutrient Intakes of Adolescents and Young Adults

N.L. Bull[1,2]

Herts, England

Contents

[1] N. Bull is now a freelance nutritionist who until 1982 worked in the Nutrition Branch of the Ministry of Agriculture, Fisheries and Food, London, England.

[2] The author is particularly grateful to Miss Susan Gatenby for her help in locating a number of the papers referred to in this review.

Introduction

Children, adolescents and young adults of today have more spending power than ever before and this is recognised by manufacturers and advertisers of everything from crisps to hi-tech toys. When it comes to food and drink, young people share a problem common to many in countries where food supply is not a limiting factor. In consequence, it is necessary to stimulate and educate the ability to choose a balanced diet where the range of items is so vast, and to select foods which will not only satisfy appetite and taste good but will fulfil nutritional requirements. Some adolescents, as part of their quest for independence, find difficulty in accepting existing values and life-styles in the home [92]. They may experiment with extremes of behaviour or rebel in other ways against traditional or current practices. Diet may be one aspect of this and in otherwise well-fed and developed Western societies there may, as a result, be young people who place themselves at particular nutritional risk by choosing to follow extreme eating patterns. These may fall into a number of categories. There are those who have a genuine concern for environmental or ecological issues but who carry their ideas to an extreme with respect to their own diets, rejecting all processed foods, all animal foods or all foods produced using anything 'artificial'. Macrobiotic, vegan or organic diets can be part of this phenomenon but the numbers of young people following such diets to extremes are relatively small and studies aimed specifically at assessing the diets of adolescents or young adults on such dietary regimes are few.

Other young people severely restrict their consumption in order to achieve or maintain a low body weight. Some, almost all of them female, develop anorexia nervosa. The development and course of this condition and studies which have been conducted with anorexic women are outside the scope of this review. Young athletes have been the subject of a number of dietary studies [11, 30, 86, 101] and in some cases such individuals have also been shown to have very low intakes of energy and some nutrients.

The most well-recognised aspect of the diets of young people is that they tend to opt for fast foods and convenience snacks, as seen on television and advertised in most major streets in towns and cities throughout the developed world. One might imagine that, for people who have yet to reach the age of 40, such a style of eating has in the last 20 years become part of their way of life. The need to establish to what extent this is so for young people, who may be adopting patterns that will endure throughout

Table I. Dietary surveys of adolescents and young adults

No.	Reference	Country	Sex	Age, years	Number of subjects	Method used	Foods	Energy	Prox.	Minerals	Vitamins	Alcohol
1	Atkinson et al. [3]	UK	M+F	students	ca. 50	3 × 7-day records	+	–	–	–	–	–
2	Beals et al. [8]	Can.	M+F	11–12, 16–17	144, 83	7-day record	+	–	–	–	–	–
3	Boggio and Klepping [12]	Fr.	M+F	9–11, 14–16	75, 198	7-day record	+	+	+	+	+	–
4	Bull [14]	UK	M+F	15–18, 19–21, 22–25	382, 224, 307	14-day record	+	+	+	+	+	+
5	Bundy et al. [17]	USA	M+F	13–18	480	7-day record	–	+	+	+	+	–
6	Cook et al. [20]	UK	M+F	13–14, 15	234, 148	7-day weighed	–	+	+	+	+	–
7	Copper et al. [21]	USA	M+F	15–17	34	3-day record	–	+	+	+	+	–
8	Creswell et al. [22]	UK	F	14–16	270	24-hour recall	+	–	–	–	–	–
9	Darke et al. [24]	UK	M+F	10–11, 14–15, 14–15	321, 177, 791	7-day weighed	–	+	+	+	+	–
10	Desaulniers et al. [29]	Can.	M+F	'adolescents'	435	2-day record	+	–	–	–	–	–
11	Durnin et al. [31]	UK	M+F	14	419	7-day weighed	+	+	+	+	–	–
12	Endres et al. [33]	USA	F	15–19	27	24-hour recall	–	+	+	+	+	–
13	Frank et al. [36]	USA	M+F	10–11, 12, 13–14	25, 22, 18	24-hour recall	–	+	+	–	–	–
14	George and Krondl [38]	Can.	M+F	14–17	135	questionnaire	+	–	–	–	–	–
15	Greger et al. [41]	USA	F	ca. 13	183	24-hour recall	–	+	+	+	+	–
16	Guzman et al. [45]	Phil.	M+F	10–19	1,535	questionnaire + 2-day recall	+	+	+	+	+	–
17	Hackett et al. [46, 50]	UK	M+F	11–14	375	5 × 3-day records	+	+	+	+	+	–
18	Hagger [51]	UK	M+F	students	109	7-day record	–	+	+	+	+	–
19	Hagman et al. [52]	Swe.	M+F	13	341	24-hour recall	+	+	+	+	+	–

20	Hitchcock and Gracey [57]	Aust.	M+F	11–15, 15–18	48, 26	24-hour recall	–	+	+	+	+	+
21	Johnson and Jensen [63]	USA	M+F	10.5	60	record + recall	–	+	+	+	+	–
22	Kaufmann et al. [65]	Isr.	M+F	17	1,178	24-hour recall	–	+	+	–	–	–
23	Kenney et al. [66]	USA	F	12–16	1,195	24-hour recall	+	+	+	+	+	–
24	Kuczmarski et al. [70]	USA	M+F	10–19	1,010	24-hour recall	+	+	+	–	–	+
25	Lai et al. [71]	USA	M+F	11–14, 15–18	282, 279	24-hour recall	–	+	+	+	+	–
26	Lee [72]	USA	M+F	12–19	118	24-hour recall	–	+	+	+	+	–
27	Rasanen et al. [104]	Fin.	M+F	12, 15, 18	324, 291, 272	48-hour recall	+	+	+	+	+	+
28	Salz et al. [107]	USA	M+F	10–14, 15–19	506, 550	24-hour recall	–	+	+	–	–	–
29	Samuelson [108]	Swe.	M+F	13	620	24-hour recall	+	+	+	+	+	–
30	Schorr et al. [109]	USA	M+F	12–18	118	3-day record	+	–	–	+	+	–
31	Seoane and Roberge [110]	Can.	M+F	10–12, 13–15, 16–18	171, 195, 134	3-day record	–	+	+	+	+	+
32	Skinner et al. [111]	USA	M+F	16–18	225	1-day record	+	+	+	+	+	–
33	Stordy and Cowhig [114]	UK	M+F	students	221	5-day record	–	+	+	+	+	–
34	Wenlock et al. [123]	UK	M+F	10–11, 14–15	1,723, 974	7-day record	+	+	+	+	+	–
35	Woodward et al. [127]	Aust.	M+F	12, 13, 14, 15	214, 263, 260, 218	24-hour recall	–	+	+	+	+	–
36	Wyn-Jones et al. [133]	UK	M+F	students	ca. 50	3 × 7-day records	–	+	+	+	+	–
Studies on young athletes												
37	Benson et al. [11]	USA	F	12–17	92	3-day record	–	+	+	+	+	–
38	Moffatt [86]	USA	F	15	13	2 × 3-day records	–	+	+	+	+	–
39	Perron and Endres [101]	USA	F	13–17	31	24-hour recall + 2-day record	+	+	–	+	+	–
40	Smeaton [112]	UK	F	17–28	6	7-day record	–	+	–	+	+	–

their adult lives, and most especially what the nutritional consequences are, has prompted considerable dietary research.

At the same time it is becoming apparent that attempts to influence dietary habits as part of preventive health care are most effective if targetted at particular sections of the population. In the UK for example, programmes have been undertaken with those approaching retirement. As these individuals spend more time in the home and concern for their own health is heightened with advancing years, they may be particularly receptive to advice about diet as their life-styles change [25, 59].

Adolescents and young adults may also be susceptible to specific nutrition education for a number of reasons [54]. Peer pressure is especially strong during adolescence [96] and achieving and maintaining a desired body weight and shape can be extremely important to a young person, with a high proportion of adolescents reporting that they are trying to lose or gain weight or change their body proportions [60]. Involvement in sports, dance, gymnastics or, for older adolescent girls and young women, pregnancy, may all initiate or heighten an interest in diet. However, if a particular population group is to be the subject of nutrition education, either through the school curriculum or national health education campaigns, then its current nutritional status, dietary habits and attitudes towards food all need to be assessed. Such assessment may also contribute to national baseline data against which the effects of changes in a country's nutrition policy can be evaluated.

During the last 20 years there have been a number of reports about the dietary status and health of a broad cross-section of young people. From much of this work, findings of improved stature and earlier maturation in adolescents indicate the considerable improvements in both standard of

Table II. Energy and nutrient intakes by young female athletes

Ref.[a]	Energy		Protein	Fat		CHO	Calcium	Iron	Zinc	Magnesium
	kcal	MJ	g	g	% kcal	g	mg	mg	mg	mg
37	1,890	7.9	72	75	35	236	933	13.4	7.7	228
38	1,923	8.0	74	82	38	222	707	11.3	7.4	202
39	1,799	7.5	na	na	na	na	772	11	na	na
40	2,360	9.9	na	na	na	na	na	13.5	11.2	321

[a] See table I.

living and nutrition that have taken place since the Second World War [40]. Such work also tends to indicate that the problems arising from adolescents' diets now are not dissimilar to those of the general population. Thus, in affluent nations, continuing weight gain leading to obesity at an early age suggests that over-nutrition may be a primary area of concern among this age group [56]. Nevertheless, there has been a progressive fall in average energy intakes, particularly of girls, over the last 50 years or more [125]. This is attributed to marked changes in physical activity. Lower energy needs, however, only accentuate the necessity of achieving a diet with appropriate nutrient density if requirements for all nutrients are to be met. It is therefore a cause for concern that these findings are accompanied by increasing evidence that young people 'habitually skip meals and satisfy their appetite by eating certain food items which could lead to a seriously unbalanced diet' [40].

It is the purpose of this review to bring together the findings of recent dietary studies among 10- to 25-year-olds and to identify any common features or dietary patterns which appear to be characteristic of young people. Table I summarises the studies which have been included, indicating where data is provided for food consumption and nutrient intakes. In some cases this data is not given in a form allowing direct comparison with strictly quantitative results. Thus, for example, food consumption results may only have been given in terms of the contribution of food groups to total nutrient intakes, rather than in weights consumed over a specified period. Similarly, some reported nutrient data are not in the form of daily intakes. Where it has been possible to derive the daily intake of nutrients from the information supplied, this has been done and the results included for comparison in nutrient tables II–VI.

Thiamin mg	Ribofl. mg	Nic.ac. Eq mg	Folate µg	Vit. B_6 mg	Vit. B_{12} µg	Vit. C mg	Vit. A ret.Eq	Vit. D µg	Vit. E mg
1.65	1.95	20.2	266	1.56	5.13	148	1,410	na	9.4
1.04	1.39	13.4	129	1.27	2.39	84	884	7.32	8.1
na	na	na	na	na	na	97	816	na	na
na	na	na	190	1.2	4.6	89	1,213	na	5.8

Table III. Energy and nutrient intakes by subjects aged approximately 10–12 years

Ref.[a]	Energy		Protein	Fat		CHO	Alcohol	Fibre	Calcium	Iron	Zinc	Thiamin	Ribofl.	Nic.ac. Eq	Folate	Vit. B_6	Vit. B_{12}	Vit. C	Vit. A	Vit. D
	kcal	MJ	g	g	% kcal	g	g	g	mg	mg	mg	mg	mg	mg	µg	mg	µg	mg	RE	µg
Males																				
3	1,995	8.3	70	88	40	228	na	na	827	11.3	na	1.07	1.50	na	na	na	na	88.1	na	na
9	2,169	9.1	62	91	38	292	na	na	899	10.8	na	1.03	1.43	na	na	1.16	na	48.5	na	1.66
25	2.654	11.1	106	106	36	340	na	na	na	na	na	na	na	na	na	na	na	na	na	na
27	2,361	9.9	83	102	39	289	0	na	1,287	17	13	1.6	2.7	32	na	na	na	97	1,238	na
28	2,621	11.0	96	111	38	328	na	na	na	na	na	na	na	na	na	na	na	na	na	na
31	2,171	9.1	79	87	36	273	0.2	na	1,095	12.1	na	1.3	2.2	17.0	na	na	na	96	934	na
34	2,070	8.7	61	88	38	274	na	na	833	10	na	1.21	1.70	26.5	na	1.17	na	49	854	1.48
35	2,366	9.9	80	98	37	291	na	na	810	13.8	na	1.50	2.6	31	na	na	na	79	900	na
Females																				
3	1,765	7.4	64	78	40	200	na	na	772	10.4	na	0.96	1.44	na	na	na	na	83.7	na	na
9	1,916	8.0	55	83	39	252	na	na	787	9.7	na	0.88	1.24	na	na	1.05	na	46.2	na	1.44
25	2,057	8.6	77	82	36	269	na	na	na	na	na	na	na	na	na	na	na	na	na	na
27	1,947	8.2	71	82	38	242	0	na	1,103	15	11	1.4	2.3	28	na	na	na	95	1,196	na
28	2,197	9.2	79	92	38	282	na	na	na	na	na	na	na	na	na	na	na	na	na	na
31	1,891	7.9	70	77	37	234	0	na	951	10.6	na	1.1	1.9	14.7	na	na	na	80	820	na
34	1,840	7.7	53	79	39	241	na	na	702	8.6	na	1.03	1.40	23.1	na	1.03	na	49	691	1.32
35	2,127	8.9	62	84	36	268	na	na	640	10.9	na	1.31	2.0	27	na	na	na	96	790	na
Both sexes																				
13	1,857	7.8	65	83	40	216	na	2.5	na	na	na	na	na	na	na	na	na	na	na	na
13	1,900	7.9	62	80	38	241	na	2.7	na	na	na	na	na	na	na	na	na	na	na	na
21	1,857	7.8	79	na	na	na	na	na	1,038	10.7	na	1.0	1.9	14.3	na	na	na	74	778	na

[a] See table I.

Methods Used in Dietary Studies of Adolescents

Dietary surveys may be conducted in a number of ways in order to arrive at an assessment of the food consumption patterns and nutrient intakes of individuals [83]. The methods most frequently used with adolescents and young adults are the dietary recall and the consumption record. In the 24-hour recall method an interviewer asks each subject to recall the foods and drinks consumed during either the previous day (12 midnight to 12 midnight for example) or the 24 h immediately preceding the interview. Recalls of more than one day are sometimes performed but the accuracy with which subjects can remember their consumption over a period of more than 3 days probably renders unreliable recalls of greater extent. Two considerable disadvantages are inherent in the recall method. First, the method depends for its quantitative accuracy on the ability of each subject to provide accurate assessments of the weights and volumes of foods and drinks, or to correctly identify with the aid of food models, the sizes of portions consumed. Second, the recall of a single day's intake may not be representative of a subject's usual eating habits [37].

The use of a consumption record overcomes this problem to some extent. It does not rely on the memory of the subject but on the recording of all occasions throughout the day when food or drink is consumed. Weighed records are considered to be the most accurate way of assessing the diets of individuals. In most cases the subjects are first trained in the use of the weighing scales and in recording their consumption in a diary. The interviewer may make contact with subjects during the weighing period to check that they are carrying out instructions properly. The weighing method relies on the literacy and numeracy of the population under study although surveys have been done where the investigator is present at each meal to weigh and record the subject's food. Such surveys are obviously very costly and labour-intensive.

Where adolescents or young adults are being studied, both the recall method and the consumption record suffer from specific drawbacks which share common origins. First, the recall method is more likely to produce a reliable estimate of intake where a regular meal pattern is adhered to. Snacking and between-meal eating may be easily omitted on recall and this has obvious disadvantages where set meals may not be the greatest contributors to food consumption. The weighing method has a similar drawback in that the meals eaten at home may be weighed relatively easily but, again, between-meal eating and snacks or meals eaten outside the home may be

Table IV. Energy and nutrient intakes by subjects aged approximately 13–15 years

Ref.[a]	Energy		Protein	Fat		CHO	Alcohol	Fibre	Calcium	Iron	Zinc	Thiamin	Ribofl.	Nic.ac. Eq	Folate	Vit. B_6	Vit. B_{12}	Vit. C	Vit. A RE	Vit. D
	kcal	MJ	g	g	% kcal	g	g	g	mg	mg	mg	mg	mg	mg	μg	μg	μg	mg		μg
Males																				
3	2,616	10.9	95	117	40	291	na	na	1,016	16.7	na	1.25	1.95	na	na	na	na	88.3	na	na
5	2,557	10.7	97	113	40	299	na	4.1	1,235	17.4	13.1	1.92	2.73	24.8	na	1.88	6.86	154	1,430	na
6	2,771	11.6	76	na	na	na	na	na	1,038	14	na	1.2	1.7	na	na	na	na	56	1,171	2.90
6	2,875	12.0	80	na	na	na	na	na	1,085	15	na	1.3	1.8	na	na	na	na	61	1,149	3.08
9	2,674	11.2	75	115	39	356	na	na	950	13.4	na	1.16	1.61	na	na	1.41	na	58.3	na	2.10
9	2,451	10.3	71	102	37	330	na	na	870	12.4	na	1.17	1.48	na	na	1.40	na	53.3	na	2.11
11	2,610	10.9	78	115	40	334	na	na	1,020	14	na	na	na	na	na	na	na	na	na	na
17	2,253	9.4	64	101	40	286	na	14.7	888	10.6	na	na	na	na	na	na	na	40.3	704	na
19	2,533	10.6	92	103	37	295	na	na	1,600	18.7	10.9	1.7	2.6	31	na	2.0	10.3	79	2,000	6.1
20	2,294	9.6	80	96	38	292	0	na	910	14.8	na	1.6	2.6	31.6	na	na	na	68	1,186	na
26[b]	2,666	11.2	99	127	43	288	na	na	1,192	13	na	1.3	2.5	18.5	na	na	na	53	1,056	na
26[c]	2,004	8.4	83	101	45	201	na	na	747	11	na	0.9	1.6	14.0	na	na	na	55	364	na
27	2,818	11.8	101	125	40	337	0	na	1,483	21	16	1.9	3.2	40	na	na	na	86	1,674	na
28	2,621	11.0	96	111	38	328	na	na	na	na	na	na	na	na	na	na	na	na	na	na
29	2,668	11.2	89	121	41	289	na	na	1,495	16.7	na	1.5	2.6	27.7	na	na	na	78	1,500	4.2
30	na	na	na	na	na	na	na	na	1,308	15.4	na	na	na	na	na	na	na	105	1,130	na
31	2,609	10.9	94	105	36	327	1.9	na	1,180	15.0	na	1.5	2.6	21.7	na	na	na	119	1,040	na
34	2,490	10.4	75	106	38	324	na	na	925	12.2	na	1.47	1.89	32.6	na	1.35	na	49	969	1.63
35	2,796	11.7	98	124	40	327	na	na	1,090	16.4	na	1.78	3.1	39	na	na	na	93	1,120	na
35	2,891	12.1	95	124	39	356	na	na	1,090	16.5	na	2.00	3.4	39	na	na	na	122	1,200	na
35	2,844	11.9	101	126	40	349	na	na	910	17.5	na	2.14	3.2	42	na	na	na	107	1,190	na

Females																				
3	2,027	8.5	72	91	40	222	na	na	763	12.2	na	1.02	1.37	na	na	na	na	72.2	na	na
5	1,912	8.0	97	85	40	229	na	3.1	961	12.7	10.3	1.54	2.06	18.1	na	1.35	5.21	120	1,168	na
6	2,067	8.6	58	na	na	na	na	na	759	12	na	0.9	1.3	na	na	na	na	54	1,037	2.68
6	2,046	8.6	59	na	na	na	na	na	777	11	na	0.9	1.3	na	na	na	na	44	935	2.18
9	2,063	8.6	60	92	40	264	na	na	705	10.9	na	0.90	1.18	na	na	1.15	na	47.2	na	2.18
9	1,911	8.0	57	85	40	243	na	na	667	10.1	na	0.92	1.13	na	na	1.17	na	48.8	na	1.81
11	2,020	8.5	62	93	41	247	na	na	796	11	na	na	na	na	na	na	na	na	na	na
15[d]	2,030	8.5	76	88	39	242	na	na	1,044	11.1	11.3	1.1	2.0	na	na	na	na	80	822	na
15[e]	1,940	8.1	73	80	37	240	na	na	994	10.6	11.3	1.1	1.9	na	na	na	na	88	695	na
17	2,023	8.5	55	92	41	256	na	13.5	778	9.4	na	na	na	na	na	na	na	39.9	604	na
19	1,924	8.1	70	77	36	225	na	na	1,230	13.9	8.2	1.2	1.9	23	na	1.5	8.0	60	1,700	4.9
20	2,019	8.5	65	88	39	249	0	na	783	12.8	na	1.3	2.2	24.7	na	na	na	65	1,195	na
23	2,017	8.4	67	88	39	257	na	na	798	11.4	9.9	1.19	1.99	28.0	173	1.18	3.94	84	859	5.23
26[b]	1,671	7.0	60	74	40	188	na	na	1,011	9	na	0.8	1.4	12.4	na	na	na	57	505	na
26[c]	1,730	7.2	68	73	38	179	na	na	822	9	na	0.9	1.7	11.8	na	na	na	87	912	na
27	1,804	7.6	63	73	36	227	0	na	974	13	10	1.3	2.0	25	na	na	na	86	1,103	na
28	2,197	9.2	79	92	38	282	na	na	na	na	na	na	na	na	na	na	na	na	na	na
29	2,194	9,2	71	102	42	235	na	na	1,232	13.5	na	1.3	2.2	22.6	na	na	na	67	1,300	3.1
30	na	na	na	na	na	na	na	na	843	8.8	na	na	na	na	na	na	na	73	711	na
31	2,059	8.6	74	83	36	255	1.0	na	1,009	11.3	na	1.2	2.0	16.6	na	na	na	101	932	na
34	1,880	7.9	56	82	39	240	na	na	692	9.3	na	1.04	1.32	24	na	1.06	na	48	801	1.24
35	2,151	9.0	74	89	37	279	na	na	700	12.3	na	1.43	2.1	30	na	na	na	103	810	na
35	2,199	9.2	76	97	40	270	na	na	720	13.1	na	1.47	2.5	31	na	na	na	91	920	na
35	2,032	8.5	74	91	40	250	na	na	730	12.2	na	1.45	2.3	29	na	na	na	97	900	na
Both sexes																				
13	2,445	10.2	86	113	42	261	na	3.3	na	na	na	na	na	na	na	na	na	na	na	na

[a] See table I; [b] White subjects; [c] Black subjects; [d] Autumn; [e] Spring.

Table V. Energy and nutrient intakes by subjects aged approximately 16–18 years

Ref.[a]	Energy		Protein	Fat		CHO	Alcohol	Fibre	Calcium	Iron	Zinc	Thiamin	Ribofl.	Nic.ac. Eq	Folate	Vit. B_6	Vit. B_{12}	Vit. C	Vit. A	Vit. D
	kcal	MJ	g	g	% kcal	g	g	g	mg	mg	mg	mg	mg	mg	µg	mg	µg	mg	RE	µg
Males																				
4	2,420	10.1	76	116	43	270	7.5	16.4	1,000	11.0	na	1.16	1.91	34.3	153	na	5.98	50	na	na
5	2,557	10.7	97	113	40	299	na	4.1	1,235	17.4	13.1	1.92	2.73	24.8	na	1.88	6.86	154	1,430	na
20	2,834	11.9	93	123	39	349	1.2	na	868	18.6	na	1.7	2.7	37.1	na	na	na	95	1,670	na
22	2,490	10.4	82	93	32	330	na	na	na	na	na	na	na	na	na	na	na	na	na	na
25	3,079	12.9	123	127	37	394	na	na	na	na	na	na	na	na	na	na	na	na	na	na
27	2,964	12.5	110	130	39	351	2	na	1,617	22	18	2.1	3.3	44	na	na	na	113	1,515	na
28	3,243	13.6	121	142	40	389	na	na	na	na	na	na	na	na	na	na	na	na	na	na
30	na	na	na	na	na	na	na	na	1,308	15.4	na	na	na	na	na	na	na	105	1,130	na
31	2,945	12.3	107	118	36	347	13.8	na	1,348	16.3	na	1.6	2.9	24.7	na	na	na	114	1,295	na
32	3,071	12.8	104	133	39	365	na	na	1,364	15.9	na	1.83	2.77	23.3	na	na	na	110	1,040	na
Females																				
4	1,860	7.8	59	90	44	210	4.1	13.1	885	8.5	na	0.90	1.51	26.1	125	na	4.63	50	na	na
5	1,912	8.0	74	85	40	229	na	3.1	961	12.7	10.3	1.54	2.06	18.1	na	1.35	5.21	120	1,168	na
12	2,107	8.8	84	na	na	na	na	na	932	15.2	na	1.5	2.3	23.2	231	1.4	na	84.8	1,027	1.88
20	1,664	7.0	54	75	41	199	0	na	590	8.5	na	1.0	1.4	19.8	na	na	na	43	880	na
22	1,611	6.7	53	63	34	208	na	na	na	na	na	na	na	na	na	na	na	na	na	na
25	2,028	8.5	76	79	35	270	na	na	na	na	na	na	na	na	na	na	na	na	na	na
27	1,827	7.7	64	78	38	225	1	na	941	13	10	1.3	1.9	26	na	na	na	89	1,047	na
28	2,020	8.5	72	87	39	249	na	na	na	na	na	na	na	na	na	na	na	na	na	na
30	na	na	na	na	na	na	na	na	843	8.8	na	na	na	na	na	na	na	73	711	na
31	1,904	8.0	68	76	36	235	4.4	na	782	10.3	na	0.9	1.6	15.8	na	na	na	87	845	na
32	2,063	8.6	65	92	40	250	na	na	746	11.0	na	1.20	1.52	15.3	na	na	na	62	546	na
Both sexes																				
7	1,947	8.1	75	77	35	238	na	5.1	998	12.4	na	1.4	2.1	19.0	na	na	na	126.2	1,421	na

[a] See table I.

Table VI. Energy and nutrient intakes by subjects aged approximately 18–25 years

Ref.[a]	Energy		Pro-tein	Fat		CHO	Alco-hol	Fibre	Calcium	Iron	Zinc	Thiamin	Ribofl.	Nic.ac. Eq	Folate	Vit. B_6	Vit. B_{12}	Vit. C	Vit. A	Vit. D
	kcal	MJ	g	g	% kcal	g	g	g	mg	mg	mg	mg	mg	mg	µg	mg	µg	mg	RE	µg
Males																				
4	2,485	10.4	83	118	43	260	16.3	16.5	1,100	11.5	na	1.17	1.98	38.3	179	na	7.65	52	na	na
4	2,470	10.3	85	119	43	250	17.1	17.0	1,125	11.6	na	1.18	2.03	38.9	186	na	8.27	54	na	na
18[b]	2,868	12.0	91	na	na	na	na	na	na	17	na	1.5	2.4	25	na	na	na	63	na	na
18[c]	3,203	13.4	103	na	na	na	na	na	na	17	na	1.6	2.1	26	na	na	na	64	na	na
33[b]	2,975	12.4	90	na	na	na	na	na	na	19	na	1.5	2.1	na	na	na	na	68	na	na
33[c]	3,001	12.6	86	na	na	na	na	na	na	17	na	1.65	2.0	na	na	na	na	57	na	na
36	2,718	11.4	83	na	na	na	na	na	na	16	na	1.29	2.04	na	na	na	na	49	na	na
Females																				
4	1,675	7.0	57	81	44	180	5.3	12.3	745	8.3	na	0.83	1.33	25.7	116	na	4.88	46	na	na
4	1,830	7.7	65	93	46	185	5.4	13.5	880	9.3	na	0.92	1.55	28.4	133	na	5.89	53	na	na
18[b]	2,294	9.6	67	na	na	na	na	na	na	12	na	1.3	1.7	20	na	na	na	63	na	na
18[c]	2,749	11.5	93	na	na	na	na	na	na	20	na	1.4	1.8	21	na	na	na	55	na	na
33[b]	2,148	9.0	67	na	na	na	na	na	na	13	na	1.2	1.2	na	na	na	na	72	na	na
33[c]	2,484	10.4	74	na	na	na	na	na	na	15	na	1.4	1.6	na	na	na	na	71	na	na
36	2,096	8.8	63	na	na	na	na	na	na	13	na	1.06	1.45	na	na	na	na	56	na	na

[a] See table I; [b] Students, self-catering; [c] Students, meals provided.

excluded from the record. In addition, the prospect of being required to weigh foods throughout the day for a period of up to a week or more may result in unwillingness to participate, with the resulting sample of young people being less typical of their population. Investigators have adopted a number of measures in attempts to alleviate these problems.

Post et al. [102] used a modified cross-check dietary history method in their 4-year longitudinal survey of Dutch adolescents. They had previously established that, in comparison with the 24-hour recall method, this gave smaller and non-significant intra-individual differences between test-retest measurements. The method was found to be less time-consuming than recall interviewing. Musgrave et al. [88] recognised the need for a method of assessing diets that would be less expensive than individual interviews and a strategy for group interviewing was introduced. A recording system was devised that provided information on the consumption of each subject over 3 days. At a morning group session the recording task was explained with the aid of food models and students recalled and recorded the breakfast eaten earlier that day. With assistance from the investigators during the school day and from parents at home they then completed the 3-day diary.

Meredith et al. [84] carried out an assessment of the ability of schoolchildren to recall their food intake. Ninety-four subjects in the age range 9–18 years recalled their school lunch and although there was considerable lack of agreement between the record of actual consumption and the record of the subject's recall, these differences were relatively small when nutrient analysis was performed. However, significant differences resulting from inaccurate recall did seem likely to occur for vitamins A and C. In the study reported by Greger et al. [42] interviewers were trained to ask questions which would prompt subjects to a full recall of their intake. The ability of schoolchildren to assess amounts of food consumed was tested by Comstock et al. [19] in a three-way comparison of assessment by trained observers, ratings by children and weighing of plate waste. They found that indirect measures of individual plate waste were highly correlated with weights. A six-point visual estimation scale (from ate/drank none through to ate/drank all) was used by the children and a similar scale for the amount left on the plate was used by the trained observers. Of the methods studied, visual estimation by trained observers was more highly correlated with the actual percentage of food waste. The indirect methods were both less expensive and less time-consuming than weighing. Samuelson [108] also reports a study which investigated the accuracy of childrens' records of school lunch consumption. Fifty-six 8-year-olds and 43 13-year-olds participated in the survey conducted in Northern Sweden and the author concluded that these groups were able to provide an acceptable estimate of their consumption of a specific meal as part of a 24-hour recall.

In a study of over 1,000 Tasmanian adolescents, Woodward [127] used a 24-hour recall procedure requiring relatively little supervision. An easily understood record form, divided into sections for 'breakfast', 'lunch', 'evening meal' and 'food eaten at other times' was completed by each subject. Each heading was followed by a list of food and drink items and spaces for 'any other foods' and all that was required was insertion of an amount in terms of specified units, e.g. cups, teaspoons, etc. The aim was to make the listing as comprehensive as possible on the assumption that subjects might fail to record items not listed on the form. A very similar approach was adopted in the design of a 2-week dietary diary for a survey of 15- to 25-year-olds carried out by the Ministry of Agriculture, Fisheries and Food (MAFF) in Great Britain [14]. In this case a pre-coded format was used in order to lessen the burden on the participants. They were required simply to indicate the amount of each food consumed in terms of a number of measures as specified, e.g. teaspoons for sugar, bowls for breakfast cereals, etc. Although less accurate from a quantitative point of view, this approach resulted in a very good response rate with very few of the subjects initially recruited failing to complete the 2-week diary successfully. This type of methodology requires good portion size data and, if possible, this information should be based upon portions consumed by the same type of subject.

Guthrie [44] has studied the ability of young adults to describe amounts of food and also the amounts which young adults select as being an average portion. For some foods, the amounts selected corresponded closely with accepted standard portion sizes, while for others larger portions were chosen. Men almost always selected larger portions than women. The ability to describe amounts chosen in a quantifiable way but without the use of measuring devices was poor. Between 8 and 68% of the 147 subjects were able to estimate individual items to within ±25% of the actual amount. The results were taken as an indication of the need to provide subjects with help in estimating portion sizes or to use methods which do not depend on the subjects' ability to describe their portion sizes accurately.

In Sweden, Hagman et al. [52] used the 24-hour recall method to assess the nutritional intake of a group of 13-year-old subjects coupled with dietary histories to obtain data on individuals' intakes. Comparisons between the two sets of results, expressed as group means, indicate that the

24-hour recall method produces lower estimates than the dietary history type of method. This finding has been reported by other workers who have studied different types of subject [1, 16] and should be borne in mind when comparisons are being made between the results of studies where different methods have been employed.

Many of the studies in the literature have been undertaken on a purely cross-sectional basis. However, in a longitudinal study carried out in England, Appleton et al. [2] found that for energy, protein, fat, carbohydrate and sugars the use of five 3-day dietary diaries, each followed by an interview and conducted over a 2-year period, was a reliable and satisfactory way of assessing the diets of subjects initially aged 11–12 years. In assessing the influences on food intake during this survey of adolescents, Hackett et al. [49] found, like Post et al. [102] in Holland, that weekdays differed from weekend days. The British workers concluded that all days of the week should be sampled in dietary studies because of the unpredictable nature of this difference.

Most of the dietary surveys carried out during the past 20 years have relied upon the development of computer based methods of data analysis. In the UK the food tables almost always used have been McCance and Widdowson's The Composition of Foods [74, 99], and computer programs have been developed which incorporate this data base. In some instances the food tables are extended by particular researchers who have collected their own analytical or manufacturers' data or by the inclusion of published additions [126]. Kuczmarski et al. [70] employed a novel approach to the analysis of their 24-hour recall data. Food groups, rather than each food item, were used to interpret the dietary intakes of over 1,000 adolescents aged 10–19. To group the foods, emphasis was placed on fat and carbohydrate content. Frequency of consumption of foods was then determined. Although the relative contributions of different food groups to the intakes of macronutrients could be assessed using this method, no estimation could be made of the daily intakes of nutrients by the subjects.

Factors Affecting Adolescent Diets

Knowledge about Diet

In Australia the nutritional knowledge of two groups of young people was assessed by questionnaire. Frequency format questions were also used to estimate usual dietary intake. It was concluded that for both the 250 undergraduate students and the 300 non-officer service recruits, health-oriented knowledge was not necessarily translated into health-oriented behaviour [4]. Cresswell et al. [22] concluded from their study that educating adolescents does not achieve its long-term potential until they are in their own homes. They found that among adolescent schoolgirls, snacking in addition to normal meals was common and the diet lacked fruit and vegetables. The roles of fat, sugar and fibre in the diet were not understood by all subjects and sources of fibre were not well recognised. These authors suggested that it would be practical to devise nutrition education aimed specifically at the snack food area, which falls largely within the financial control of adolescents themselves. They also recommended that efforts should be made to increase the availability of better snack foods, with lower fat and sugar and higher fibre.

In his review of the factors affecting food selection and preferences, Khan [67] reports that older children are influenced more by social or external pressures, especially at school, and that knowledge of a friend's preferences is influential, while for younger children the home environment is more important. This is borne out by the findings of the survey conducted for the British Ministry of Agriculture, Fisheries and Food [14]. Parents and friends were mentioned as sources of dietary information by equal proportions of 19- to 21-year-olds whereas more of the 15- to 18-year-olds mentioned parents and more of the 22- to 25-year-olds mentioned friends.

A survey among Israeli 13- and 14-year-olds revealed fairly sound knowledge of basic nutrition [64]. In general it was the overweight and obese adolescents who had better knowledge of the nutritive values of food and the causes of obesity. This was reflected in their reported eating habits; the overweight and obese were more conscious of their food intake and more likely to limit or avoid foods believed to promote obesity. A common misconception among this age group is illustrated by the finding that two thirds of all the subjects did not realise that to prevent obesity all kinds of foods may be eaten but in limited amounts. In addition, only one third recognised that lack of physical exercise is a cause of obesity.

Curry [23] studied the awareness of 11- to 16-year-olds with respect to cultural influences on their diets. British and American traditions were seen to have had an important effect on the food habits of adolescents in New Zealand, England and America and there was little sign that adolescent children of minority groups in these countries had retained their traditional habits.

Perron and Endres [101] found that nutrition knowledge and attitudes were positively and significantly correlated, suggesting that the more knowledgeable the subject was about nutrition, the more positive her attitudes towards nutrition were likely to be. However, among the subjects in their study, 13- to 17-year-old athletic girls, there was no correlation between varying nutrition knowledge and variations in any of the nutrient values of their diets. As an example of this, the vast majority of subjects knew that milk was a good source of calcium yet relatively few had diets meeting the recommended dietary allowance (RDA) for calcium.

The major nutritional concerns of American adolescents were identified by Mapes [81] using a questionnaire. The top five in order, as selected from 12 options were: (1) How can I improve my figure or physique? (2) What diet should I use to lose weight fast? (3) Is snacking bad? (4) Are organic foods healthier? (5) Is there anything I'm eating that causes acne?

Similar concerns were among the dietary issues reported as being most important to 15- to 25-year-olds in the British study of approximately 1,000 young adults [14].

Overweight

Miller and Binns [85] provided suggestive evidence that lack of physical activity is more important than excess energy consumption in childhood overweight. They assessed energy intake by 24-hour recall and also recorded TV viewing habits, age, weight, height and triceps skinfold thicknesses for 129 Australian children born to Italian migrants and 188 born to Australian parents. Average energy intakes were lower than recommended levels for both ethnic groups and both sexes yet Italian boys and girls and Australian girls were heavier for their age and height than the standards. These differences in anthropometric measurements showed the same trends as differences in amounts of daytime TV viewing. The same phenomenon has been recognised in North America. Environment and heredity both appear to play a part in the development of adolescent obesity and inadequate physical exercise is also an important factor as many obese adolescents do not appear to overeat [93]. Childhood obesity is a major problem in developed countries and its importance in relation to adult health can be seen in the estimates of Stunkard and Burt [116] that the odds against an obese child becoming a normal weight adult are more than 4:1 at age 12 but rise to approximately 28:1 if weight has not been reduced by the end of adolescence.

Dieting and Meal-Skipping

Dieting is a common practice among adolescent females and is not confined to those who are actually overweight. Dwyer et al. [32] found that many more girls dieted to lose weight than would be objectively classified as obese or even nearing obesity. Dieting first started at around age 14–15 and the omission of certain foods or of snacks were the most common features. Although knowledge of calorie values was low across female adolescents as a whole, it was greater among the dieters and the overweight.

Macdonald et al. [76] attempted to identify the variables that differentiate between adolescent girls with poor dietary intakes and those with good dietary intakes. It was hypothesized that those with poor diets would be less active, have lower self-esteem and a larger body image perception. Twenty-four-hour recalls were collected from 276 subjects aged 14–18, together with socioeconomic data, weights, heights, skinfold thicknesses and information on body image, dieting and physical activity. When divided into two groups on the basis of dietary quality, it was seen that the group with poorer quality diets was significantly heavier, skipped meals more often, spent more hours sleeping, sitting or standing at rest and was dieting or had dieted more often. Using discriminant function analysis to identify the combination of variables which contributed most to the difference between the two groups, it was found that subjects who spent more hours per day in inactive pursuits, had dieted more times in the past and selected an ecto-mesomorphic 'ideal' body image were more likely to have poorer quality diets. Storz and Greene [115] also studied body weight and body image and, in addition, the perceived desirability of fad diets among 203 adolescent girls. Most were within or below the average range for body weight yet most wanted to lose weight and expressed dissatisfaction with their own physique. Most of the subjects rated more healthy methods of weight reduction higher than fad diets but many nevertheless reported that they had tried one or more fad-type diets. The authors concluded that adolescent girls should be a target audience for nutrition education, particularly with reference to weight control. Among 15- to 25-year-old women in Britain the prevalence of self-assessed overweight was found to be lower among 15- to 18-year-olds (26%) than among 19- to 21-year-olds (40%) and 22- to 25-year-olds (38%) [6].

Meal-skipping and unstructured meal patterns are perhaps inevitable features of modern life-styles. When so much can be done at short notice and at high speed, the time needed for sitting down to a prearranged meal may not be afforded a high priority. For adolescents there may also be some reaction against the set meal seen as a family occasion. Lee [72] reported the incidence of meal-skipping amongst both black and white adolescents in Kentucky. With the exception of white boys, meals were omitted more often by those who smoked. In addition, the higher incidence of meal-skipping among black adolescents (82% of boys and 67% of girls reported skipping meals) was considered to be partially responsible for their less satisfactory food intake. Earlier American work done in the mid-1960s showed that adolescents tended to eat more than three times a day but that they ate breakfast less regularly after the age of about 16 and omitted lunch more often than other meals. As a result of omitting meals, the consumption of between-meal snacks improved nutrient intakes [53, 61]. Meal-skipping in the UK has been assessed in a number of studies and a comparison of the findings is reported by McGuffin [78]. In the Republic of Ireland, McSweeney and Kevany [80] conducted 24-hour recalls with 507 subjects, the majority of whom were aged 15–16. Questions were also asked about dietary habits. The National Dairy Council [89] also used 24-hour recalls with 1,748 subjects aged 5–18. The results from their 14–18 age group, together with those of McSweeney and Kevany [80] and those of McGuffin from Northern Ireland, who questioned over 2,000 15- to 16-year-olds [1979, unpublished], are summarised below:

	Northern Ireland	Irish Republic	England and Wales
Cooked breakfast, %	22	16	9
Cereal/bread based, %	60	63	67
No breakfast, %	4	4.5	20
Nothing at midday, %	2	4.5	5

Breakfast consumption was studied in France by Boggio and Klepping [12] who found that breakfast played a decreasing role in the diet with increasing age. Morgan et al. [87] used the American Nationwide Food Consumption Survey to evaluate the breakfast consumption patterns of both children and adolescents. Their results also showed that breakfast skipping increased with age and that the habit was most prevalent among female adolescents. In addition it was shown that in this group in particular, omission of breakfast detracted from the quality of the diet. It was concluded that breakfast, especially when containing ready-to-eat cereal, made a valuable contribution to the nutritional quality of the diets of children and adolescents. As long ago as 1952 it was reported from the USA that adolescents who always ate breakfast more nearly met the recommended allowances of energy and nutrients for their age than did those who missed breakfast once a week or more [113].

Walker et al. [122] studied the breakfast habits of different racial groups of adolescents in South Africa. They found that breakfast was omitted by between 13 and 21% of the groups of 16- to 18-year-olds. In the groups studied, however, the omission of breakfast did not appear to have a significant influence on weight, height, academic record or frequency of absence from school.

The Nutrition Committee of the Canadian Paediatric Society [92] recommended that adolescents eat a breakfast including a fortified cereal plus a serving of fruit or juice rich in vitamin C. This recommendation was especially aimed at addressing the problem of low dietary iron intakes among female adolescents.

Skinner et al. [111] found that 34% of the 225 American 16- to 18-year-olds in their study had skipped breakfast on the day of recording. Those who omitted breakfast had lower average intakes of energy and nutrients than those who ate breakfast. Quantitative and qualitative differences in the diets of those eating breakfast and those who did not eat it suggested that breakfast eaters made better food choices throughout the day and that those who omitted breakfast failed to compensate at other eating occasions. Of those who ate breakfast, 67 adolescents who prepared their own meal had lower average intakes of several nutrients than those whose mothers had prepared their breakfasts. On the survey day, 23% of the adolescents had prepared their own evening meal. Evening meals prepared by subjects were of lower average nutrient density than those prepared by mothers. They were also more likely to include a sandwich and less likely to include vegetables than meals prepared by mothers.

In a school meals survey conducted in 1970–1971, questions relating to the consumption of breakfast and of school milk showed that omitting breakfast and refusing school milk both became more common with increasing age from infant through to junior and senior school. In the senior schools (11–12 years and over) 13.6% had no breakfast [10].

Snacking and Fast Foods

In a study of the snacking habits of 15- to 18-year-olds it was seen that the quality of snacks varied throughout the day, with morning snacks, mostly from school shops and vending machines, tending to be confectionery and salty snack foods lower in nutrient density than snacks eaten at home in the afternoon or evening [34]. Snacks may contribute more energy to the total daily intake than breakfast. This situation could be altered if breakfast at home was encouraged. Study of the intakes of fat and of sugar and starch among 10- to 14-year-old Americans tended to suggest that by the age of 12 they had reached a peak of confectionery and soft drink consumption and begun to choose hamburgers, pizzas and chips as snack foods instead [36].

Musgrave [88] found few studies with definitive data on which adolescents snack most, when they snack, what foods they eat when they snack or how these foods contribute to the nutrient intake in relation to the overall diet. One hundred and forty-two students aged 10–16 were studied in an attempt to measure their snacking patterns and to develop a strategy for answering some of these questions. It was found that only 5 of the 142 subjects did not snack at all in a 3-day recording period. Most students ate three meals a day plus one or two snacks. On the whole, meals were not omitted in favour of snacks. Ten-year-olds snacked most often and the 10- to 13-year-olds snacked more often than the 14- to 16-year-olds. However, adolescents ate a greater variety of snack foods than did the 10- or 11-year-olds and females a greater variety and more snacks than males.

In a study of between-meal eating, Beals et al. [8] found that biscuits, fruit, milk, soft drinks and sweets were the five foods most often chosen. In general, 16- to 17-year-olds ate more snacks than either 5- to 6- or 11- to 12-year-olds and they also showed more differences between boys and girls than did the younger groups. The 16- to 17-year-old boys chose sandwiches and soft drinks more often while the girls more frequently ate chewing gum, doughnuts and coffee or tea.

Fast foods have a considerable role in modern diets, either as snacks or as meals, especially for young people, and their promotion as contributors to the diet often rests upon the nutrient content of a standard meal, usually hamburger, chips and milkshake, for example. It is probable, however, that this combination is by no means the one most frequently selected. Greecher and Shannon [39] found that 280 interviewees at two fast food outlets had ordered only 19 milkshakes and 13 glasses of milk compared with 115 soft drinks and 80 cups of coffee. Fast food, as consumed, is therefore not as nutritionally balanced an element in the diet as its advertising may suggest. In practice, the high consumption of chips, in particular, contributes significantly to high fat intakes.

Sport and Diet

Table II summarises the nutritional findings from four surveys of young athletes. These studies were all conducted with female subjects. There do not appear to have been dietary surveys directed specifically at the male adolescent athlete.

In a study of 92 female ballet school pupils aged 12–17, 3-day histories were used to assess their dietary intakes. Poor dietary habits were revealed, with low energy and nutrient intakes. It was suggested that the dancers' desire for a 'sylphlike' figure makes them unwilling to eat sufficient for health and that there is therefore a role for nutrition education as part of the curriculum in the professional dance schools [11]. In other studies, with smaller groups of subjects, even lower average intakes of energy and nutrients have been found. Moffatt [86] studied 13 female gymnasts who were all involved in training regularly. Nutrient intakes were assessed on the basis of two 3-day food records. Although the group was small, several nutrients were judged to be generally inadequate on the basis that one fourth or more of the sample failed to consume at least 50% of the RDA. Nutrients so judged as inadequate were vitamin B_6, folate, zinc and magnesium. The mean nutrient density of the gymnasts' diets was low and the average energy intake was marginally below the RDA. This RDA does not take into account the additional energy expenditure of perhaps 300 kcal ascribable to approximately 1.5 h physical training per day.

Perron and Endres [101] studied the diets and attitudes of 31 female athletes aged 13–17 who were all members of a volleyball team. Diets were similar to those of other adolescent girls in the USA. Mean energy intake was below the RDA and may have been inadequate for these active subjects. Average intakes of vitamins A and C exceeded RDA while those for calcium and iron were less than two thirds of the RDA.

In the UK, Smeaton [112] found that the self-selected diets of six top female athletes failed to meet recommended levels for a number of vitamins and minerals. Over a 7-day recording period none of the 6 subjects, whose ages were between 17 and 28, achieved recommended average daily intakes for vitamin E, vitamin B_6 [35] or biotin [97].

Brown et al. [13] found that the iron status of adolescent female athletes was significantly poorer than that of non-athletes. Dietary intake was assessed in addition to biochemical measurements and it was concluded that female adolescent athletes may be at greater risk of iron-deficiency anaemia than their peers.

There are many myths surrounding appropriate diets for sportsmen and women. The Nutrition Committee of the Canadian Paediatric Society [94] recommended that athletes of all ages are best advised to have a balanced normal diet. Supplements are not necessary because the additional nutrients will be present in the extra food eaten to meet the energy needs consistent with increased activity.

The Role of the School Meal

A survey of the midday eating habits of 11- to 18-year-olds in London, England, in the early 1970s, indicated that 41% ate a school meal, 31% bought food outside school, 20% brought food from home, 4% ate at home and a further 4% ate nothing. There was a marked fall in school meal uptake with age, from almost 60% at age 11 to less than 20% at 16. The reverse was seen for consumption of food bought outside school. Of all the available options the school meal provided most energy and protein. Those who ate at home had a meal which compared favourably with the school meal but contributed fewer calories. For those who brought food from home or bought lunch outside school, lunchtime consumption was found to be low in protein, iron and calcium and high in sugar [105]. More recently, the British DHSS survey [123] has shown that where school meals are taken they still provide about one third of total energy intake although no specific nutritional standard to this effect has applied since the Education Act 1980 was passed. Some concern was expressed, however, about particular groups of children, and Wharton [124] has suggested that objective evidence could be gathered on the importance of school meals. If, for example, iron intakes are lower for adolescent girls eating out of school, then their haemoglobin concentrations, in comparison with those of girls who eat school meals, should be assessed. Wharton [124] also ascribes educational and social value to the provision of school meals but acknowledges that they need to be presented in an attractive way to ensure that they are actually eaten.

However, in a survey of over 400 14-year-olds in Scotland, no significant differences were found in the levels of energy or nutrient intakes between those eating school meals and those who did not [31]. In the southeast of England it was found that subjects who had school meals achieved higher weekday lunchtime nutrient intakes during term time than those who did not [20]. Again, in an American study of the influence of their midday meal on the nutrient intakes of 10-year-olds, Johnson and Jensen [63] found that school lunches and lunches eaten at home were nutritionally superior to lunches brought from home to be eaten at school.

In their longitudinal study in Holland, Post et al. [102] found that adolescent girls aged between 12 and 17 had a constant energy intake with age, but consistently higher intakes on weekend days than on school days. Boys had slightly higher energy intakes on weekend days and their intakes increased gradually with age both for school days and weekend days.

Living Accommodation

Stordy and Cowhig [114] assessed the differences in diets of students according to their type of term-time accommodation. For women rather more than for men it appeared that self-catering accommodation was linked to lower intakes of energy and some nutrients. More of the women living in a flat or bed-sitting room had intakes below the recommended levels for energy, protein, iron, thiamin and vitamin C. Very similar findings were recorded by Hagger [51] who also studied students and concluded that self-catering accommodation, although allowing students much freedom in life-style and diets, also made it easy for them to adopt an inferior diet when compared with the traditional halls of residence where all meals were provided. The British survey of 15- to 25-year-olds [15] also suggested links between diet and type of living accommodation, with lower intakes of energy and most nutrients for both men and women who lived alone compared with those who lived either with their parents or with a partner.

In the UK it has been suggested that young adults may be among the groups particularly at risk of consuming an inadequate diet for economic reasons [18]. However, it would seem that for young adults who have left home and are catering for themselves for the first time, an inadequate diet may result from lack of experience in planning meals, or general lack of interest in food, as much as from financial constraints.

Other Factors

Woodward [128] used non-parametric statistical techniques to evaluate the influence (in statistical terms) of a variety of personal characteristics, upon the energy and nutrient intakes of adolescents in Tasmania. Some of these influences were those which might have been expected and which have been demonstrated by other studies, for example the differences between the sexes and the effect of age among boys. Woodward [128] also demonstrated that the consumption of more food by boys does not uniformly embrace all types of food. They eat more dairy, meat and cereal foods but not necessarily more fruit and vegetables. However, Woodward also showed that alcohol usage, smoking and the use of vitamin supplements appeared to influence the diets of some groups of adolescents. Thus, older boys who regularly drank alcohol had higher energy and fat intakes, the former not being attributed to the energy content of the drinks consumed. Among the younger boys (mostly those under 14 years) greater intakes of thiamin and nicotinic acid equivalents were related to smoking more than 10 cigarettes per week. The thiamin and nicotinic acid intakes of these subjects were associated with greater consumption of fruit and vegetables. For girls, regular usage of vitamin supplements was associated with higher intake of calcium, this not being attributable to any calcium included in the supplements.

Schorr et al. [109] assessed the complexity of the diets of subjects aged 12–18. They found that complexity increased significantly in relation to father's and mother's occupational level and mother's educational level but was not related to the age of the subject, sex, family size or the number of sources of nutrition information the subject identified. Dietary complexity was associated with greater intakes of calcium, iron, vitamin C and vitamin A. In this study the subjects were also asked to list their favourite foods and their most disliked foods. Carbonated beverages, milk, steak, hamburgers and pizza received the most mentions as favourite foods. Liver was the least favourite, followed by fish. Spinach and cabbage were also among the least liked foods. Similar likes and dislikes were expressed by young adults interviewed during the British MAFF study [14].

Krehl [69] identified a number of dietary patterns common to adolescents which he considered to be of significance in relation to their nutritional status. First, the omission of breakfast and its replacement with a mid-morning 'empty-calorie' type of snack. Second, non-compulsory school lunches with consequent replacement of lunch by confectionery, soft drinks, crisps or similar items and third, the fact that adolescents are often found to dislike fruits, vegetables or salads.

In a paper by Marktl [82], it is suggested that some of the feelings and patterns of behaviour, related to food and occurring in adolescence, may have their roots in problems arising during the integration of eating, nutrition and emotion in the very first phases of life. The establishing of successful infant feeding thus has important implications for the diets of adolescents.

Twenty years ago, Leverton [73] recognised that those with professional responsibilities in the areas of nutrition and dietetics should make more effort to recognise and respect the complex range of needs and problems in the world of the adolescent. She lists a number of reasons why adolescents may not follow nutritional recommendations. For example, they have too often been given the idea that nutrition means 'eating what you don't like because it's good for you'; they do not immediately experience the nutritional disaster that adults are telling them will result from poor food habits; and food is only one element in their busy lives, while what they need and will eat is not always available at the appropriate places and times. Leverton [73] suggested, on the positive side, that good habits established in childhood are just as difficult to break as bad habits and that this can be used to advantage in the encouraging of good eating habits early in life. She further suggested that school timetables should take into account the need for meals and snacks because allocating too little time for eating may encourage schoolchildren to grab any food they can during school hours.

Food Consumption Patterns

As a result of the different methodologies employed in dietary surveys of adolescents and young adults and because such surveys have been conducted with varying objectives, it is not possible to construct a comparative table showing food consumption results. Where results have been presented for consumption of foods they have often been grouped in different ways or expressed in different units. For example, in many of the North American studies data on consumption of foods, where given, is in terms of number of servings. This has often been done to facilitate comparison with recommendations under the four food groups system but for the purposes of this review the lack of truly quantitative data in the literature renders comparison with the results of other studies very difficult in terms of food consumption patterns.

A number of studies of adolescents' diets have focussed on the habit of snacking or eating between meals. In some cases it has been found that the foods most often associated with snacking are largely of the 'empty-calorie' type, for example carbonated beverages, confectionery and crisps and other potato or corn snacks. Lai et al. [71] reported that in general the nutritional quality of schoolchildren's diets decreased with age and that a relatively high energy contribution came from snacks and sugar rich foods. Thomas and Call [117], however, looked at the actual amount of seven nutrients supplied per 100 kcal by the snack foods which 12- to 17-year-old Americans had reported eating. Comparison with their RDA, also expressed on a 'per 100-kcal' basis, led the authors to conclude that between-meal foods were supplying a relatively good balance of nutrients, with the exceptions of calcium and iron. Data for these nutrients are given below (mg/100 kcal):

	Meals	Between meal foods	Total	RDA
Ca				
males	46.2	39.1	44.6	50
females	43.1	34.3	41.0	55.3
Fe				
males	0.61	0.33	0.55	0.64
females	0.59	0.34	0.53	0.77

These findings lend support to the suggestions made by others that, rather than discourage between-meal eating by adolescents, young people should be directed towards appropriate foods and that suitable between-meal snacks, rich in iron and calcium, should be made available.

Truswell and Darnton-Hill [119] suggested that growing adolescents need the energy provided by soft drinks and that these are innocuous examples of 'fun foods' as described by McKenzie [79]. Soft drinks, especially carbonated beverages, are undoubtedly popular with young people but as a result of her recent study Guenther [43] has reached a rather different conclusion regarding their nutritional impact. Scrutiny of the beverage consumption reported by adolescents who had participated in the American Nationwide Food Consumption Survey led to an assessment of the nutritional impact of soft drinks. It was concluded that by replacing more nutrient dense beverages, and milk in particular, soft drinks may depress overall intakes of calcium, magnesium, riboflavin, vitamin A and vitamin C.

Musgrave et al. [88] found that the foods selected most often as snacks by American 10- to 16-year-olds were 'empty calorie' items but the 142 subjects did not snack exclusively on foods of low nutrient density. Raisins and peanuts were chosen more often than crisps. However, the widespread belief that children consume large amounts of refined sugar in their snacks was supported. The top ten choices of snack foods, in descending order, were biscuits, confectionery, cakes etc., fruit, bread or crackers, milk, ice cream, carbonated beverages, chewing gum, nuts and peanut butter. This study did not support the suggestion of Frank et al. [36] that consumption of confectionery and soft drinks as snacks probably peaks at about age 12 as there was no shift in snack food choices with increasing maturity. In the British study of 15- to 25-year-olds there was an apparent decline in the consumption of confectionery and soft drinks with increasing age; average consumptions falling from 35 to 20 and 40 to 25 g of confectionery per day and from 200 to 155 and 220 to 145 g of soft drinks per day for female and male subjects, respectively [14]. In the British survey of schoolchildren, however [123], a decline in soft drink consumption was seen between the 10–11 age group and the 14–15 age group. It also appeared that 10- to 11-year-old girls ate more confectionery than the older girls but for boys there did not appear to be a difference in consumption between the two age groups. These findings may reflect the fact that by 14–15 years the girls are becoming more diet-conscious while for many boys this age coincides with the period of maximum adolescent growth rate and energy intakes are high, reflecting increased appetite.

Differences between the sexes have been shown for other types of foods as well as for snacks. For example, in a study of 50 student volunteers Atkinson et al. [3] found that there were distinct differences between the sexes in the consumption of the main food groups. Thus, females ate more citrus fruit and cheese but less meat, bread and potatoes.

From a large study of Tasmanian adolescents aged 11-16, Woodward [129] has reported the relative influences of physical, behavioural and socio-economic characteristics on intakes of five broad categories of foods (cereals, meats, dairy, fruit and vegetables, miscellaneous). The pattern of influences varied considerably from food to food. Sex differences were strong for cereals, meats and dairy foods. Intakes of cereals increased with age for boys. Woodward [130, 131] also found that fatter girls were more likely to have low intakes (below the 25th percentile for the girls studied) of 'empty energy' foods and less likely to have high intakes (above the 75th percentile for the girls studied) of meat and 'empty energy' foods. In a more detailed analysis of the factors affecting consumption of specific foods, Woodward [132] has shown that with increasing fatness girls actually consume less milk, potatoes, cakes and desserts. At the same time, boys who reported higher levels of alcohol consumption ate more red meats and confectionery. For both sexes higher social class was associated with greater consumption of citrus and berry fruits. In a food frequency study reported by Bailey et al. [5] low intakes of both fresh fruit and vegetables were found among adolescents in low income households.

Hackett et al. [50] also concluded that social class differences in diet can be seen for adolescents. In their study, for example, the children of lower social class had more 'undesirable' eating habits, with the highest consumption of chips and the lowest of brown breads. There was also some evidence that these children had a greater consumption of sugar and of confectionery and lower intakes of fruit and vegetables (other than potatoes).

Finland has a high incidence of coronary heart disease and fat accounts for about 38% of the total energy intake of Finnish children and adolescents [104]. The traditional Finnish diet is rich in fat, especially from high fat milk products. Dietary recommendations for Finland, as for other Western nations, include limiting fat calories to 30–35% and increasing the ratio of polyunsaturated to saturated fats. In practice this means limiting consumption of animal fats and high fat milk products. Prattala et al. [103] studied consumption patterns every 2 years between 1977 and 1985 among 12- to 18-year-olds, with questionnaires covering the frequency of use and sizes of portions of a number of foods. Their results indicate decreases in the use of high fat milk and butter among Finnish adolescents during the period of the study. However, socio-economic and regional differences in consumption patterns persisted over the 8-year period with adolescents from farming families, those from lower social classes and those from an Eastern province continuing to use high fat milk and butter more than those from white collar families and those from the more urbanised South and Southwest. The authors suggested that when these adolescents reach the age of 40–60 the risk of coronary heart disease may be lower than among adults today but that inequalities between subgroups may remain.

The consumption of dairy products by Canadian adolescents was studied by Desaulniers et al. [29]. More than half of the total daily consumption of 21.6 oz was milk, while average consumption of cheese was only 0.5 oz. Cheese was also found to account for only a very small part of the consumption of dairy foods in the study of British schoolchildren reported by Wenlock et al. [123], with average daily consumptions of less than 0.5 oz by both boys and girls aged 10–11 and 14–15. For 15- to 25-year-olds in Britain cheese consumption averaged approximately 1 oz and was highest for those in the 22- to 25-year-old groups [14].

Durnin et al. [31] found that cheese, fish and eggs contributed surprisingly little to the diets of the 14-year-olds they studied and that the milk consumption of this age group as recorded in 1971 was lower than that found in 1964. Hackett et al. [50] made comparisons with Durnin's findings in reporting their longitudinal study of more than 400 British adolescents initially aged 11.5. They suggested that downward trends were possibly shown for consumption of milk, bread and cakes and biscuits among adolescents, with an upward trend in the contribution of potato products to energy intakes. They found that potatoes (largely chips and crisps) were the largest single source of energy in the diets of 11- to 14-year-olds.

Reduction in the consumption of sugars is recommended for most population groups in developed countries and is likely to have benefits for dental health and the avoidance of obesity. Rugg-Gunn et al. [106], also reporting on the longitudinal study of British adolescents, showed that confectionery, table sugar and soft drinks accounted for 71% of the 'added' sugars intake in adolescents' diets, with milk, fruit and fruit products providing most of the natural sugars. A high proportion of the sugars consumed by the subjects in this study were in foods eaten between meals. Snacks accounted for 65% of the sugars intake and snacking was therefore a component of their eating habits which would require particular attention in any attempt to reduce the consumption of sugars [48]. Such a reduction could be achieved by reducing the consumption of a relatively small number of groups of foods of low nutrient density. It was recommended by the authors [106] that labelling of foods with their sugars content would enable consumers to make prudent choices. This tends to presuppose that adolescents are interested enough to read and act upon the information supplied on food labels. In the study of British 15- to 25-year-olds, carried out for the Ministry of Agriculture, Fisheries and Food, only 21% of subjects reported that they often read food labels [14].

A large study of adolescent girls in the Southern States of America indicated that there are some differences in food consumption patterns between urban and rural groups. Urban girls derived more energy from carbonated beverages, desserts and confectionery and more carbohydrates from cooked starchy foods and breakfast cereals than did rural girls. There was an age related decline in consumption of dairy products between 12 and 16 years. This decline was less marked for black girls who consumed less dairy produce at all ages. The authors noted that lactose intolerance may have contributed to this racial difference [66]. Analysis by income indicated that as income increased so did consumption of breakfast cereals and fruit, while consumption of eggs decreased.

In a study of households with young mothers it was found that consumption levels of milk, vegetables and fruits were low where the mother was aged between 15 and 19. As a result it was suggested that intakes of protein, iron and vitamin C might be less than adequate in such families and that young mothers should be the subject of nutrition education programmes aimed at improving diets with particular reference to these nutrients [120].

In the recent large study of British schoolchildren [123] it was found that almost all subjects, aged 10–11 and 14–15, consumed potatoes and/or potato products, notably chips, and cereal products during the survey week. The older boys ate the most chips while the younger boys ate the most cakes and biscuits. In the British MAFF survey of 15- to 25-year-olds a similar pattern was seen, with average consumption of desserts and cakes and of sweet biscuits declining with age among the male subjects and consumption of vegetables increasing with age. Among all groups of 15- to 25-year-olds, potatoes accounted for approximately half the vegetables eaten, with chips as the most popular form of potatoes [14]. Both surveys reinforced the general conclusion of many other workers that consumption of many foods varies by age and sex. Milk was drunk by almost all 10- to 11-and 14- to 15-year-olds, with boys consuming more on average than girls. Lower levels of consumption were found among 15-to 25-year-olds but for both male and female participants, consumption was greater at 15–18 than at 22–25 and was higher for men than for women. Both surveys found that, on average, boys ate more breakfast cereals and less fruit than girls. In the youngest age group (10–11) boys and girls had approximately equal average consumption of confectionery while at all other ages up to 25 the female subjects consumed, on average, less chocolate and other confectionery than male subjects of the same age.

Nutrient Intakes

Tables II–VI summarise the nutritional findings from a number of surveys of adolescents and young adults conducted during the last 20 years. For ease of reference these studies are identified by the consecutive numbers given to them in table I. Studies particularly directed at athletes have been grouped separately in table II and have been discussed above in connection with factors affecting adolescents' diets. The remaining nutritional results have been divided into four tables according to the ages of the subjects. In some cases, where the age range of subjects studied falls into two of the ranges in the tables, results are shown in both tables.

In the majority of cases the data given here are as presented in the original work. However, in some instances it has been necessary to convert results for vitamins A and D from international units into retinol equivalents and micrograms, respectively. Table VII gives the current RDA in use in the UK, the USA, Canada and Australia for the age ranges covered by this review. Where the national RDA have been used to assess dietary adequacy in different countries, the same nutrients have nevertheless often been considered to be lacking in adolescents' diets despite, in some instances, quite considerable differences in the RDA for those nutrients.

The findings of the studies detailed in tables III–VI are discussed below, together with data from other work where appropriate. It has not been possible to cover the tables strictly in order, from the younger subjects to the older ones, because of the number of studies including two or more age groups.

Considering first those studies which have included subjects aged 10, 11 or 12, a French survey of 9- to 11- and 14- to 16-year-olds has shown energy intakes lower than recommended levels and low iron and calcium intakes among adolescent girls. This survey used a 7-day record technique. The contributions of protein, fat and carbohydrate to energy intakes were the same, on average, for 9- to 11-year-olds and for 14- to 16-year-olds (14.5, 40 and 45.5%, respectively) [12]. Studies of schoolchildren carried out by the British Department of Health & Social Security (DHSS) [24] indicated that many subjects had nutrient intakes lower than the recommendations without showing any signs of malnutrition. Calcium, iron, vitamin A, thiamin, riboflavin and vitamin C were all mentioned in this context. However, mean intakes of all nutrients either approximated to or were greater than the RDA. The energy intakes of adolescents, along with those of other groups, appear to have fallen steadily over the years [31] and

Table VII. Recommended daily allowances

	Energy		Protein	Calcium	Iron	Zinc	Thiamin	Ribofl.	Nic.ac. Eq	Folate	Vit. B_6	Vit. B_{12}	Vit. C	Vit. A	Vit. D
	kcal	MJ	g	mg	mg	mg	mg	mg	mg	µg	mg	µg	mg	ret.Eq	µg
Males															
ca. 10–12															
UK	2,280	9.5	57	700	12	–	0.9	1.2	14	–	–	–	25	575	(10)[a]
USA	2,700	11.3	45	1,200	18	15	1.4	1.6	18	400	1.8	3.0	50	1,000 (600)[b]	10
Can.	2,500	10.4	38	900	10	7	1.0	1.3	18	170	0.6	1.0	40	800	2.5
Aust.	2,900	12.1	51–87	600–1,400	12	12–18	1.2	1.5	19	200	1.4–2.1	2.0	40	725	–
ca. 13–15															
UK	2,640	11.0	66	700	12	–	1.1	1.4	16	–	–	–	25	725	(10)[a]
USA	2,700	11.3	45	1,200	18	15	1.4	1.6	18	400	1.8	3.0	50	1,000 (700)[b]	10
Can.	2,800	12.0	49	1,100	12	9	1.1	1.4	20	160	0.7	1.5	50	900	2.5
Aust.	2,900	12.1	51–87	600–1,400	12	12–18	1.2	1.5	19	200	1.4–2.1	2.0	40	725	–
ca. 16–18															
UK	2,880	12.0	72	600	12	–	1.2	1.7	19	–	–	–	30	750	(10)[a]
USA	2,800	11.8	56	1,200	18	15	1.4	1.7	18	400	2.0	3.0	60	1,000 (700)[b]	10
Can.	3,200	13.2	54	900	10	9	1.3	1.6	23	190	0.8	1.9	55	1,000	2.5
Aust.	3,000	12.6	67–90	500–1,400	12	12–18	1.2	1.5	20	200	1.5–2.2	2.0	50	750	–
18+															
UK	2,900	12.0	72	500	10	–	1.2	1.6	18	–	–	–	30	750	–
USA	2,900	12.2	56	800	10	15	1.5	1.7	19	400	2.2	3.0	60	1,000 (700)[b]	7.5
Can.	3,000	12.4	57	800	8	9	1.2	1.5	22	210	0.9	2.0	60	1,000	2.5
Aust.	2,800	11.7	70	400–800	10	12–16	1.1	1.4	18	200	1.3–1.9	2.0	30	750	–

Females															
ca. 10–12															
UK	2,050	8.5	51	700	12	–	0.8	1.2	14	–	–	–	25	575	(10)[a]
USA	2,200	9.2	46	1,200	18	15	1.1	1.3	15	400	1.8	3.0	50	800 (600)[b]	10
Can.	2,200	9.2	39	1,000	10	7	0.9	1.1	16	170	0.6	1.0	40	800	2.5
Aust.	2,500	10.5	52–75	600–1,300	12	12–18	1.0	1.3	17	200	1.2–1.8	2.0	40	725	–
ca. 13–15															
UK	2,150	9.0	53	700	12	–	0.9	1.4	16	–	–	–	25	725	(10)[a]
USA	2,200	9.2	46	1,200	18	15	1.1	1.3	15	400	1.8	3.0	50	800 (600)[b]	10
Can.	2,200	9.2	43	800	13	8	0.9	1.1	16	160	0.6	1.5	45	800	2.5
Aust.	2,500	10.5	52–75	600–1,300	12	12–18	1.0	1.3	17	200	1.2–1.8	2.0	40	725	–
ca. 16–18															
UK	2,150	9.0	53	600	12	–	0.9	1.7	19	–	–	–	30	750	(10)[a]
USA	2,100	8.8	46	1,200	18	15	1.1	1.3	14	400	2.0	3.0	60	800 (600)[b]	10
Can.	2,100	8.8	47	700	14	8	0.8	1.1	15	160	0.7	1.9	45	800	2.5
Aust.	2,200	9.2	60–66	500–1,300	12	12–18	0.9	1.1	15	200	1.1–1.6	2.0	50	750	–
18+															
UK	2,150	9.0	54	500	12	–	0.9	1.3	15	–	–	–	30	750	–
USA	2,100	8.8	44	800	18	15	1.1	1.3	14	400	2.0	3.0	60	800 (600)[b]	7.5
Can.	2,100	8.8	41	700	14	8	0.8	1.1	15	165	0.6	2.0	45	800	2.5
Aust.	2,000	8.4	58	400–800	12	12–16	0.8	1.0	13	200	0.9–1.4	2.0	30	750	–

UK: DHSS [1979]; USA: Natn. Res. Co./Natn. Acad. Sci. [1980]; Can.: Dept. Natn. Health & Welfare [1983]; Aust.: Natn. Health & Med. Res. Co. [1979].

[a] No dietary sources may be necessary with sufficient exposure to sunlight but supplementation by this amount is recommended for children and adolescents during the winter.

[b] See Olson [1987].

the widespread finding of lower energy intakes unaccompanied by any growth failure or deficiency symptoms has resulted in reductions to the recommended amounts of energy for young people [26].

In a study of 10- to 14-year-olds in America, at least 45% of the girls failed to meet two thirds of the RDA for vitamin A, vitamin C, iron, calcium, thiamin and nicotinic acid [36]. Although boys did better, at least one third of them also failed to achieve intakes of two thirds RDA for these nutrients. A detailed 24-hour recall procedure was used in the study. Similarly, a large study of American adolescent girls reported by McCoy et al. [75] indicated that the nutrients most often lacking in the diet were iron, calcium, zinc, magnesium, vitamin B_6, folate, vitamin A and vitamin D. In their survey of American 10-year-olds, Johnson and Jensen [63] found that average intakes of most nutrients met the RDA. The exceptions were energy intake, thiamin and nicotinic acid. However, intakes of calcium, iron, vitamin A and vitamin C were highly variable, with some subjects consuming as little as 30% of the RDA and others having intakes in excess of 250%. These very wide ranges in intakes displayed by young subjects led the authors of this report to conclude that increased attention should be focussed on the intakes of individuals rather than on group averages, if those nutritionally at risk are to be identified.

Lai et al. [71] in Hawaii found that many school students, aged approximately 11–14, had 24-hour recalls indicating daily intakes of less than two thirds RDA for iron, calcium, thiamin and vitamins A and C. There were also high intakes of sodium, cholesterol and saturated fatty acids. The same findings applied to the subjects in the 15- to 18-year-old age range. Again in the USA, Salz et al. [107] studied 24-hour recalls of 10- to 19-year-olds. They found that boys' average energy intake rose considerably between the 10- to 14-year-olds and the 15- to 19-year-olds while girls' average energy intake peaked at 10–14 years at approximately 2,200 kcal. Protein intake by the older boys provided 15% of energy while for girls protein provided an average of 14% of dietary energy for both age ranges. Fat calories were 38% for the younger girls and boys, rising to 39% for girls and 40% for boys aged 15–19. Boys consumed more cholesterol, total fat and saturated fat than girls. In contrast, Kuczmarski et al. [70] report that a 24-hour recall study of over 1,000 American adolescents indicated that the contributions of fat, protein and carbohydrate to energy intakes were similar for both male and female subjects.

In Canada, Seoane and Roberge [110] used a 3-day record method to study 500 10- to 18-year-olds. Iron intakes were low in their three female groups (10- to 12-, 13- to 15- and 16- to 18-year-olds) and thiamin was also low on average in the oldest group. Carbohydrate provided proportionately more calories in the diets of male subjects in the two younger groups. When concentrated sugar sources (table sugar, syrup, honey, etc.) were evaluated separately, their energy contribution was significantly higher for 10- to 12-year-old boys than for girls of the same age. The boys aged 16–18 obtained significantly more calories from alcohol than did females of the same age. This finding is similar to that reported by Bull [14].

In the study of schoolchildren carried out for the British DHSS [123], energy intakes were found to be, on average, approximately 10% lower than recommended levels for 10- to 11- and 14- to 15-year-olds. This was also found for older adolescents and young adults in the study carried out for the MAFF in Britain [14]. In the former study, data on heights and weights were also collected and the authors were therefore able to demonstrate that these lower intakes did not necessarily imply any risk to health as no evidence of undernutrition was found. Energy requirements then, appeared to be less than the recommended energy allowances for the age groups studied. Among the 10- to 11- and 14- to 15-year-olds protein provided 12% of energy on average. For 15- to 25-year-olds protein contributed 13–14% of calories. The DHSS RDA is based on protein providing 10% of dietary energy and protein intakes were therefore found to be more than adequate for all these age ranges. Both surveys found that fat contributed more energy than the 35% maximum recommended by the COMA Panel on Diet and Cardiovascular Disease [27]. For 10- to 11-year-olds fat contributed on average 37% of calories for boys and 38% for girls with corresponding values for 14- to 15-year-olds of 38 and 39%. The older age groups studied by the MAFF had greater intakes of fat, particularly among the male subjects. However, the lower energy intakes of the older females in these groups resulted in apparent energy contributions from fat which were even higher for women than for men. These results are shown below:

	Percentage of energy from fat		
	15–18	19–21	22–25
Male	42	42	42
Female	43	43	45

Both these recent British surveys found that iron was the nutrient most likely to be lacking in the diets of young people and they both suggested that the female adolescents, especially those dieting to lose weight, were the most vulnerable. The study of schoolchildren concluded that the school meal provided a valuable contribution to the overall diet and that the older subjects, aged 14–15, who did not have school lunches (i.e. who consumed a 'self-selected' diet) had the poorer diets in terms of overall nutritional quality. The survey of older adolescents and young adults tended to confirm this, with the high fat and low iron intakes being even more pronounced in the over-15-year-olds.

Woodward [130, 131] has used a statistical technique based on analysis of the 25th and 75th percentiles to examine the characteristics affecting the prevalence of low or high intakes of energy and nutrients among a large group of 11- to 16-year-olds. The 25th and 75th percentiles can be regarded as the averages of those with below- or above-average intakes and analysis of survey results as described by Woodward provides insight into the characteristics of adolescents who are more likely to have either below- or above-average intakes of energy and nutrients. He found that among girls, those who were fatter were more likely to have low intakes (below the 25th percentile for girls) of energy, carbohydrate, iron, calcium and nicotinic acid equivalents. Lack of exercise was the most influential factor related to low intake of protein and the type of school attended the most influential in relation to low intakes of fat, riboflavin and vitamin A. By contrast, the prevalence of high intakes (above the 75th percentile for girls) of energy and most nutrients was not affected by any of the characteristics studied. However, girls from small families were less likely to have high calcium intakes, while those from state schools were less likely to have high thiamin intakes. For boys, height and age had the greatest influence on the prevalence of low intakes (below the 25th percentile for boys) of energy and almost all nutrients with the taller, older boys less likely to have low intakes. Age also had the greatest influence on the prevalence of high intakes (above the 75th percentile for boys), with older boys more likely to have high intakes of energy and most nutrients. High fat intakes, however, were associated with alcohol usage, being common among boys who reported having drunk more than five glasses of alcoholic drink in the preceding week. In addition, high calcium intakes were more common among those taking more exercise.

From surveys where the majority of participants were over the age of 13, as with those concentrating on younger subjects, it has been widely found that boys have greater intakes of energy and all nutrients than girls. An American study of 225 16- to 18-year-olds, who each completed one-day food records, indicated that the girls' average intakes of vitamin A, calcium and iron were low at all eating occasions throughout the day. Boys' average intakes of iron were low at breakfast, lunch and snacks and their vitamin A intakes were low from snacks. When intakes were analysed per 1,000 kcal, there was a significant difference between boys and girls only for riboflavin, supporting the assumption that the nutrient intakes of boys are more likely to be adequate simply because they consume more food [111].

In a large-scale nationwide study of 13- to 18-year-olds in the USA, the results of 7-day diaries indicated mean intakes of zinc, magnesium and energy below the RDA, with some adolescents consuming less than two thirds of the RDA for energy, vitamin A, vitamin C and phosphorus. It was found that snacks contributed significantly to the intakes of energy, vitamin B_6, iron and magnesium for both male and female adolescents [17].

In a survey of the nutritional status of schoolchildren in southeast England, described by Topp et al. [118] and carried out between 1968 and 1970, sex, age and weight were all found to be associated with significant differences in average daily nutrient intakes, for almost all nutrients [20]. Social class, number of siblings and mother's work status were not generally associated with significant differences in the average daily nutrient intakes of the 13- to 15-year-olds studied, although children from higher social classes did have higher intakes of all nutrients except carbohydrate and sugar, on a per 1,000 kcal basis. This was taken to indicate that these groups had a better quality of diet. It was also found that only children had significantly higher intakes of many nutrients, and of nutrients per 1,000 kcal, than children with siblings [62].

Adolescents at a Seventh-Day Adventist boarding school in the USA were assessed in relation to cardiovascular risk factors. Their diet was found to contribute 34% of calories as fat, with 11% derived from saturated fat [21]. These findings compare very favourably with current dietary recommendations and it was concluded that if their dietary habits continued into adult life then the incidence of premature coronary heart disease for the group was likely to be reduced compared with other Americans.

Dietary recalls conducted with adolescent girls in the USA led to estimated average iron consumption of only 60% of the RDA with average energy intakes also rather lower than recommended levels [41]. In the Philippines also, the iron intakes of most of the public high school girls studied were less than 70% of the RDA. Iron intakes for the male students were found to average 90% or more of the RDA [45].

It is particularly during the adolescent growth spurt that the dietary supply of another important mineral, calcium, may become limiting and although milk and dairy products are recognised as the major contributors of this nutrient, Hackett et al. [47] have shown that in the UK the maintenance of a policy of flour fortification is also an important element in achieving adequate levels of calcium in the diets of adolescents. For individuals with a large skeletal mass, a dietary intake well in excess of some of the lower recommendations (e.g. the current British RDA) might be required during the rapid bone growth of adolescence. This would be particularly necessary where calcium sources are such that the lower ranges of calcium absorption prevail. From earlier work, conducted in the 1960s, it was found that in the diets of American adolescent girls the intakes of iron and calcium were lowest compared to RDA, in that order, with the same nutrients but in the reverse order, lowest for boys. The next nutrient most likely to be in short supply in the diet was vitamin C [53, 61].

The study of Australian families conducted by Hitchcock and Gracey [57] resulted in a very similar pattern for Australian adolescents as that found in the UK and the USA. That is, energy intakes were lower on average than recommended levels, intakes of most nutrients were adequate but with a rather high proportion of energy from fat. In addition, dietary iron intakes by adolescent females were very low compared with recommendations. From their study of British adolescents, Hackett et al. [46] suggested that for girls it is their low intakes of energy that are limiting iron intakes. Although this would seem to be supported by the findings from many other studies the authors point out that the use of food tables in dietary analysis can give rise to poor estimates of iron intake. Adolescents are particularly susceptible to iron deficiency anaemia because of the increased need for dietary iron during the growth spurt, when both blood volume and muscle mass are increasing [40]. The pattern of food selection displayed by adolescents in a number of studies, with low consumption of fruits and vegetables [42], may result in reduced intake of vitamin C [40], and because of the interrelationship between vitamin C and absorption of iron it is especially important to establish the dietary patterns as well as simply the amounts of food consumed over the whole period of a dietary study.

Clinical studies are undoubtedly necessary before iron deficiency anaemia can be diagnosed in any group of subjects and such studies would be a valuable indicator as to the usefulness of the current recommended daily amounts [7].

In comparisons with American RDA, Lee [72] found grossly deficient intakes of calcium, iron and vitamin A among both black and white female adolescents in Kentucky. The contribution of fat to dietary energy was high for all groups (42 and 40% for white boys and girls, 46 and 38% for black boys and girls, respectively). Biochemical and clinical findings from this study, together with the dietary and meal pattern data, revealed the prevalence of coronary heart disease risk factors such as smoking, high blood pressure, raised serum lipid levels and obesity in addition to the nutritional problems associated with a high incidence of anaemia, low intakes of calcium, vitamins A and C and irregular eating habits. Schorr et al. [109] studied the diets of 118 12- to 18-year-olds in the USA. They found that the percentages of subjects having intakes lower than two thirds of the RDA for vitamin C, calcium, vitamin A and iron were 21, 44, 51 and 69, respectively.

In an area of England with many Asian immigrants, rickets was found to occur among the adolescent girls. Dietary interviews with 100 girls aged 12–17 indicated that 99% were taking less than the then recommended intake of vitamin D [100]. Although RDA for vitamin D are now only given in the UK for the under-fives, and for pregnancy and lactation, it is nevertheless suggested that in winter children and adolescents should receive 10 μg daily, as sunlight exposure may be insufficient. In the case of Asian children and adolescents the combination of dietary habits and social customs, especially traditional clothing, are important factors in the causation of rickets. The inclusion of fortified margarine in the daily diets of Asian children, in order to increase their vitamin D intakes, has been encouraged and generally accepted.

The Dutch longitudinal study of Post et al. [102] revealed adequate intakes of vitamins and minerals for 12- to 17-year-olds with the exception of iron intakes which were borderline for the female subjects. Weekdays and weekend days were studied separately and results presented only in graphical form so that the inclusion of the Dutch results in a comparative table is not possible. However, in many respects the study reinforced the findings of both recent British national surveys [14, 123] by highlighting low iron intakes by girls, high fat (especially cholesterol) intakes and the level of alcohol consumption by boys as areas of possible concern. Post et al. [102] found that alcohol intake increased with age and that the consumption of alcoholic drinks on schooldays, as opposed to only at weekends, started at the age of about 15–16. Consumption was greater on weekend days, reaching 7.1 g alcohol/day for girls and 19.6 g/day for boys by age 17–18. If non-drinkers are excluded these figures rise to 11 and 29 g, respectively.

Heald et al. [55] reviewed dietary studies of adolescents prior to 1960 and concluded that the energy and nutrient requirements for boys and girls are very closely linked, not to their chronological age but to the stage of physiological development. Thus, the peak energy need for boys is at an average age of 16 years but may occur at any age between 11 and 17. For girls, however, the situation is very different, with average energy intake peaking at approximately age 12; the female growth spurt occurring before the onset of menarche. The stage of physiological development of subjects is therefore an important factor to be taken into consideration, particularly in studies with small numbers of subjects.

Where studies of small groups of subjects are being considered, the conclusions reached by Darke et al. [24] should also be borne in mind. In drawing together results from dietary surveys among different age groups in the UK, they showed that within a group many individuals may be found to consume less than the recommended amounts of energy or nutrients without showing any signs of deficiency. At the same time the average intake for the group may approximate to, or exceed, the RDA. This led to the suggestion for modification of the definition of the UK RDA as 'the average amount of the nutrient which should be provided per head in a group of healthy people if the needs of practically all members of the group are to be met', and it should therefore be stressed that low average intakes across small groups do not necessarily reflect a low intake among the larger population from which the group has been chosen. Nevertheless, many of the studies included in this review have had relatively large groups of subjects drawn from the adolescent population and there is therefore some reason to suppose that the findings common to so many of these studies may reflect a widespread pattern among adolescents. In addition, Hodges [58] draws on findings from the American Ten State survey to demonstrate that there are imperfect but nevertheless important interrelationships between dietary findings and the results of physical and biochemical assessment. Thus, low iron intakes have in some instances been correlated with a high prevalence of low haemoglobin values in particular groups of adolescent females.

The need to consider the results of dietary surveys, whenever possible, in terms other than the average intakes over a group of subjects is reinforced by the longitudinal study reported by Wyn-Jones et al. [133]. This work indicated that even where the group mean intakes reach the standards set by RDA, this may mask very wide ranges in nutrient intake even within quite small groups of subjects. For example, when students had completed three 7-day food records in different months of the year, the overall mean daily intake of iron by female subjects was 13 mg whereas the ranges of intake were 4–18, 5–19 and 6–18 mg in the 3 months studied. Furthermore, it was found that in each month it was generally the same students who had intakes at the extreme ends of the range for a particular nutrient.

In Israel, Kaufmann et al. [65] found that the nutrient intake of young people in Jerusalem differed markedly from that of young populations in other Western countries. The subjects were 17 years old and their energy intakes were lower than recommended for that age but, when related to body weight, intakes were only low for girls. Fat contributed 32 and 34% of calories for boys and girls, respectively, according rather well with current recommendations for optimum health and in marked contrast with many of the findings reported from the UK and the USA. It was noted that boys whose fathers were born in Israel or Europe had higher intakes of fat and cholesterol, and both boys and girls had higher intakes of saturated fatty acids, and lower intakes of carbohydrate and starch, than their counterparts whose fathers were born in Asia or North Africa.

An American study looking at the effect of pregnancy on the diets of adolescents suggested that the energy and nutrient intakes of pregnant adolescents, while not significantly different from those of other groups of older pregnant women and of non-pregnant adolescents, were nevertheless significantly lower than these groups when expressed as percentages of the appropriate RDA [33]. In table V the results shown from this work, for comparison with other adolescents, are those of the non-pregnant group. King et al. [68] compared the diets of 18 pregnant adolescents with those of 5 never-pregnant girls. The never-pregnant girls consumed significantly less energy, protein, carbohydrate, calcium, phosphorus, potassium and thiamin than the pregnant girls. It appeared that among American adolescents, the group studied had responded to pregnancy by consuming more food although they nevertheless failed in a number of cases to satisfy recommended levels of intake. The nutrient intakes most improved during pregnancy were phosphorus, calcium, iron and vitamin C. In almost half the cases significant improvements in intake of a number of nutrients were largely brought about by the inclusion of vitamin and mineral supplements during pregnancy. The nutrients which were most poorly supplied by the diets, both during and after pregnancy and despite the improvements mentioned above, were calcium, iron, vitamin A and energy. Van de Mark and Wright [121] also found that the energy intakes of non-pregnant adolescents were generally lower than those of pregnant girls but that the diets of adolescent girls as a whole were below the RDA for iron and folate as well as energy. Requirements for vitamin B_6 and folate may be elevated as a result of oral contraceptive use. This led the Nutrition Committee of the Canadian Paediatric Society [95] to recommend that adolescent girls taking oral contraceptives should pay particular attention to their diets and should avoid meal-skipping and the generally rather poor dietary patterns seen among some of their peers. These nutrients should be ingested in sufficient amounts if a balanced diet is eaten, containing dairy products, meat, poultry, fish, vegetables and fruit.

In the USA there have been recommendations that cholesterol consumption should not exceed 300 mg/day and fat should not contribute more than 30–35% calories, with less than 10% of calories derived from saturated fat. This 'prudent diet' applies not only to adults but just as much to adolescents, who are establishing their 'long-term life-style habits' [9]. It is echoed in recommendations made in most other developed countries in recent years. There is, moreover, an accumulation of evidence now suggesting that adolescence is a fruitful time to establish practices aimed at preventing atherosclerotic vascular disease in later life. McGandy et al. [77] carried out a study in the USA which indicated that blood cholesterol, an important risk factor for atherosclerotic disease, could be readily and appreciably lowered among adolescent boys by realistic and acceptable dietary modifications.

Conclusions

From the work reviewed here it is seen that adolescents and young adults in a range of Western nations have adopted very similar eating habits and display remarkably similar patterns of energy and nutrient intakes. Adolescents are 'snackers' and there is no evidence to suggest that frequent eating per se is detrimental to health. However, in this context, the availability of nutritious snack foods, both in the home and elsewhere, is of great importance and despite recommendations to this effect made two decades ago, most vending machines still offer only confectionery or other low nutrient density snacks. Low iron intakes and high fat intakes characterise the adolescent diet as studied over the past 20 years. The significance of the former cannot properly be assessed without large-scale biochemical studies but the importance of reducing fat consumption as a measure to reduce the risk of coronary heart disease is well documented.

It has been pointed out that adolescence frequently heralds the start of alcohol consumption and yet the amount of alcohol consumed and the patterns of alcohol consumption have often been ignored in dietary surveys. This is all the more surprising when it is realised that alcohol is probably involved in more adolescent fatalities than any other single factor [119].

A number of studies reviewed here have included recommendations for ways in which adolescents and young adults could be encouraged towards dietary change and these have been mentioned briefly. To a great extent the responsibility for implementation of these recommendations rests with the policy makers of industry and government and with school caterers and the producers of snack foods. As steps are taken to encourage the development of healthy eating patterns among adolescents and young adults the dietary habits and nutrient intakes of selected groups should continue to be monitored.

References

1 Acheson, K.J.; Campbell, I.T.; Edholm, O.G.; Miller, D.S.; Stock, M.J.: The measurement of food and energy intake in man – an evaluation of some techniques. Am. J. clin. Nutr. *33:* 1147–1154 (1980).

2 Appleton, D.R.; Hackett, A.F.; Rugg-Gunn, A.J.; Eastoe, J.E.: The reliability of the diary and interview method of estimating nutrient intakes of children. Proc. Nutr. Soc. *42:* 107A (1983).

3 Atkinson, S.J.; Nicholas, P.; Wyn-Jones, C.: Consumption of major food groups by students over a 3-month period. Proc. Nutr. Soc. *31:* 82A (1972).

4 Baghurst, K.I.; McMichael, A.J.: Nutritional knowledge and its relationship to dietary intake in two young Australian populations. Proc. Nutr. Soc. Aust. *4:* 121 (1979).

5 Bailey, L.B.; Wagner, P.A.; Davis, C.G.; Dinning, J.S.: Food frequency related to folacin status in adolescents. J. Am. diet. Ass. *84:* 801–804 (1984).

6 Barber, S.A.; Bull, N.L.: Food and nutrient intakes by British women aged 15–25 years, with particular reference to dieting habits and iron intakes. Ecol. Fd Nutr. *16:* 161–169 (1985).

7 Barber, S.A.; Bull, N.L.; Buss, D.H.: Low iron intakes among young women in Britain. Br. med. J. *290:* 743–744 (1985).

8 Beals, T.L.; Anderson, G.H.; Peterson, R.D.; Thompson, G.W.; Hargreaves, J.A.: Between meal eating by Ontario children and teenagers. J. Can. diet. Ass. *42:* 242–247 (1981).

9 Belmaker, E.; Cohen, J.D.: The advisability of the prudent diet in adolescence. J. Adolesc. Hlth Care *6:* 224–232 (1985).

10 Bender, A.E.; Magee, P.; Nash, A.H.: Survey of school meals. Br. med. J. *ii:* 383–385 (1972).

11 Benson, J.; Gillien, D.M.; Bourdet, K.; Loosli, A.R.: Inadequate nutrition and chronic calorie restriction in adolescent ballerinas. Phys. Sportsmed. *13:* 79–90 (1985).

12 Boggio, V.; Klepping, J.: Results of dietary surveys in 5, 10 and 15 year old children. Archs fr. Pédiat. *38:* 679–686 (1981).

13 Brown, R.T.; McIntosh, S.M.; Seabolt, V.R.; Daniel, W.A.: Iron status of adolescent female athletes. J. Adolesc. Hlth Care *6:* 349–352 (1985).

14 Bull, N.L.: Dietary habits of 15-to 25-year-olds. Hum. Nutr. appl. Nutr. *39A:* suppl. 1, pp. 1–68 (1985).

15 Bull, N.L.; Barber, S.A.: Food habits of 15–25 year olds. II. Living accommodation and social class as factors affecting the diet. Health Visitor *58:* 9–11 (1985).

16 Bull, N.L.; Wheeler, E.F.: A study of different dietary survey methods among 30 civil servants. Hum. Nutr. appl. Nutr. *40A:* 60–66 (1986).

17 Bundy, K.T.; Morgan, K.J.; Zabik, M.E.: Nutritional adequacy of snacks and sources of total sugar intake among US adolescents. J. Can. diet. Ass. *43:* 358–365, 374 (1982).

18 Cole-Hamilton, I.; Lang, T.: Tightening belts: a report on the impact of poverty on food (London Food Commission, London 1986).

19 Comstock, E.M.; St-Pierre, R.G.; Mackiernan, Y.D.: Measuring individual plate waste in school lunches. J. Am. diet. Ass. *79:* 290–296 (1981).

20 Cook, J.; Altman, D.G.; Moore, D.M.C.; Topp, S.G.; Holland, W.W.; Elliott, A.: A survey of the nutritional status of schoolchildren. Relation between nutrient intake and socio-economic factors. Br. J. prev. soc. Med. *27:* 91–99 (1973).

21 Cooper, R.; Allen, A.; Goldberg, R.; Trevisan, M.; Horn, L. van; Liu, K.; Steinhauer, M.; Rubenstein, A.; Stamler, J.: Seventh-day Adventist adolescents – life-style patterns and cardiovascular risk factors. West. J. Med. *140:* 471–477 (1984).

22 Cresswell, J.; Busby, A.; Young, H.; Inglis, V.: Dietary patterns of third-year secondary schoolgirls in Glasgow. Hum. Nutr. appl. Nutr. *37A:* 301–306 (1983).

23 Curry, K.R.: Cultural aspects of food habits: teenager awareness in New Zealand, England and the United States. J. N.Z. diet. Ass. *38:* 38–50 (1984).

24 Darke, S.J.; Disselduff, M.M.; Try, G.P.: Frequency distributions of mean daily intakes of food energy and selected nutrients obtained during nutrition surveys of different groups of people in Great Britain between 1968 and 1971. Br. J. Nutr. *44:* 243–252 (1980).

25 Davies, L.; Holdsworth, M.D.: Nutrition and health at retirement age in the United Kingdom. Hum. Nutr. appl. Nutr. *39A:* 315–332 (1985).

26 Department of Health and Social Security: Recommended daily amounts of food energy and nutrients for groups of people in the UK. Reports on health and social subjects, No. 15 (HMSO, London 1979).

27 Department of Health and Social Security: Diet and cardiovascular disease. Reports on health and social subjects, No. 28 (HMSO, London 1984).
28 Department of National Health and Welfare: Recommended nutrient intakes for Canadians (Ottawa 1983).
29 Desaulniers, M.; Sauvagean, C.; Gilbert, M.; Saladin, G.; Sevigny, J.: Consumption of dairy products by adolescents in Quebec. J. Can. diet. Ass. *43:* 55–63 (1982).
30 Douglas, P.D.; Douglas, J.G.: Nutrition knowledge and food practices of high school athletes. J. Am. diet. Ass. *84:* 1198–1202 (1984).
31 Durnin, J.V.G.A.; Lonergan, M.E.; Good, J.; Ewan, A.: A cross-sectional nutritional and anthropometric study, with an interval of 7 years, on 611 young adolescent schoolchildren. Br. J. Nutr. *32:* 169–179 (1974).
32 Dwyer, J.T.; Feldman, J.J.; Mayer, J.: Adolescent dieters: Who are they? Physical characteristics, attitudes and dieting practices of adolescent girls. Am. J. clin. Nutr. *20:* 1045–1056 (1967).
33 Endres, J.M.; Poell-Odenwald, K.; Sawicki, M.; Welch, P.: Dietary assessment of pregnant adolescents participating in a supplemental food program. J. reprod. Med. *30:* 10–17 (1985).
34 Ezell, J.M.; Skinner, J.D.; Penfield, M.P.: Appalachian adolescents' snack patterns: morning, afternoon and evening snacks. J. Am. diet. Ass. *85:* 1450–1454 (1985).
35 Food and Agriculture Organisation: Report of the Codex Alimentarius Commission. ALINORM 85/22A (FAO, Roma 1985).
36 Frank, G.C.; Voors, A.W.; Schilling, P.E.; Berenson, G.S.: Dietary studies of rural schoolchildren in a cardiovascular survey. J. Am. diet. Ass. *71:* 31–35 (1977).
37 Garn, S.M.; Larkin, F.A.; Cole, P.E.: The problem with one-day dietary intakes. Ecol. Fd Nutr. *5:* 245–247 (1976).
38 George, R.S.; Krondl, M.: Perceptions and food use of adolescent boys and girls. Nutr. Behav. *1:* 115–125 (1983).
39 Greecher, C.P.; Shannon, B.: Impact of fast food meals on nutrient intake of two groups. J. Am. diet. Ass. *70:* 368–372 (1977).
40 Greenwood, C.T.: Richardson, D.P.: Nutrition during adolescence. Wld Rev. Nutr. Diet., vol. 33, pp. 1–41 (Karger, Basel 1979).
41 Greger, J.L.; Higgins, M.M.; Abernathy, R.P.; Kirksey, A.; DeCorso, M.B.; Baliger, P.: Nutritional status of adolescent girls in regard to zinc, copper and iron. Am. J. clin. Nutr. *31:* 269–275 (1978).
42 Greger, J.L.; Divilbiss, L.; Aschenbeck, S.K.; Dietary habits of adolescent females. Ecol. Fd Nutr. *7:* 213–218 (1979).
43 Guenther, P.M.: Beverages in the diets of American teenagers. J. Am. diet. Ass. *86:* 493–499 (1986).
44 Guthrie, H.A.: Selection and quantification of typical food portions by young adults. J. Am. diet. Ass. *84:* 1440–1444 (1984).
45 Guzman, M.P.E. de; Donato, D.S.; Jandayan, M.O.; Abanto, Z.U.; Agustin, C.P.: Nutritional evaluation of the food intake, dietary pattern and food habits of public high school students in Central Luzon. Phil. J. Nutr. *34:* 147–159 (1981).
46 Hackett, A.F.; Rugg-Gunn, A.J.; Appleton, D.R.; Eastoe, J.E.; Jenkins, G.N.: A 2-year longitudinal nutritional study of 405 Northumberland children initially aged 11.5 years. Br. J. Nutr. *51:* 67–75 (1984).
47 Hackett, A.F.; Rugg-Gunn, A.J.; Allinson, M.; Robinson, C.J.; Appleton, D.R.; Eas-

toe, J.E.: The importance of fortification of flour with calcium and the sources of Ca in the diet of 375 English adolescents. Br. J. Nutr. *51:* 193–197 (1984).

48 Hackett, A.F.; Rugg-Gunn, A.J.; Appleton, D.R.; Allinson, M.; Eastoe, J.E.: Sugar-eating habits of 405 11- to 14-year-old English children. Br. J. Nutr. *51:* 347–356 (1984).

49 Hackett, A.F.; Appleton, D.R.; Rugg-Gunn, A.J.; Eastoe, J.E.: Some influences on the measurement of food intake during a dietary survey of adolescents. Hum. Nutr. appl. Nutr. *39A:167–177* (1985).

50 Hackett, A.F.; Rugg-Gunn, A.J.; Appleton, D.R.; Coombs, A.: Dietary sources of energy, protein, fat and fibre in 375 English adolescents. Hum. Nutr. appl. Nutr. *40A:* 176–184 (1986).

51 Hagger, D.L.: Nutrient intakes of students in two different types of residences. Proc. Nutr. Soc. *34:* 119A (1975).

52 Hagman, U.; Bruce, A.; Persson, L.-A.; Samuelson, G.; Sjolin, S.: Food habits and nutrient intake in childhood in relation to health and socio-economic conditions. A Swedish multi-centre study 1980–81. Acta paediatr. scand. suppl. 328 (1986).

53 Hampton, M.C.; Huenemann, R.L.; Shapiro, L.R.; Mitchell, B.W.: Caloric and nutrient intakes of teen-agers. J. Am. diet. Ass. *50:* 385–396 (1967).

54 Harper, A.E.: Science and the consumer. J. Nutr. Educ. *11:* 171–175 (1979).

55 Heald, F.P.; Remmell, P.S.; Mayer, J.: Caloric, protein and fat intakes in children and adolescents; in Heald, Adolescent nutrition and growth, pp. 17–35 (Meredith Corp., New York 1969).

56 Henderson, L.M.: Nutritional problems growing out of new patterns of food consumption. Am. J. publ. Hlth *62:* 1194–1198 (1972).

57 Hitchcock, N.E.; Gracey, M.: Nutrient consumption patterns of families in Busseltown, Western Australia. Med. J. Aust. *1:* 359–362 (1978).

58 Hodges, R.E.: Vitamin and mineral requirements in adolescence; in McKigney, Munro, Nutrient requirements in adolescence, pp. 127–136 (MIT Press, Cambridge 1976).

59 Holdsworth, M.D.; Davies, L.: Nutrition education for the elderly. Hum. Nutr. appl. Nutr. *36A:* 22–27 (1982).

60 Huenemann, R.L.; Hampton, M.C.; Shapiro, L.R.; Behnke, A.R.: Adolescent food practices associated with obesity. Fed. Proc. *25:* 4–10 (1966).

61 Huenemann, R.L.; Shapiro, L.R.; Hampton, M.C.; Mitchell, B.W.: Food and eating practices of teen-agers. J. Am. diet. Ass. *53:* 17–24 (1968).

62 Jacoby, A.; Altman, D.G.; Cook, J.; Holland, W.W.; Elliott, A.: Influence of some social and environmental factors on the nutrient intake and nutritional status of schoolchildren. Br. J. prev. Soc. Med. *29:* 116–120 (1975).

63 Johnson, W.A.; Jensen, J.R.: Influence of noon meal on nutrient intakes and meal patterns of selected fifth grade students. J. Am. diet. Ass. *84:* 919–923 (1984).

64 Kaufmann, N.A.; Poznanski, R.; Guggenheim, K.: Eating habits and opinions of teenagers on nutrition and obesity. J. Am. diet. Ass. *66:* 264–268 (1975).

65 Kaufmann, N.A.; Friedlander, Y.; Halfon, S.T.; Slater, P.E.; Dennis, B.H.; McClish, D.; Eisenberg, S.; Stein, Y.: Nutrient intake in Jerusalem – consumption in 17-year-olds. Israel J. Med. Scis *18:* 1167–1182 (1982).

66 Kenney, M.A.; McCoy, J.H.; Kirby, A.L.; Carter, E.; Clark, A.J.; Disney, G.W.; Floyd, C.D.; Glover, E.E.; Korslund, M.K.; Lewis, H.; Liebman, M.; Moak, S.W.;

Ritchey, S.J.; Stallings, S.F.: Nutrients supplied by food groups in diets of teenaged girls. J. Am. diet. Ass. *86:* 1549–1555 (1986).
67 Khan, M.A.: Evaluation of food selection patterns and preferences. CRC crit. Rev. Fd Sci. Nutr. *14:* 129–153 (1981).
68 King, J.C.; Cohenour, S.H.; Calloway, D.H.; Jacobson, H.N.: Assessment of nutritional status of teenage pregnant girls. I. Nutrient intake and pregnancy. Am. J. clin. Nutr. *25:* 916–925 (1972).
69 Krehl, W.A.: Nutrition of the low socio-economic class adolescents; in Heald, Adolescent nutrition and growth, pp. 95–99 (Meredith Corp., New York 1969).
70 Kuczmarski, R.J.; Brewer, E.R.; Cronin, F.J.; Dennis, B.; Groves, K.; Haynes, S.: Food choices among white adolescents: the Lipid Research Clinics Prevalence Study. Pediat. Res. *20:* 309–315 (1986).
71 Lai, M.K.; Shimabukuro, S.K.; Wenkam, N.S.; Raman, S.P.: A nutrient analysis of students' diets in the state of Hawaii. J. Nutr. Educ. *14:* 67–70 (1981).
72 Lee, C. Ja: Nutritional status of selected teenagers in Kentucky. Am. J. clin. Nutr. *31:* 1453–1464 (1978).
73 Leverton, R.M.: The paradox of teen-age nutrition. J. Am. diet. Ass. *53:* 13–16 (1968).
74 McCance, R.A.; Widdowson, E.M.: The composition of foods. MRC spec. rep. ser., No. 297 (MRC, London 1967).
75 McCoy, J.H.; Kenney, M.A.; Kirby, A.; Disney, G.; Ercanli, F.G.; Glover, E.; Korslund, M.; Lewis, H.; Liebman, M.; Livant, E.: Nutrient intakes of female adolescents from eight southern states. J. Am. diet. Ass. *84:* 1453–1460 (1984).
76 Macdonald, L.A.; Wearring, G.A.; Moase, O.: Factors affecting the dietary quality of adolescent girls. J. Am. diet. Ass. *82:* 260–263 (1983).
77 McGandy, R.B.; Hall, B.; Ford, C.; Stare, F.J.: Dietary regulation of blood cholesterol in adolescent males: a pilot study. Am. J. clin. Nutr. *25:* 61–66 (1972).
78 McGuffin, S.J.: Food fashions. Nutr. Fd. Sci. *81:* 6–7 (1983).
79 McKenzie, J.: Food is not just for eating; in Hollingsworth, Morse, People and food tomorrow, p. 21 (Applied Science Publishers, London 1976).
80 McSweeney, M.; Kevany, J.: Nutrition beliefs and practices in Ireland (Health Education Bureau, Dublin 1981).
81 Mapes, M.C.: Gulp – an alternative method for reaching teens. J. Nutr. Educ. *9:* 12–16 (1977).
82 Marktl, W.: The interrelationship between nutrition and social development in adolescence. Ernährung *6:* 226-227 (1982).
83 Marr, J.W.: Individual dietary surveys: purposes and methods. Wld Rev. Nutr. Diet., vol. 13, pp. 105–164 (Karger, Basel 1971).
84 Meredith, A.; Matthews, A.; Zickefoose, M.; Weagley, E.; Wayave, M.; Brown, E.G.: How well do schoolchildren recall what they have eaten? J. Am. diet. Ass. *27:* 749–751 (1951).
85 Miller, M.R.; Binns, C.W.: Cultural differences in children's TV viewing habits and implication for nutritional status. Proc. Nutr. Soc. Aust. *4:* 120 (1979).
86 Moffatt, R.J.: Dietary status of elite female high school gymnasts: inadequacy of vitamin and mineral intake. J. Am. diet. Ass. *84:* 1361–1363 (1984).
87 Morgan, K.J.; Zabik, M.E.; Stampley, G.L.: Breakfast consumption patterns of US children and adolescents. Nutr. Res. *6:* 635–646 (1986).

88 Musgrave, K.O.; Achterberg, C.L.; Thornbury, M.: Strategies for measuring adolescent snacking patterns. Nutr. Rep. int. *24:* 557–573 (1981).
89 National Dairy Council: What are children eating these days? (NDC, London 1982).
90 National Health and Medical Research Council: Dietary allowances for use in Australia (Australian Govt. Publ. Serv., Canberra 1979).
91 National Research Council: Recommended dietary allowance; 8th ed. (revised) (Natn. Academy of Science, Washington 1980).
92 Nutrition Committee, Canadian Paediatric Society: Adolescent nutrition. 2. Normal nutritional requirements. Can. med. Ass. J. *129:* 420–422 (1983).
93 Nutrition Committee, Canadian Paediatric Society: Adolescent nutrition. 3. Obesity. Can. med. Ass. J. *129:* 549–551 (1983).
94 Nutrition Committee, Canadian Paediatric Society: Adolescent nutrition. 4. Sports and diet. Can. med. Ass. J. *129:* 552–553 (1983).
95 Nutrition Committee, Canadian Paediatric Society: Adolescent nutrition. 5. Pregnancy and diet. Can. med. Ass. J. *129:* 691–692 (1983).
96 Nutrition Committee, Canadian Paediatric Society: Adolescent nutrition. 6. Fast foods, food fads and the educational challenge. Can. med. Ass. J. *129:* 692–695 (1983).
97 Office of the Federal Register: Code of Federal Regulations 21 (US Govt. Printing Office, Washington 1984).
98 Olson, J.A.: Recommended dietary intakes (RDI) of vitamin A in humans. Am. J. clin. Nutr. *45:* 704–716 (1987).
99 Paul, A.A.; Southgate, D.A.T.: McCance and Widdowson's The Composition of Foods. MRC spec. rep., No. 297 (HMSO, London 1978).
100 Pearson, D.; Burns, S.; Cunningham, K.: Dietary survey of immigrant schoolgirls in Leicester. J. hum. Nutr. *31:* 362–364 (1977).
101 Perron, M.; Endres, J.: Knowledge, attitudes and dietary practices of female athletes. J. Am. diet. Ass. *85:* 573–576 (1985).
102 Post, B.; Kemper, H.C.G.; Storm-van-Essen, L.: Longitudinal changes in nutritional habits of teenagers: differences in intake between schooldays and weekend days. Br. J. Nutr. *57:* 161–176 (1987).
103 Prattala, R.; Rahkonen, O.; Rimpela, M.: Consumption patterns of critical fat sources among adolescents in 1977–1985. Nutr. Res. *6:* 485–498 (1986).
104 Rasanen, L.; Ahola, M.; Kara, R.; Uhari, M.: Atherosclerosis precursors in Finnish children and adolescents. VIII. Food consumption and nutrient intakes. Acta paediat. scand. *74:* suppl. 318, pp. 135–153 (1985).
105 Richardson, D.P.; Lawson, M.: Nutritional value of midday meals of senior schoolchildren. Br. med. J. *iv:* 697–699 (1972).
106 Rugg-Gunn, A.J.; Hackett, A.F.; Appleton, D.R.; Moynihan, P.J.: The dietary intake of added and natural sugars in 405 English adolescents. Hum. Nutr. appl. Nutr. *40A:* 115–124 (1986).
107 Salz, K.M.; Tamir, I.; Ernst, N.; Kwiterovich, P.; Glueck, C.; Christensen, B.; Larsen, R.; Pirhonen, D.; Prewitt, T.E.; Scott, L.W.: Selected nutrient intakes of free-living white children ages 6–19 years. The Lipid Research Clinics Program Prevalence Study. Pediat. Res. *17:* 124–130 (1983).

108 Samuelson, G.: An epidemiological study of child health and nutrition in a Northern Swedish county. I. Food consumption survey. Acta Paediat. scand. suppl. 214, pp. 5–44 (1971).
109 Schorr, B.C.; Sanjur, D.; Erickson, E.C.: Teen-age food habits. J. Am. diet. Ass. *61:* 415–420 (1972).
110 Seoane, N.A.; Roberge, A.G.: Caloric and nutrient intake of adolescents in the Quebec City region. Can. J. publ. Hlth *74:* 110–116 (1983).
111 Skinner, J.D.; Salvetti, N.N.; Ezell, J.M.; Penfield, M.P.; Costello, C.A.: Appalachian adolescents' eating patterns and nutrient intakes. J. Am. diet. Ass. *85:* 1093–1099 (1985).
112 Smeaton, I.: Nutrient intake of six elite women athletes. Proc. Nutr. Soc. *47:* 20A (1988).
113 Steele, B.F.; Clayton, M.M.; Tucker, R.E.: Role of breakfast and of between-meal foods in adolescents' nutrient intake. J. Am. diet. Ass. *28:* 1054–1057 (1952).
114 Stordy, B.J.; Cowhig, J.R.: Nutrient intake of students in various types of accommodation. Proc. Nutr. Soc. *31:* 81A (1972).
115 Storz, N.S.; Greene, W.H.: Body weight, body image and perception of fad diets in adolescent girls. J. Nutr. Educ. *15:* 15–18 (1983).
116 Stunkard, A.J.; Burt, V.: Obesity and the body image. II. Age at onset of disturbances in the body image. Am. J. Psychiat. *123:* 1443–1447 (1967).
117 Thomas, J.A.; Call, D.L.: Eating between meals – a nutrition problem among teenagers? Nutr. Rev. *31:* 137–139 (1973).
118 Topp, S.G.; Cook, J.; Elliott, A.: Measurement of nutritional intake among schoolchildren. Br. J. prev. soc. Med. *26:* 106 (1972).
119 Truswell, A.S.; Darnton-Hill, I.: Food habits of adolescents. Nutr. Rev. *39:* 73–88 (1981).
120 Van de Mark, M.S.; Underwood, V.R.S.: Dietary habits and food consumption patterns of teenage families. J. Home Econ. *63:* 540–544 (1971).
121 Van de Mark, M.S.; Wright, A.C.: Hemoglobin and folate levels of pregnant teenagers. J. Am. diet. Ass. *61:* 511–516 (1972).
122 Walker, A.R.P.; Walker, B.F.; Jones, J.; Ncongwane, J.: Breakfast habits of adolescents in four South African populations. Am. J. clin. Nutr. *36:* 650–656 (1982).
123 Wenlock, R.W.; Disselduff, M.M.; Skinner, R.K.; Knight, I.: The diets of British schoolchildren: preliminary report of a nutritional analysis of a nationwide dietary survey of British schoolchildren (DHSS, London 1986).
124 Wharton, B.A.: School dinners. Br. med. J. *294:* 1635 (1987).
125 Whitehead, R.G.; Cole, T.J.: Trends in food energy intakes throughout childhood from one to 18 years. Hum. Nutr. appl. Nutr. *36A:* 57-62 (1982).
126 Wiles, S.J.; Nettleton, P.A.; Black, A.E.; Paul, A.A.: The nutrient composition of some cooked dishes eaten in Britain: a supplementary food composition table. J. hum. Nutr. *34:* 189–223 (1980).
127 Woodward, D.R.; Lynch, P.P.; Waters, M.J.; Maclean, A.R.; Ruddock, W.E.; Rataj, J.W.; Lemoh, J.N.: Dietary studies on Tasmanian high school students: intakes of energy and nutrients. Aust. paediat. J. *17:* 196–201 (1981).
128 Woodward, D.R.: Major influences on median energy and nutrient intakes among teenagers: a Tasmanian survey. Br. J. Nutr. *52:* 21–32 (1984).

129 Woodward, D.R.: Teenagers and their food: the effects of physical, behavioural and socio-economic characteristics on intakes of five food categories in Tasmania. J. Fd Nutr. *42:* 7–12 (1985).
130 Woodward, D.R.; What sort of teenager has low intakes of energy nutrients? Br. J. Nutr. *53:* 241–249 (1985).
131 Woodward, D.R.: What sort of teenager has high intakes of energy and nutrients? Br. J. Nutr. *54:* 325–333 (1985).
132 Woodward, D.R.: What influences adolescent food intakes? Hum. Nutr. appl. Nutr. *40A:* 185–194 (1986).
133 Wyn-Jones, C.; Atkinson, S.J.; Nicholas, P.: Nutrient intake by students over a 3-month period. Proc. Nutr. Soc. *31:* 83A (1972).

N.L. Bull, MA, MSc, CBiol, MIBol, FRSH, Ferndale, 84 Grove Road, Tring, HP23 5PB Herts (England)

Wld Rev. Nutr. Diet., vol. 57, pp. 75–94 (Karger, Basel 1988)

Energy Expenditure of Preschool Children in a Subtropical Area[1]

Zhi-chien Ho, He Mei Zi, Luan Bo, He Ping

Department of Clinical Nutrition, Sun Yet-sen University of Medical Sciences, Guangzhou, People's Republic of China

Contents

Energy expenditure and energy needs for the human body are basic aspects for worldwide consideration. Many related works have concerned adults in different situations and some involved children [1–4]. The conditions of subtropical environments raise some questions, especially for preschool children, i.e. if we use food consumption as a measure of energy expenditure, the results may often prove contradictory. To meet the energy needs for growing children in the subtropics where many developing countries are located is a matter of health for millions in the future and is closely related to the world's food consumption.

[1] This work was supported by UNICEF.

The Recommendation of Dietary Allowance (RDA) for energy had some small differences among many countries for the age group of 4- to 6-year-olds. The Joint FAO/WHO Expert Group set 1830 kcal daily for this age in 1973; this figure may be considered as very safe, in order to cover worldwide variations for children in various situations [3]. Nutritionists of some countries in the tropical area have set a lower caloric recommendation for children in this age group, and it may be reasonable and suitable for their needs, because there are so many differences between the northern and southern hemispheres [5]. The Chinese Society of Nutrition set a figure of 1,600 kcal as recommendation for this age group in 1981.

Caloric and protein intakes are of great importance. Incorrect caloric intake leads to signs of malnutrition, such as marasmus or stunted growth. However, overfeeding has been a problem lately in areas where surpluses of cereal grain and sugar exist. An old concept is the tendency to fill the stomach to a feeling of satiety; this feeling might be reasonable in certain cases but may not be reasonable for children. The emphasis of an incorrect energy intake may consequently lead one to overlook the use of protein-rich foods [6], and the risk of degenerative diseases may be present in later childhood.

The aim of this study is try to find an optimum energy intake for growing children in whom the growth speed is either slower than in young children or slower than in adolescents, an energy intake supportive of the fitness required for further development in the conditions of the subtropics. To this aim a series of investigations was carried out, including some of the basic measurements, i.e. body surface and basal metabolism.

Materials and Methods

Subjects

181 healthy 5-year-old children in a Guangzhou kindergarten were chosen after clinical examinations verified normal height and weight for both sexes against the growth chart. The children come from families of different kinds, such as workers, cadres, and numerous professionals. The number of subjects in the study are randomized according to needs. Before the experiments, the doctors taking part organized joint activities with the children in order to make a familiar and friendly working atmosphere.

Dietary Records

The dietary records of the children were collected, and monitored and estimated when needed. The daily activity schedule of the kindergarten remained the same without any disturbance. An air-conditioned room was set in the kindergarten with all the instruments needed for efficiency and accuracy. The nurses and teachers of the kindergarten were trained for recognizing the goals of the study and its requirements.

The duration of the study is 1.5 years; thus, the children are observed throughout at least four seasons. Actually, there are only two seasons in Guangzhou, i.e. the winter-spring season and the summer-autumn season. The age of the subjects is approaching 6 years by the end of the investigation.

Measurements

The method of body surface area measurement is basically the same as Du Bois' [7], but modified materials were used: very thin and specially made cotton clothing, including underwear, socks and gloves. A well-fitting mask was put on each subject before the use of bandages, which was what Du Bois [7] did. The clothes give an elastic fitting to the body and the bandages are made with a thin layer of adhesive glue so that they can assume all kinds of shapes except the face, which is covered in cotton cloth and glue. All parts of the materials covering the body were carefully removed by cutting along a mid line. The material was then cut into pieces and flattened into its original shape. The inner face of the materials was then placed on a standard area-counting paper which has an accuracy to 1 mm^3. The total area was then calculated. The height and weight of the subject was measured in the nude with an electric balance accurate to 10 g, and the skinfold thickness was also taken. The data were put into a computer and processed. For this study, 30 children were chosen, half of whom females.

The basal metabolism for 156 children of 5 years old, including 71 males and 85 females, was measured under specific conditions [8]. The subjects were mostly boarding at kindergarten. A 12-hour fast should be made before measurement, including 9 h for sleeping and a 30-min period lying relaxed in bed before collecting the respiratory air using a fitted mask and a Douglas bag for the open circular method. The analysis of room and expired air for this method is done using a Beckman OM-11 paramagnetic analyser and a Beckman LB-2 infrared carbon dioxide analyser.

Each subject was measured once or twice for one season, i.e. four or more times in a year at least, except those who have to recheck for assurance.

The temperature of the measurement room was kept constant at around 21 °C for the whole year. The room remained quiet and the bed was comfortable. Any influence that could affect the basal metabolism test was avoided, including feelings and sentiment. A preliminary practice for each child was required, including expired air collection.

The meteorological records were collected from the city's record station. The variations of temperature between seasons is not high, the coldest day is in the early spring and is about 10 °C on average; the hottest day is in the summer and is around 34 °C on average. There is no heating habit or air conditioning at home for the people and so the children are exposed to the temperatures above during all four seasons; the difference of temperature between indoors and outdoors is about 3–5 °C in extreme climates. The basal metabolic rate (BMR) was calculated against body weight per kilogram or body surface per square meter using the equation made from the study above.

Measurement of Energy Expenditure

The energy expenditure of children 5–6 years old was measured. There are 21 items of activities in the daily life of children in the kindergarten. 30 children were randomly selected from 181. The sexes were divided equally. The measurements used an indirect method through a specially made mask and light thin plastic Douglas bag for expired air collection during all activities, which the exception of eating, sleeping and singing, etc. For those activities, we used a respiratory chamber which is a specially made small tent with a small ventilator fan. The total space inside the tent is 3.375 m^3 where the subject may live; this method is basically from Taylor [9]. The concentration of oxygen and carbon dioxide in the sealed compartment was analysed through a sampling tube before and after certain activities, and was estimated by the changes of oxygen and carbon dioxide concentration during 30 min just as the indirect method mentioned above.

A daily activity record was obtained from a 24-hour follow-up study of 10 children; the time and motion calculations were compared with the results of energy expended for each item estimated above. Another daily activity record for the total number of children in the kindergarten was also obtained from seasonal and weekly schedules of activity; both of the records were calculated and the energy spent obtained.

The dietary records were collected carefully so the calorie intake could be compared to the output from the daily activity in a 7-day observation in the moderate autumn season. The energy obtained from foods was calculated from the Chinese food table.

The daily habitual energy spent in the kindergarten was estimated either by a combination of both sexes or for boys and girls separately in a weekly pattern. Because of the active schedule in the kindergarten and the opportunity for children being good enough for the different requirements of physical and mental development, it is thought to be typically representative of children of the same age living at home.

The Specific Dynamic Action of Food for Children

The specific dynamic actions of eight kinds of the most common foods were studied in children using the same methods as Forbes [11] and Lusk [10]. The method of measurement of energy spent after meals is the same as that mentioned above. The energy expended during fasting or basal metabolism was compared to the energy spent after the ingestion of a specific food in this study, because there is a 3-hour interval between children's meals, so the observation time was limited to 3 h in 18 children.

The food items tested included refined sugar, starch, egg white, beef made into a ball shape with 3% starch, lean beef, skim milk powder, margarine, and a common mixed diet that consisted of fried egg and rice (table I).

Results

Body Surface

The results of body measurement on 30 children for skinfold thickness is 2.95 ± 0.84 cm on average in the location of subscapular and 3.05 ± 1.02 cm in the cross line of nipple and umbilicus; there is no significant difference between the two sexes ($p > 0.05$). The average body weight is 16.7 ± 2.1 kg, and height 108.3 ± 5.5 cm. These figures are in the normal ranges for this age but just a little higher than the 50th percentile of the growth chart.

Table I. The composition of food tested for SDA

Food	Intake g	Protein	Fat	Carbo-hydrate	kcal	Percentage of cal from protein
Sugar	52.5	0	0	52.0	208.0	0
Starch	48.1	0.2	0	41.4	166.4	0
Egg white	186.7	18.7	0.2	2.4	85.9	87.1
Beef ball	152.9	20.8	6.3	14.8	199.1	41.8
Lean beef	100.0	20.3	6.2	1.7	144.0	56.3
Skim milk	32.6	19.6	0.3	9.5	119.1	65.8
Margarin	25.5	0	20.4	0	178.2	0
Fried rice with egg, oil	64.2	7.0	7.5	23.3	188.5	14.8

The quantity of those food eaten in the test is based on the assumption of a morning meal according to they can eat and satiety after meal in the cooking form the subjects like to have.

On the body weight and height above, the mean body surface is 7,224.5 cm^2 (range from 6,406 to 8,832.3 cm^2), and the parts of body surfaces are (cm^2): (1) head and neck, 1,154.5 ± 65.1; (2) trunk, 1,838.9 ± 252.1; (3) arms, 948.5 ± 99.1; (4) hands, 242.3 ± 43.8 cm^2; (5) legs, 2,285.6 ± 274.7, and (6) feet, 572.5 ± 57.1 (table II).

The coefficient based on each subject's height, weight and body surface is in good correlation with $R = 0.9422$. The equation was developed from 30 children's height, weight and body surface:

$$S \text{ (surface in cm}^2) = 42.3556 \times H + 175.6882 \times W - 272.2716.$$

H is the height in cm and W is the weight in kg in the formula. The theoretical value for all the 30 children is 7,248.8 cm^2 which is 24.2 cm^2 lower than the practical measurement. By using the Du Bois equation for these 30 children, the result of calculation is 7,096.3 cm^2, which is 128.2 cm^2 lower than the practical measurement, but there is no significant difference between the results of our equation and that of Du Bois ($p > 0.05$).

Two formulae had checked with the theoretical and practical values for all subjects. The result of $[\Sigma(Y - \hat{Y})^2]$ is much larger in Du Bois's formula (value 1,989,908) than in our formula (value 1,295,002). This means that our formula made a better coverage of the children.

Table II. Body surface area for preschool children

No.	Sex	Age	Height cm	Weight kg	Head and neck		Trunk		Arms	
					cm²	%	cm²	%	cm²	%
001	F	5	107.0	18.4	1,183.95	16.5	1,577.60	21.9	964.70	13.4
002	F	5	103.2	16.7	1,074.75	15.5	1,448.11	20.9	1,056.16	15.3
003	M	5	101.5	15.5	1,141.15	16.9	1,531.81	22.6	846.41	12.5
004	M	5	104.5	14.0	1,071.68	16.7	1,408.36	22.0	846.52	13.2
005	F	5	105.9	15.0	1,217.95	18.2	1,199.63	17.9	873.96	13.0
006	M	5	102.1	14.5	1,072.49	16.6	1,771.65	27.5	836.30	13.0
007	M	5	102.8	15.2	1,180.40	17.2	1,820.97	26.5	941.70	13.7
008	F	5	96.2	13.6	1,087.10	17.0	1,714.35	26.8	798.97	12.5
009	F	5	103.8	16.0	1,105.52	16.0	1,832.60	26.5	890.60	12.9
011	F	5	108.3	16.0	1,097.83	16.3	1,776.11	26.3	839.40	12.4
012	M	6	115.4	18.2	1,214.60	15.4	2,211.00	28.1	1,009.20	12.8
013	F	6	114.2	18.3	1,227.16	15.9	1,957.09	25.3	1,036.60	13.4
014	M	5	110.8	18.0	1,194.10	15.7	2,087.70	27.4	978.00	12.8
015	F	5	119.0	22.0	1,239.90	14.0	2,223.70	25.2	1,114.50	12.6
016	M	5	110.2	17.5	1,245.90	16.2	2,057.40	26.8	987.70	12.9
017	F	5	116.0	18.5	1,194.70	15.7	1,974.90	26.0	1,066.96	14.0
018	M	5	110.5	19.0	1,241.50	15.8	2,173.70	27.7	920.10	11.7
019	M	5	113.5	18.5	1,281.60	16.0	2,219.90	27.6	1,045.90	13.0
020	M	5	107.5	16.0	1,102.90	15.7	1,849.60	26.4	902.30	12.9
021	F	5	103.8	14.6	1,186.70	18.1	1,731.70	26.4	827.05	12.6
022	M	5	109.4	15.0	1,131.40	15.8	1,820.70	25.5	886.20	12.4
023	F	5	112.0	18.7	1,195.45	15.6	1,887.20	24.6	1,126.30	14.7
024	F	5	101.5	14.8	1,129.90	16.9	1,652.80	24.8	852.80	12.8
025	M	5	112.9	17.8	1,053.80	13.9	1,982.20	26.2	1,010.99	13.4
026	M	5	108.5	16.0	1,124.20	15.9	1,779.30	25.1	925.10	13.1
027	F	6	119.5	21.5	1,200.40	14.2	2,095.10	24.7	1,180.80	13.9
028	F	5	105.0	15.6	1,042.50	15.3	1,745.80	25.6	907.90	13.3
029	F	5	107.5	15.8	1,140.80	15.8	2,097.80	29.0	904.40	12.5
030	F	5	110.0	16.0	1,098.10	15.8	1,748.60	25.2	999.60	14.4
031	M	5	106.4	14.5	1,157.30	16.6	1,790.75	25.6	879.80	12.6
$\overline{X} \pm SD$			108.4 ± 5.5	16.7 ± 2.1	1,154.52 ± 65.10	16.0	1,838.94 ± 252.19	25.5	948.56 ± 99.15	13.1

[a] Formula: body surface area cm² = $\log^{-1}$ (log W × 0.425 + log H × 0.725 + 1.8564).

Hands		Legs		Feet		Total		By Du Bois' formula[a]
cm²	%	cm²	%	cm²	%	cm²	%	cm²
402.90	5.6	2,499.00	34.7	563.88	7.8	7,192.03	100	7,332.48
401.90	5,8	2,294.74	33.2	643.82	9.3	6,919.48	100	6,854.44
512.68	7.6	2,123.95	31.4	615.20	9.1	6,771.20	100	6,561.13
405.86	6.3	1,971.16	30.8	705.88	11.0	6,409.46	100	6,417.47
402.12	6.0	2,437.56	36.4	568.76	8.5	6,699.98	100	6,672.50
388.12	6.0	1,798.06	27.9	580.86	9.0	6,447.48	100	6,405.09
406.10	5.9	1,978.65	28.8	536.50	7.8	6,864.32	100	6,567.17
375.99	5.9	1,952.06	30.5	477.95	7.5	6,406.42	100	5,969.75
397.33	5.8	2,149.85	31.1	533.19	7.7	6,909.09	100	6,759.18
394.30	5.8	2,122.00	31.4	523.30	7.7	6,752.94	100	6,970.38
401.70	5.1	2,380.10	30.2	657.30	8.3	7,873.90	100	7,709.56
442.40	5.7	2,489.80	32.2	586.50	7.6	7,739.55	100	7,669.19
452.60	5.9	2,297.50	30.1	610.60	8.0	7,620.50	100	7,450.44
472.80	5.4	3,138.20	35.5	643.20	7.3	8,832.30	100	8,544.79
466.10	6.1	2,345.00	30.6	565.60	7.4	7,667.70	100	7,332.85
293.20	3.9	2,498.60	32.9	574.50	7.6	7,602.86	100	7,792.56
456.10	5.8	2,459.78	31.4	584.80	7.5	7,835.98	100	7,608.66
475.70	5.9	2,389.10	29.7	620.40	7.7	8,032.60	100	7,670.44
465.98	6.6	2,184.80	31.2	502.50	7.2	7,008.08	100	6,933.01
366.50	5.6	1,959.45	29.9	482.00	7.4	6,553.40	100	6,501.19
480.00	6.7	2,228.90	31.2	597.80	8.4	7,145.00	100	6,831.66
423.30	5.5	2,514.40	32.7	535.40	7.0	7,682.05	100	7.631.60
427.50	6.4	2,141.20	32.1	469.60	7.0	6,673.80	100	6,433.53
449.30	5.9	2,496.20	33.0	578.03	7.6	7,570.52	100	7,516.78
426.80	6.0	2,266.60	32.0	559.20	7.9	7,081.20	100	6,979.71
474.90	5.6	2,852.90	33.7	661.04	7.8	8,465.14	100	8,487.47
443.30	6.5	2,116.00	31.0	560.80	8.2	6,816.30	100	6,742.80
408.40	5.7	2,124.70	29.4	549.40	7.6	7,225.50	100	6,896.05
381.60	5.5	2,220.80	31.9	503.70	7.2	6,952.40	100	7,049.54
434.10	6.2	2,139.70	30.6	584.60	8.4	6,986.25	100	6,599.55
424.32 ± 43.83	5.9	2,285.69 ± 274.76	31.6	572.54 ± 57.14	7.9	7,224.58 ± 608.90	100.0	7,096.36 ± 615.17

Basal Metabolic Rate

There is no significant difference in the values of respiration, pulse rate and body temperature between the sexes in the children studied ($p > 0.05$), but there is a difference for BMR between female and male. The average BMR value is 45.5 ± 3.08 kcal/m²/h or 1.97 ± 0.17 kcal/kg/h or 34.1 ± 3.01 kcal/h for 151 boys, and 43.2 ± 2.65 kcal/m²/h or 1.97 ± 0.17 kcal/kg/h or 32.0 ± 2.99 kcal/h for 187 girls in the whole calculation for the four seasons.

Considering the longest season, the summer-autumn season lasted about 7–8 months; the average BMR value is 43.6 ± 2.57 kcal/m²/h for boys and 41.9 ± 2.19 kcal/m²/h for girls. These figures were a little lower than the total average above. Conversely, about 7% of the calories are higher in the winter-spring season than the average over the four seasons. In all, if the average for the four seasons is taken as a standard value, it will be more accurate to add 4% for boys and 3% for girls in the winter-spring season. Conversely, accuracy is achieved by a reduction of 4% for boys and 3% for girls in the summer-autumn season (table III).

The BMR value in both sexes had variations either calculated by body surface or body weight, but less than 10%. The difference between the BMR values for winter and spring, or summer and autumn in both sexes were not significant when analysed by χ^2 test, but there is a significant difference ($p < 0.05$) between male and female in this study – about 4–7% higher for boys (5% on average).

Using the multiple regression analysis for nine items, such as the age, height, weight, pulse rate, respiratory rate, body surface, oxygen consumption, and the carbon dioxide production, respiratory quotient, etc., the BMR had the highest correlation with oxygen consumption followed by carbon dioxide production, the R value being 0.9824 and 0.8186, respectively. Body weight is correlated well with BMR also, the R value is 0.6928 for boys and 0.7590 for girls; similarly, the correlation between body surface and BMR is also statistically significant in both sexes, the R for boys is 0.6668, and 0.7247 for girls.

Because the body weight of children is most easy to obtain in the field works, so the equation by body weight can use stepwise regression analysis as follows:

BMR for boys = 17.8938–0.8701 W
BMR for girls = 16.7551–0.8548 W
(the unit for BMR is kcal/h, and W is body weight in kg)

Table III. Basal metabolism values during four seasons

Season	Cases	Sex	Age	Body weight	Body surface	Basal metabolism value		
						kcal/m²/h mean ± SD	kcal/kg/h mean ± SD	kcal/h mean ± SD
Winter	22	M	5.3	16.7	0.726	46.5 ± 3.67	2.03 ± 0.17	33.8 ± 3.96
	29	F	5.3	16.2	0.718	44.0 ± 3.81	1.96 ± 0.17	31.6 ± 3.71
Spring	35	M	5.6	17.2	0.743	47.4 ± 4.16	2.06 ± 0.21	35.2 ± 3.74
	40	F	5.5	16.6	0.730	44.4 ± 3.04	1.96 ± 0.23	32.3 ± 2.86
Summer	31	M	5.8	17.5	0.757	44.5 ± 2.16	1.93 ± 0.13	33.7 ± 2.46
	44	F	5.7	17.2	0.747	42.3 ± 2.17	1.85 ± 0.14	31.7 ± 3.54
Autumn	63	M	5.8	18.3	0.776	43.6 ± 2.57	1.86 ± 0.15	33.8 ± 2.53
	74	F	5.7	18.1	0.769	41.9 ± 2.19	1.80 ± 0.12	32.2 ± 2.49
Total	151	M	–	–	–	45.5 ± 3.08	1.97 ± 0.17	34.1 ± 3.01
	187	F				43.2 ± 2.65	1.89 ± 0.17	32.0 ± 2.99

The difference between calculation by the formulae above and the actual measurements for all subjects is not statistically significant ($p > 0.05$) and, using the body surface figure for these calculations, produces the same results (table IV).

Habitual Energy Expenditures

The measurements of energy expenditure were defined by the modes of each activity as follows: (1) basal metabolism, as described above; (2) rest lying on the bed quietly during daytime; (3) sitting on a bench freely; (4) walking freely at a speed of about 50 m/min; (5) running slowly at a speed of about 80 m/min; (6) running quickly at a speed of about 210 m/min; (7) running up and down stairs at about 90 steps/min; (8) running up and down stairs quickly at a speed of about 130–150 steps/min; (9) writing or drawing: sitting and working at a table freely with a color pencil; (10) playing on the ground: kneeling on the ground and playing with light toys, such as a jigsaw puzzle or a top, or playing with sand; (11) physical exercise: a series of exercises including the movement of upper arms, spread-out arms, kicking legs, turning the trunk and waist or callisthenics; (12) dancing: sets of dancing with series of movements with hands and legs in music, generally at moderate speed; (13) riding a tricycle: a small child's

Table IV. Comparisons of the calculated and measured values

No.	Calculated	Measured	No.	Calculated	Measured	No.	Calculated	Measured
1	31.2929	35.06	22	34.9471	32.58	43	32.9112	33.51
2	31.9889	30.80	23	33.9901	35.26	44	34.5817	35.78
3	31.1188	31.32	24	33.8161	32.48	45	34.6861	36.20
4	35.3822	36.15	25	30.9448	29.02	46	34.2511	33.09
5	35.5991	33.37	26	32.5109	31.39	47	38.8972	38.07
6	32.859	34.44	27	32.8591	32.36	48	34.5991	36.26
7	33.468	31.48	28	34.3381	36.32	49	33.7116	36.36
8	33.9901	33.74	29	35.3822	35.64	50	31.4843	28.73
9	33.468	36.53	30	35.0341	36.28	51	36.3218	34.99
10	33.9901	34.21	31	32.5880	28.82	52	40.3416	41.67
11	34.4251	34.71	32	33.2070	36.45	53	36.2696	34.64
12	33.642	36.03	33	33.5550	31.78	54	34.4947	36.07
13	31.3799	29.85	34	32.8590	31.31	55	33.9379	34.64
14	33.468	33.37	35	33.8683	31.48	56	31.9019	32.13
15	32.772	32.28	36	36.6003	38.33	57	32.8590	31.28
16	32.3369	33.61	37	32.8590	34.06	58	32.0759	35.54
17	34.6861	32.28	38	33.8683	31.70	59	35.7998	32.13
18	33.9901	33.10	39	36.1304	38.65	60	34.7035	32.94
19	33.8161	32.28	40	31.6235	32.58	61	33.3375	31.71
20	34.5121	33.53	41	33.2418	30.40	62	33.9727	36.72
21	33.381	33.96	42	34.5121	35.57	63	32.6850	32.06

$t = 0.0861$; $p > 0.90$.
The calculated value indicates the value from the equation and the measured value is the practical value from the study.

tricycle, riding level at a speed of about 200 m/min freely; (14) playing swing: single swing with two hand ropes, swinging to and fro about 8–13 times/min freely; (15) playing on a slide: walking up by stairs to the top of slide and slipping down; the slope of the slide is about 0.75 degrees; (16) playing with a skipping rope: using the rope personally and jumping about 40–80 times/min; (17) standing at rest without movements; (18) making the bedding tidy personally after rising from bed in the morning or afternoon after sleeping or napping; (19) sleeping: relaxed (measured in the tent); (20) singing: singing in a sitting position with a little movement of hands for expression (measured in the tent); (21) eating the usual meals (measured in the tent).

Table V. Energy expenditures for habitual activities for children (average for males and females)

Kinds of activities	Subjects	kcal/min mean ± SD	kcal/m²/min mean ± SD	cal/kg/min mean ± SD	Ratio to RMR
Basal metabolism	33	0.561–0.047	0.709–0.039	29.62–2.18	0.81
Lie in bed	24	0.597–0.009	0.759–0.11	31.74–4.90	0.85
Sitting	47	0.684–0.109	0.885–0.114	37.38–6.60	1.00
Play while kneeling	25	1.102–0.043	1.385–0.253	56.60–10.90	1.35
Standing	30	0.821–0.140	1.080–0.161	45.30–6.78	1.22
Walking	29	1.547–0.347	1.892–0.383	76.00–14.5	2.14
Running slowly	25	1.906–0.427	2.400–0.506	101.56–24.9	2.71
Running rapidly	28	3.799–0.601	4.762–0.683	195.74–27.75	5.38
Up and down stairs					
90 steps/min	32	2.090–0.307	2.623–0.345	106.45–14.88	2.96
130–150 steps/min	31	3.485–0.398	4.393–0.498	180.20–22.5	4.96
Writing	30	0.922–0.117	1.151–0.138	46.91–6.35	1.61
Singing	14	1.060–0.189	1.423–0.245	59.48–9.43	2.00
Eating meals	18	0.838–0.125	1.053–0.164	44.37–7.44	1.19
Tidy the bedding	23	1.270–0.226	1.582–0.281	63.63–12.30	1.79
Playing on swing	30	2.151–0.405	2.647–0.502	107.15–22.87	2.99
Playing on slide	30	3.126–0.582	3.828–0.604	154.48–25.77	4.33
Riding tricycle	29	2.452–0.638	3.050–0.697	123.86–28.10	3.45
Skipping	30	3.109–0.614	3.781–0.633	153.69–25.78	4.27
Physical exercise	33	1.489–0.253	1.851–0.259	75.05–10.27	2.09
Dancing	27	1.680–0.267	2.091–0.297	85.65–13.15	2.36
Asleep (1st hour)	9	0.512–0.020	0.651–0.053	26.87–2.74	0.74
Asleep (4th hour)	9	0.501–0.062	0.639–0.100	26.20–4.66	0.72

The average body weight of 30 subjects in the energy expediture study is 18.1 kg at the beginning of measurement and 20.26 kg at the end. Because the experiment lasted more than a year, the height increased from 110.3 to 116.1 ± 4.0 cm on average at the end. About 2.16 kg weight increase and 5.8 cm height increase was gained in one year with children's ages ranging from 5.2 to 6.1 years at the start of the study. The body surface was estimated simultaneously using the same formula.

The energy expenditures of various activities measured (table V) are on a basis of the average of a group of children. The lowest energy spent is in sleeping, and the highest spent is in rapid running; the values are 0.709 and 4.762 kcal/m²/min, respectively, the latter is about 6.7-fold

Table VI. The different of energy expenditures between boys and girls

Activities	Energy expenditure, cal/kg/min				Ratio	p
	boys	n	girls	n		
Basal metabolism	29.57	16	26.46	17	1.12	–
Asleep 1st hour	27.45	4	26.41	5	1.04	–
Lie in bed	33.85	12	29.63	12	1.14	*
Sitting	39.48	22	34.20	25	1.15	**
Standing	47.59	15	43.09	15	1.10	–
Walking	78.70	13	73.79	16	1.07	–
Run slowly	114.94	14	84.53	13	1.36	**
Run rapidly	210.03	13	183.37	15	1.15	**
Up and down stairs						
90 steps/min	108.46	15	104.67	17	1.04	–
130–150 steps/min	180.74	16	179.63	15	1.01	–
Singing	65.59	7	53.37	7	1.23	**
Eating meal	43.58	9	45.16	9	0.97	–
Writing	48.48	15	45.33	15	1.07	–
Play during kneeling	59.34	13	56.31	15	1.05	–
Physical exercise	78.62	17	67.05	16	1.17	*
Dancing	90.12	13	81.43	14	1.11	–
Playing on swing	107.43	15	103.53	15	1.04	–
Playing on slide	167.01	15	141.90	15	1.18	**
Skipping	163.86	15	143.52	15	1.14	*
Tidy the bedding	66.97	10	61.05	13	1.10	–
Riding tricycle	143.20	14	105.82	15	1.35	**

* Statistically significant $p < 0.05$; ** statistically significant $p < 0.01$; – = not significant.

of the former. Boys spend a little more calories than girls in the same activity but only some of the values are statistically significant (table VI). It is thought that the intensity of actions may be higher in boys in our observation.

The total daily energy expenditure was estimated in 5 boys and 5 girls selected at random from a class and carefully followed up by a time and motion study (table VII). The total amount of energy expended is 1,049.08 ± 44 kcal/day on average in 10 samples, but when using the daily activity schedule of the kindergarten's original set as routine during a season for all

Table VII. Total daily estimated energy expenditure in children

Case No.	Body surface, m^2	Energy expenditure in 24 h										Average kcal
		sleep and nap				habitual activities				total		
		1*		2*		1*		2*		1*	2*	
		min	kcal	min	kcal	min	kcal	min	kcal	kcal	kcal	
Boys												
1	0.7734	850	488	777	436	590	563.6	663	650.6	1,078.1	1,099.3	1,088.7
2	0.7583	842	464	865	476	598	755.3	575	593.6	1,062.0	1,051.2	1,056.6
3	0.8058	826	483	861	504	614	689.7	579	631.0	1,097.2	1,082.9	1,090.1
4	0.7072	840	431	857	440	600	454.0	583	607.4	1,031.1	1,023.0	1,027.1
5	0.8568	838	521	828	515	602	736.0	612	746.6	1,123.3	1,127.0	1,125.2
Girls												
6	0.7685	844	451	837	447	596	563.6	603	562.0	1,014.1	1,009.1	1,011.6
7	0.8002	853	477	850	475	587	553.9	590	587.2	1,031.0	1,062.6	1,064.8
8	0.7695	842	452	859	460	598	617.9	581	530.4	1,070.8	990.3	1,030.6
9	0.7361	846	435	780	401	594	551.2	660	533.9	986.5	935.2	960.9
10	0.7642	838	448	861	460	602	545.3	579	640.0	1,005.2	1,099.9	1,052.6

Average energy expenditure (kcal): for boys 1,077.6 ± 37.0; for girls 1,020.5 ± 36.9; for boys and girls 1,049.1 ± 43.7.
* 1 and 2 are the numbers of samples for follow-up recording.

Table VIII. Maximum energy expenditure according to schedule of kindergarten

Activities	Time min	Energy expenditure kcal	Percent of active activity in daytime[1]
Personal hygiene, including morning and evening	80	86.15	
Physical exercise, including morning and evening	40	89.50	6.3
Meals time including 4 meals	130	108.94	
Outdoor playing including slide, skipping, swing, tricycle, etc.	80	199.67	12.6
Free activity indoor or outdoor	90	111.72	14.28
Classroom learning, drawing, writing, singing and listening to a story, etc.	60	86.45	
Sleep and nap	810	454.41	
Walking around	45	69.62	7.1
Watching TV or listening to a story	45	30.83	
Other resting, mostly sitting			
Sitting at rest	60	41.04	
Total	1,440	1,278.3	40.8

[1] The total daytime is about 630 min.

the children, the energy spent is estimated to be 1,278 kcal/day. It is reasonable to determine that this figure may cover the level of expenditure for all children in the state of maximum activity (table VIII).

The average caloric intakes for 4 meals per day for children at 5 years of age in this study is estimated to be 1,281 kcal during 7 days dietary study in the same season and was checked by direct estimation of the group observed (table IX). This figure is quite close to the energy spent estimated on a group scale and is higher by about 8.2% than the results from follow-up records.

Table IX. Estimated energy intake of the children studied

Day	Protein g	Fats g	Carbo-hydrates g	Calories kcal	Percent of calories in total caloric intakes		
					protein	fats	carbohydrates
1	34.6	59.4	150.9	1,276.6	10.8	41.9	47.3
2	32.7	48.5	156.9	1,194.7	10.9	36.0	52.5
3	43.8	51.8	149.8	1,240.6	14.1	37.6	48.3
4	37.2	42.3	157.8	1,160.8	12.8	32.8	54.4
5	35.7	63.3	197.5	1,502.6	9.5	37.9	52.6
6	28.5	50.1	131.2	1,089.7	10.5	41.4	48.1
7	35.7	63.3	197.5	1,502.6	9.5	37.9	52.6
Average	35.5	54.1	163.1	1,281.0	11.1	37.9	51.0

Specific Dynamic Actions of Foods

The results of specific dynamic actions (SDA) for food tested in children revealed that there are some differences between the values from studies on animals and adults, but a similarity is that protein produces the higher heat spent and sugar produces the lowest (table X). From the time of eating a specific food to about 200 min afterwards, the peak of heat output is different for a variety of foods: for sugar, 50 min; for starch, 100 min; for egg white and skim milk, 150 min; for margarine it nearly maintained a plateau from 50 to 180 min; but the mixed diet composed of fried egg, rice and peanut oil raised a peak at 50 min which remained to about 150 min.

It is quite clear that food from sugar only gave a respiratory quotient (RQ) of 0.86 at the start, reaching 1.0 after 45 min, but starch maintained a level from 0.83 to 0.89 at 180 min. The remaining foods tested gave an RQ mostly around 0.84–0.94 throughout 180 min.

The fried egg rice with oil had a caloric contribution from nutrients similar to the daily diets of the kindergarten; the proportion of calories provided from protein is about 11.4%, fats 38.0% and carbohydrates 50.6%. This means about 10% (9.84%) of SDA in a mixed diet. Given a total caloric intake of about 1,281 kcal in this study, the SDA will be approximately 128 kcal and is roughly a little more than 10% of the daily energy expended.

Table X. The specific dynamic actions of foods tested in children

Food	Number of cases			Specific dynamic action, %		t-test
	total	male	female	mean	SD	
Egg white	15	8	7	22.95	10.75	*
Lean beef	8	4	4	22.22	9.13	*
Skim milk	8	4	4	20.90	8.31	*
Beef ball	14	6	8	18.93	8.25	*
Margarine	6	2	4	12.37	7.55	**
Sugar	18	10	8	10.73	4.44	**
Fried egg rice with oil	8	4	4	9.84	4.12	**
Starch	15	7	8	8.95	4.55	**

* The statistical difference is significant with starch, fried egg rice with oil and sugar ($p < 0.05$).
** The statistical difference is significant in starch, fried egg rice with oil, sugar and margarine ($p < 0.05$) before and after meal.

Discussion

A series of studies on a group of children was designed to limit the variation and undesirable errors in the working processes of the study, but it is hard for us to compare our results with similar data obtained in subtropical areas.

The equation to obtain body surface from body weight and height by Du Bois' method seemed suitable for the children of around 5 years old in the subtropics even though Stevenson [12] had modified the Du Bois formula for Chinese adults, and even our formula achieved a little more accuracy in the 5-year-old group.

It may be important to point out that the results of basal metabolism for 5-year-old children in subtropical conditions is quite different from the figures from the Western world. We have considered that the lower BMR in the children tested may arise from an error in the study, but the same results were obtained from a careful repeat test with the same subject. There are similarities with the data for many studies, mainly: the difference between the sexes was found at 5 years of age, and the seasonal variation for BMR is similar for the observation by Suzuki [15] in Japanese

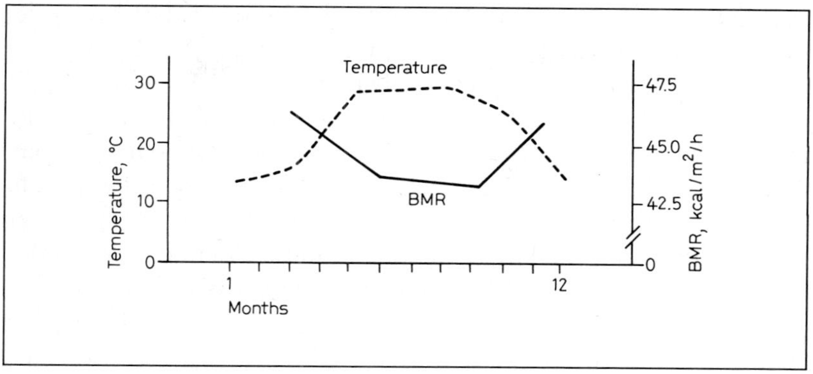

Fig. 1. The seasonal changes of BMR and temperatures.

adults. It is also worth mentioning that the results of Benedict and Ghrven [13] estimated in North China are quite close to these findings (fig. 1). The figures of Fleisch or Boothby [14], commonly used before, are much higher than those of our findings; for example, Boothby's data give 56.3 kcal/m^2/h for males and 53.0 kcal/m^2/h for females in 5-year-old children. This is 10.8 kcal higher for boys and 9.8 kcal higher for girls against our findings in this study. Thus, we overestimated 240 kcal in a period of 24 h.

The lower BMR in our study compared with previous data may arise from variations found in our study, and the number of subjects studied may be important. We assumed that our finding of a lower BMR compared to the Western World may come from the effects of climate rather than genetics.

The specific dynamic actions of foods in children appeared quite similar to those findings of Suzuki [15], in Japanese adults, who found that about 16–17% of heat is spent with a high-protein diet and only 6–7% with a high-fat diet. Suzuki [15] found about 7–8% of total SDA for total caloric intakes in a mixed diet and in our study it was 10%.

The energy expenditure of children in various activities is hard to compare with that of adults because of different body shape, the intensity of actions or the growth situation. A daily habitual activity in kindergarten for 5-year-old children will be a little higher than for those living at home where the playarea is limited, expecially in urbanized areas, or those who just stay at home under the care of their grandparents. On the other hand, in the situations of rural areas, the activity may be a little more or a little less. In the case of living in a kindergarten, even just a day-care center in a township, the activity is still quite similar to that in this study [16]. Children spend about 9 h sleeping at night and about 2 h napping at noon; children of 5 years old even sleep earlier in rural areas. In rural conditions, most of the children may have more space to play outdoors and may perform some household chores, especially girls. If a boy or girl walked for 1 h instead of sitting at home and if their body weight is 18 kg, the energy requirement will be 42 kcal more than in those children living in the city; thus, 42 kcal added to 1,278 kcal makes 1,320 kcal at maximum.

It is worth considering that an improper calorie intake may limit a child's activity. Torún and Viteri [17] observed that the children spent more energy in physical activities with the highest level of intake but there is no change in their behavior or in the pattern and intensity of their activities; they also found that there was no difference in energy balance with different levels of dietary energy intake from 90 to 106 kcal/kg/day. Their finding agrees well with our observations. We can say that the energy is basically balanced in this study with an increase of body weight of about 2.16 kg in a year.

The caloric intake for the children in this study is about 1,281 kcal and this figure is quite similar to that for our nutrition surveys in township kindergarten [16], and a similar observation has been reported in the USA [20]. The children's appetite and the density of food provided need to be known when using food consumption as a measure of energy expenditure. As rice and wheat are basic staple foods in China, the effect on children of these foods' bulk should be considered. There are 4 meals daily in this study for children, and the energy contents of their food is 37% from fat, 12% from protein, and about 51% included sugar from carbohydrates. Rice seemed not too bulky for their stomachs. The children observed in this study are mostly active; stunted or lazy children are rare.

To set up an RDA for one nutrient it is reasonable to consider safety factors and to cover almost all individuals in a given population. It is understood that the RDA for protein added 2 SD to the mean requirement and to consider the available of food protein, but might not all the same in the case of energy supported even the ideas is controversial.

The safety level for energy recommended for a population should be taken into account in the situation of developing countries. The reason at least is to consider that the urban and rural situations are quite different and so the variations might be larger in those children in developed countries. In our cases studied in the subtropics, we followed up 10 subjects for intensive observations. The total energy expenditure was 1,049 ± 44 kcal/day, and if 2 SD was added, it woud be 1,138 kcal/day. The digestibility of a mixed diet on the basis of rice was assumed to be 90%, for a diet based on corn it is about 88% [4], and if this is taken into consideration, total energy needs will be only about 1,251 kcal.

The body weight increase for the 30 subjects in a year is about 2.16 kg, thus an increase of 6 g/day; if 5 kcal were needed for 1 g of body weight growth [3], about 35 kcal may be added to the energy intake. Even if the spent calories were already included in what we measured in all the activities of children in the study, then the total caloric support would be 1,251 ± 35, equal to 1,286 kcal.

If using the estimation from the whole group of children observed by their seasonal scheduled activity, i.e. 1,278 kcal, and if adding 2 SD it will be 1,366 kcal, then a 90% digestibility for food calories added will be 1,502 kcal or, if the energy for growth is still included, the total will be 1,537 kcal at most, but this kind of consideration may not be appropriate for the majority of 5- to 6-year-olds, because if this higher figure is used as a recommendation, the probability of adding from 1 to 2 SD in the caloric intake is only 0.07 according to Beaton [18] and Anderson et al. [19], even using the mean requirement. On the other hand, the regulations of caloric intake concerned with the feeding practices of children may affect the appetite of a small percentage of them.

The heat losses from other sources have been considered, such as losses from sweat, urine or feces; these losses have not been included in the measurements as they are so small.

We suggest that the mean energy expenditure and the basis of an energy intake recommendation for this whole group of 5-year-old children observed in this subtropical study – i.e. 1,278 kcal plus 35 kcal for growth needs and an additional 10% for the absorption of food energy – totals 1,444 kcal. About 12 h sleeping in bed in the kindergarten is our observation, but this may be reduced for those who live elsewhere. This should be considered especially in the case of rural areas, and some calories may be added for compensations; thus, an RDA of 1,500 kcal/day should be acceptable.

The success of birth control as well as the 'one family one child policy' in China has led some of the parents to force-feed their singleton child; this would not be an advantage for the next generations. Conversely, a balanced diet and a proper caloric intake may be suitable for such a large population.

References

1 Andersen, K.L.; Masironi, R.; Rutenfranz, J.; Seliger, V.: Habitual physical activity and health. WHO Regional Publications, Eur. Ser., No. 6, Copenhagen 1978, pp. 1–35.
2 Zhi-chien, Ho: The energy expenditure of three categories of labourers in South China. Food Nutr. Bull., suppl. 10, pp. 193–197 (1984).
3 WHO/FAO: Energy and protein requirements. Report of a Joint FAO/WHO Ad Hoc Expert Committee. Tech. Rep. Ser., No. 522 (WHO, Genève 1973).
4 Torún, B.; Viteri, F.E.: Energy requirement of preschool children and effects of varying energy intakes on protein metabolism. Food Nutr. Bull., suppl. 5, pp. 229–236 (1981).
5 Devadas, R.P.; Murthy, N.K.: Nutrition of the preschool child in India. Wld Rev. Nutr. Diet., vol. 27, pp. 1–33 (Karger, Basel 1977).
6 Kemmerow, F.A.: Optimum nutrition through better planning of world agriculture. Wld Rev. Nutr. Diet., vol. 45, pp. 1–41 (Karger, Basel 1985).
7 Du Bois, E.F.: The estimation of the surface area of the body in basal metabolism in health and disease, pp. 25–38 (Lea & Febiger, Philadelphia 1936).
8 Consolazio, C.F.: Physiological measurements of metabolic functions in man (McGraw-Hill, New York 1963).
9 Taylor, C.M.: The energy expenditure of 9- to 11-year old boys and girls (1) standing, drawing and (2) dressing and undressing. J. Nutr. *36:* 123–136 (1948).
10 Lusk, G.: The specific dynamic action. J. Nutr. *3:* 519–523 (1931).
11 Forbes, E.B.: Dynamic effects and net energy value of protein carbohydrate and fat. J. Nutr. *18:* 57–62 (1939).
12 Stevenson, P.H.: Calculation of the body surface area of Chinese. Chin. J. Physiol. Rep. Ser. *1:* 13–24 (1928).
13 Benedict, F.G.; Ghrven, H.S.D.: The basal metabolism of male Chinese in Manchuria. Chin. J. Physiol. *10:* 141–147 (1936).
14 Spector, W.S.: Handbook of biological data, p. 259 (Saunders, Philadelphia 1956).
15 Suzuki, S.: Basal metabolism in the Japanese population. Wld Rev. Nutr. Diet., vol. 1, pp. 103–124 (Karger, Basel 1959).
16 Zhi-chien, Ho: To be published.
17 Torún, B.; Viteri, F.E.: Capacity of habitual Guatemalan diets to safety protein requirements of preschool children with adequate dietary energy intakes. Food Nutr. Bull., suppl. 5, pp. 210–228 (1981).
18 Beaton, G.H.: The use of nutritional requirements and allowances; in White, Selvey, Proc. Western Hemisphere Nutrition Congr. III, pp. 356–363 (Futura, New York 1981).
19 Anderson, H.; Peterson, D.; Beaton, G.H.: Estimating nutrient deficiencies in a population from dietary records: the use of probability analyses. Nutr. Res. *2:* 409–415 (1982).
20 Owen, G.M.: A study of nutritional status of preschool children in the United States. Pediatrics *53:* 597–607 (1974).

Zhi-chien Ho, MD, Head, Department of Clinical Nutrition, Sun Yet-sen University of Medical Sciences, Guangzhou (People's Republic of China)

Wld Rev. Nutr. Diet., vol. 57, pp. 95–125 (Karger, Basel 1988)

Vitamin Requirements in Normal Human Pregnancy

H. van den Berg[a], *H.W. Bruinse*[b]

[a] TNO-CIVO Toxicology and Nutrition Institute Zeist, Utrecht,
[b] Department of Obstetrics and Gynaecology, University Hospital, Utrecht, The Netherlands

Contents

Introduction

Maternal diet and nutritional status are considered to be important factors influencing foetal growth. Under normal conditions 5–6 kg new tissue is produced during the process of pregnancy. Changes observed in biochemical indices of the nutritional status in the course of pregnancy, simulating biochemical evidence of malnutrition, seem to emphasize increased nutrient needs. Especially in the older studies evidence has been reported suggesting a relationship between specific nutritional deficiencies and obstetric complications.

In general, estimates of vitamin requirements during pregnancy are based on data on dietary vitamin intake or biochemical parameters of the vitamin and general health status in relation to data on specific pathology and functional outcome, and/or on vitamin supplementation and intervention studies [1, 2].

Based on the available information advisory committees recommend daily intakes for pregnant and lactating women [3–5]. As illustrated in table I, these recommendations are in general higher for pregnant than for non-pregnant women.

Only more recently it has been recognized that changes in dietary, biochemical and clinical indices of the nutritional status observed in the course of pregnancy should be considered against the background of the changes in body composition and maternal physiology [2, 6]. Studies in women using hormonal contraceptives indicate that hormones may influence nutrient metabolism. During pregnancy increasing amounts of various steroid and peptide hormones are produced by the foeto-placental unit. The subsequent changes in hormonal balance may affect both the maternal nutrient requirement and the nutrient supply to the foetus. Also changes in organ function, like decreased gastro-intestinal motility and gastric secretion rate, increased renal plasma flow and glomerular filtration rate, as well as haemodynamic changes like increase in the circulating blood volume, may interact with the body's nutrient economy and affect nutrient metabolism. Many excellent books and reviews on the physiological and metabolic changes occurring in the course of pregnancy are available [6, 7].

In this review some relevant aspects of these pregnancy induced 'adjustments' in maternal physiology with respect to vitamin metabolism and requirements will be discussed.

Approaches To Estimate Nutrient (Vitamin) Requirements in Pregnancy

For the production of new foetal and placental tissues and the enlargement of the maternal reproductive organs extra energy and nutrients are needed. These extra nutrient needs are calculated with the so-called factorial approach using data on body composition and daily losses of the nutrient. This approach is only feasible when solid knowledge on body composition and nutrient retention is available. However, for most vitamins these data are limited [1].

A second approach is the nutrition survey or the epidemiology in which data on the usual dietary intake are matched with clinical and laboratory findings in order to arrive at an intake which ensures that the majority of subjects will fall within the 'normal' range of a selected biochemical index of the nutritional status and will show no clinical evidence of deficiency. In this approach the most serious difficulty is probably the accurate estimation of representative dietary nutrient intake. Also the specificity and sensitivity of the biochemical or clinical criterion used should be considered. Usually biochemical indices are more early signs and therefore more sensitive than clinical signs and may lead to higher estimations of the requirement. Interpretation criteria based on observations in non-pregnant reference populations are frequently used. However, as already mentioned, it should be realized that the specificity of the parameters used may be different in the pregnant as compared with the non-pregnant state, as a result of the so-called physiological adjustments of pregnancy [2].

Because of obvious practical and ethical reasons, experimental methods like the balance technique or depletion/repletion studies in a controlled environment are generally not feasible. Furthermore, the balance technique has its intrinsic drawbacks [8].

An approach which has proved to be very useful in estimating vitamin requirements is the method in which a specific metabolic, biochemical or physiological response is measured after controlled supplementation with the specific vitamin. This method was successfully used by Dempsey [9] with respect to vitamin B_6 and by Bates [10, 11, 154] concerning vitamin C and riboflavin requirements in pregnant and lactating Gambian women. However, also with this approach the possibility of a different specificity of the parameter used should be considered.

Beaton [2] has outlined a desirable theoretical approach to define nutrient requirements in pregnancy. In his view nutrient intake should be related with functional outcome. The maternal organism should be considered at the entry and exit of the reproductive cycle to determine whether net changes have occurred. However, also in this approach accurate knowledge of the body composition is essential.

Requirements can be considered as the minimal intake or supply to prevent (or correct) certain pathology, or to maintain 'normal' function, e.g. 'biochemical normality'. Recommended daily allowances (RDA) are generally based on knowledge of (minimal) requirements taking into account the (supposed) variability within the population, utilization from the diet, etc., to cover the needs of nearly all members of the population [4]. Considering all the different approaches to assess nutrient requirement and the uncertainties in defining safety factors, it is not surprising that a considerable diversity in recommended dietary allowances occurs [12].

Table I. Recommended daily dietary allowances for pregnant (second and third trimester) and non-pregnant females

	Energy kcal	Energy (MJ)	Protein g	Vit. A[a] µg	Vit. D µg	Vit. B_1 mg	Vit. B_2 mg	Vit. B_6 mg	Niacin mg	Folacin µg	Vit. B_{12} µg	Vit. C mg
WHO [3]												
Adult women	2,200	(9.2)	29	750	2.5	0.9[b]	1.3[c]	–	14.5[d]	200[e]	2.0	30
Pregnant	2,550	(10.7)	38	750	10	1.0[b]	1.5[c]	–	17	400[e]	3.0	30
DHSS (UK) [5]												
Non-pregnant	2,150	(9.0)	54	750	–	0.9	1.3	–	15	300[f]	–	30
Pregnant	2,400	(10.1)	60	750	10	1.0	1.6	–	18	500[f]	–	60
NAS/NRC (USA) [4]												
Non-pregnant	2,000	(8.4)	44	800	5	1.0	1.2	2.0	13	400[f]	3.0	60
Pregnant	2,300	(9.6)	74	1,000	10	1.4	1.5	2.5	15	800[f]	4.0	60

[a] 1 µg retinol = 6 µg β-carotene = 12 µg carotenoids.
[b] 0.4 mg/1,000 kcal (4.2 MJ).
[c] 0.55 mg/1,000 kcal (4.2 MJ).
[d] 6.6 mg/1,000 kcal (4.2 MJ).
[e] Expressed as free folacin.
[f] Total folacin.
– = No recommendations given.

The recommendations from the joint WHO/FAO Expert group [3], the Department of Health and Social Security [5] and from the Committee on Dietary Allowances from the National Academy of Sciences and the National Research Council [4] for both pregnant and non-pregnant women (23–50 years) are summarized in table I.

Vitamin Intake from the Diet During Pregnancy

The higher amounts of vitamins needed during pregnancy can be derived from a higher dietary intake. In table II a number of reported data [13–19] on nutrient intake of women at different stages of pregnancy are summarized. This summary is far from complete but is intended to show estimated average nutrient intake levels of pregnant women living in rather privileged (industrial) societies. The methods of measurement used in many surveys, especially those involving recall, are likely to be inaccurate.

Only for a number of vitamins intake data are available, as most food composition tables include only data on vitamin A, thiamine, riboflavin, vitamin C, and some also on niacin, while data on vitamin B_6, folacin and vitamin D are mostly lacking.

Generally, vitamin intake from the diet tends to be slightly higher during pregnancy, in parallel with the increased caloric intake. However, differences with non-pregnant controls are relatively small. Some discrepancy seems apparent between dietary practice and recommendations. The higher recommendations for pregnant women are generally related to the second and third trimester. Appetite actually increases towards the end of the first trimester, but decreases again during the third trimester. In our longitudinal study with 85 healthy pregnant women [19, 162] we observed a significantly higher mean energy and vitamin intake, estimated using a dietary history method, at week 16 of pregnancy as compared with the data obtained at week 34 and 6 months postpartum (table II). Between the data from week 34 and that from 6 months postpartum differences were no longer significant for vitamin A, niacin and vitamin D, as well as the energy intake.

Data on folacin intake are scarce and probably unreliable due to still unresolved analytical problems with the folacin assay [20]. However, several studies indicate a dietary folacin intake below recommended standards [18, 21].

Table II. Mean daily energy and vitamin intake by pregnant women, reported from several studies

Authors	Subjects	Stage	n	Energy kcal[a]	Protein g	Vit. A µg RE	Thiamine mg	Riboflavin mg	Niacin mg	Ascorbic acid, mg	Survey method
Gräfe [13] (1961, DDR)	normal preg.	5th month	89	2,753	77	2,580	1.57	1.85	15	79	7-day record
		8th month		2,755	77	2,400	1.63	1.97	16	95	
Lunell et al. [14] (1969, Sweden)	healthy women	1st trim.	58	2,035	65	790	1.3	1.7	11.5	91	24-hour recall
		2nd trim.		2,185	70	680	1.2	1.8	10	103	
		3rd trim.		2,137	73	680	1.5	2.2	11	116	
Smithells et al. [15] (1977, UK)	healthy women	1st trim.	168	2,010	70	1,000	0.99	1.53	12	68	weighed 7-day record
Darke et al. [16] (1980, UK)	healthy women	3rd trim.	435	2,152	70	1,270	1.04	1.60	14	55	weighed 7-day record
Doyle et al. [17] (1982)	healthy women (low socio-economic status)	1st trim.	76	1,613	66	1,415	0.99	1.63	13.7	64	weighed 7-day record
		2nd trim.	67	1,723	68	1,325	1.04	1.63	13.8	73	
		3rd trim.	63	1,772	69	1,421	1.08	1.80	14.3	70	
Papoz et al. [18] (1981, France)	healthy women	1st trim.	156	2,307	82	670	1.40	1.83	–	172	recall
		3rd trim.		2,121	79	660	1.32	1.85	–	173	
Van den Berg and Bruinse [19] (1983, Holland)	healthy women	16 weeks	68	2,405	83	1,240	1.22	1.96	13	144	dietary history
		34 weeks	67	2,245	76	1,130	1.16	1.95	12	121	
		6 m pp	62	2,175	76	1,120	1.07	1.69	12	78	

[a] 1 kcal = 4.18 kJ.

Reported estimates of vitamin B_6 during pregnancy vary between 1 and 2 mg/day, which is also below recommended standards [15, 18, 19, 22, 107]. The same seems true for vitamin D as only a limited number of natural food products contain significant amounts of vitamin D. However, under conditions of normal solar exposure, endogenous production by the epidermal layer of the skin is amply sufficient to meet the body's requirements, although the amount obtained in this way cannot be readily assessed [23].

Effect of Pregnancy on Maternal Vitamin Metabolism and Vitamin Status – Vitamin-Related Pathology in Pregnancy

Vitamin A

Vitamin Metabolism and Status During Pregnancy. During pregnancy additional vitamin A is needed for a number of special metabolic processes, such as foetal development and storage in the liver, formation of colostrum and storage for lactation and possibly for hormone synthesis. Vitamin A is transported across the placenta as its retinol-retinol-binding protein (RBP) complex [24]. At birth livers of normal Indian and Thai infants contain rather low concentrations of vitamin A (< 50 µg/g), even if the mother is well nourished [25, 26]. Data on livers of British infants near term varied between 10 and 150 µg/g [27]. From these data it can be estimated that about 5 mg is stored in the foetal compartment. This amount constitutes about 2% of normal maternal reserves [28].

In most studies a decrease in the maternal serum retinol content during the course of pregnancy has been recorded (most of the relevant studies have been summarized by Rodriguez and Irwin [29]. However, it is doubtful whether this decrease should be interpreted as indicative of a depletion of the maternal stores. First of all the serum retinol content is a poor index of vitamin A body (liver) stores [30]. Also other factors like protein and/or zinc deficiency, hormonal changes and acute diseases may secondarily affect serum retinol content. We [19] observed a spontaneous 'recovery' towards values in the non-pregnant reference range within the first days after delivery (table III).

In general, serum total carotenoid levels show an upward trend during pregnancy [31, 32], although in some studies a progressive fall was observed [33]. Retinol and carotene levels in the foetal circulation and in cord blood are generally lower than those in the maternal circulation [34, 67].

Table III. Changes in some vitamin status parameters during and after an uncomplicated pregnancy. Data taken from Van den Berg and Bruinse [19] (n = 70)

	Period										Significance $p < 0.05$	
	wk 16 (T_1)		wk 34 (T_3)		partus (T_4)		6 w pp (T_6)		6 m pp (T_7)			
	$\overline{X}$	SD	$\overline{X}$	SD	$\overline{X}$	SD	$\overline{X}$	SD	$\overline{X}$	SD	T_1–T_3	T_1–T_7
Retinol (S) (µmol/l)	1.01	0.34	0.78	0.24	0.48	0.31	1.18	0.49	1.30	0.50	+	+
25-OH-vit. D (S) (nmol/l)	50	21	53	26	50	22	50	21	62	27	n.s.	+
ETK activity (E) (U/mmol Hb)	9.1	1.8	7.8	2.1	7.5	1.9	9.3	2.2	10.8	2.2	+	+
ETK stimulation (E) (U/U)	1.14	0.10	1.17	0.14	1.14	0.12	1.09	0.08	1.13	0.08	n.s.	n.s.
Riboflavin (B) (µmol/l)	0.30	0.04	0.31	0.03	0.35	0.05	0.32	0.05	0.32	0.04	+	+
EGR activity (E) (U/mmol Hb)	88	19	81	18	89	20	93	22	99	22	+	+
EGR stimulation (E) (U/U)	1.16	0.15	1.18	0.21	1.14	0.22	1.11	0.15	1.12	0.14	n.s.	n.s.
Pyridoxal 5′-phosphate (P) (nmol/l)	15	5	9	4	8	3	18	6	24	15	+	+
EGOT activity (E) (U/mmol Hb)	64	11	61	17	61	18	61	15	68	14	n.s.	+
EGOT stimulation (E) (U/U)	1.98	0.15	2.03	0.28	2.05	0.31	1.98	0.22	1.87	0.18	n.s.	+
Vitamin B_{12} (S) (pmol/l)	391	97	322	92	342	101	448	127	421	114	+	+
Folacin (S) (nmol/l)	6.5	2.4	3.8	2.0	3.8	1.8	4.1	2.2	4.4	2.4	+	+

S = Serum, E = erythrocytes, B = whole blood, P = plasma.

Vitamin-A-Related Pathology in Pregnancy. Animal experiments have shown profound effects of vitamin A deficiency on reproductive efficiency [24, 35]. In humans there is actually no sound evidence for vitamin-A-related pathology in pregnancy. In one (Indian) study a coincidence of low serum retinol levels with pre-eclamptic toxaemia was reported [36], while Sharma et al. [37] observed low serum retinol levels in patients with abruptio placentae. Kübler and Moch [32] found a significant positive relationship between maternal serum retinol level in the second and third trimester and birth weight.

Requirements. An extensive literature review on vitamin A requirements has been compiled by Rodriguez and Irwin [29]. Based on the data on foetal vitamin A storage an extra increase in the RDA for pregnant women between 100 and 200 μg/day as retinol, or retinol equivalents, was considered by NAS/NRC [4]. WHO [3] concluded that the daily foetal needs could be met without seriously affecting maternal body stores and therefore did not discriminate between pregnant and non-pregnant women (table I). For non-pregnant women NAS/NRC recommends 800 μg/day, WHO 750 μg/day.

Studies in The Gambia [38] indicate that dietary carotenoids can effectively replace preformed retinol, possibly with an even higher efficiency than the generally accepted 6:1 conversion ratio for β-carotene to retinol equivalents.

Vitamin D

Vitamin Metabolism and Status During Pregnancy. Pregnancy induces massive shifts in calcium; about 30 g of calcium, i.e. about 2.5% of the total maternal store, is transferred from the mother to the foetus. This change in calcium homeostasis is regulated by vitamin D. Maternal serum 1,25-$(OH)_2$-vitamin D (1,25-DHD) content increases during pregnancy, concurrent with a decrease in serum ionized calcium and a secondary hyperparathyroidism [39]. Which factors are responsible for this pregnancy induced increase in serum DHD content has not yet been fully elucidated. Both placenta and foetal kidneys can synthesize 1,25-DHD [40, 41].

Maternal serum 25-OH-vitamin D (25-OHD), the most abundant circulating metabolite of vitamin D, shows the normal seasonal variation during pregnancy with no specific pregnancy-induced trend [42]. However, in some cross-sectional studies a slight decrease during pregnancy was reported [43].

Maternal serum 24,25-$(OH)_2$-vitamin D (24,25-DHD) content is not affected, or is slightly lower than in non-pregnant controls [39, 44]. The vitamin D binding protein (DBP) content in serum increases more or less in parallel with the increase in the serum 1,25-DHD content [45].

Both 25-OHD and 1,25-DHD can cross the placenta. Cord blood 25-OHD levels are about 20% lower than the corresponding maternal level and a significant correlation between paired maternal and cord blood levels has been demonstrated [46]. Foetal DBP is about half the maternal level. Foetal 1,25-DHD serum content is lower than the corresponding maternal level, but due to the lower DBP level, the 'free' 1,25-DHD level in the foetus is identical to that of its mother or even higher [47].

A positive correlation between the maternal and foetal 1,25-DHD levels was found in some, but not all, studies [47, 48]. Cord 24,25-DHD levels are relatively high. Although vitamin D_2 and D_3 are considered to have the same biopotency, Markestad et al. [49] reported a higher 1,25-DHD_2 to 1,25-DHD_3 ratio than the corresponding 25-OHD_2 to 25-OHD_3 ratio in both the maternal and the cord serum after supplementation with 400 IU vitamin D_2 per day during pregnancy.

Vitamin-D-Related Pathology in Pregnancy. No specific maternal pathology in pregnancy has been related to vitamin D deficiency. Maternal vitamin D deficiency may be an aetiologic factor in primary dental hypoplasia [50] and be related with neonatal hypocalcemia in prematures [51].

Requirements. Based on the physiological stress on calcium metabolism during pregnancy, NAS/NRC [4] as well as WHO [3] recommend an increase of the daily allowance with 5 μg (200 IU) during pregnancy. For non-pregnant women the RDA are 5 and 2.5 μg, respectively. As already noted on page 101, diet is not the main source of vitamin D and it would therefore be difficult to cover the higher requirement solely by the diet. Regular solar exposure seems adequate, although the amount obtained this way cannot be readily assessed. This is supported by the observation that under conditions of regular solar exposure serum 25-OHD content is not seriously affected during pregnancy. However, serum 25-OHD levels in the deficient range were reported for pregnant women with heavily pigmented skins, living in areas with limited direct sunlight. For such populations vitamin D supplementation is recommendable.

Vitamin E

Vitamin Metabolism and Status During Pregnancy. Maternal serum vitamin E levels rise during pregnancy by 50% of the non-pregnant value [52, 53]. This increase in serum level parallels the increase in serum lipid concentration. The insignificant effects of vitamin E supplementation on the serum vitamin E level [54] confirms that, also in the pregnant state, the serum vitamin E level is controlled by other metabolic factors as well [55]. Cord blood levels are considerably lower than the corresponding maternal serum levels. A significant correlation between both compartments was observed in some [160], but not in all studies [56]. The lower vitamin E cord serum level probably reflects limited transport capacity, rather than impaired placental transfer [57].

Vitamin-E-Related Pathology in Pregnancy. In some older studies a relationship between serum vitamin E levels and pregnancy outcome has been reported, but the data are equivocal and were not confirmed in more recent studies [57, 58]. Vitamin E deficiency is related with the occurrence of haemolytic anaemia, intraventricular haemorrhage and retrolental fibroplasia in preterms, although Haga and Lunde [56] observed no significant difference in vitamin serum level between preterm and term infants. Low levels of serum vitamin E were reported in patients with abruptio placentae [37].

Requirements. There is no sound basis to conclude that vitamin E requirements are increased during pregnancy. NAS/NRC [4] recommends 7–13 mg α-tocopherol equivalents per day for adults. This requirement may be slightly higher for people ingesting diets with a high polyunsaturated fat content. Vegetable oils usually contain this extra tocopherol. It is expected that the increased caloric intake through a normal diet during pregnancy will supply sufficient additional vitamin E to compensate for the amount deposited in the foetus.

Vitamin K

Vitamin K deficiency is uncommon in adults, due to the significant contribution of the intestinal flora to cover vitamin K requirements. There is a growing interest in this vitamin as a (latent) deficiency may occur in new-borns when breast-fed, or fed certain (non-milk-based) formulas [59, 60]. Only recently analytical techniques with sufficient sensitivity to measure vitamin K in plasma and human milk have become available [61].

Maternal plasma vitamin K levels during pregnancy seem slightly lower than in non-pregnant women. In cord plasma vitamin K levels are very low, or even undetectable. Together with the clinical evidence of vitamin K deficiency symptoms in (preterm) babies, it seems that vitamin K uptake by the foetus is very low, which may be caused by limited transport capacity [61].

Requirements. Vitamin K is synthesized by the intestinal flora. The NAS/NRC [4] considers an intake of 70–140 μg as 'safe and adequate'. This recommendation is based on an estimated requirement of 2 μg/kg of body weight, of which about one half is contributed by bacterial synthesis.

Thiamine

Thiamine Metabolism and Status During Pregnancy. Urinary thiamine excretion, and to a lesser extent also the thiamine blood level, is reduced during pregnancy [54, 62, 63]. Cord blood thiamine levels are about two times higher than maternal levels. The erythrocyte transketolase (ETK) stimulation ratio is reported to be increased (> 1.20) in 15–50% of cases during pregnancy [19, 32, 63–65]. However, the changes in the basal, unstimulated ETK activity seem not to be related to the occurrence of thiamine deficiency [63, 66]. ETK saturation in cord blood is higher as compared with maternal blood, i.e. stimulation ratios are lower [67]. Also for placental tissue ETK saturation with the thiamine diphosphate (ThDp) coenzyme is higher as compared with that in maternal and in cord blood erythrocytes as was reported from a study performed in Kenya, suggesting some storage capacity in the placenta [68].

Thiamine-Related Pathology in Pregnancy. Hyperemesis gravidarum [69] and toxaemia [70] have been related with maternal thiamine deficiency, but these 'incidental' observations may be the (secondary) result rather than cause of the disease.

Requirements. NAS/NRC [4] recommends an additional 0.4 mg/day (0.6 mg/1,000 kcal as compared with 0.4 mg/1,000 kcal for non-pregnant women) throughout lactation to compensate for the increased requirements, as evidenced by the changes in biochemical indices of the thiamine status. WHO [3] does not differentiate between pregnant and non-pregnant women and recommends 0.4 mg/1,000 kcal for both groups. Assuming an increased energy intake of about 300 kcal/day and a thiamine content of 0.4 mg/1,000 kcal, the absolute daily thiamine intake will increase with about 0.12 mg.

Riboflavin

Riboflavin Metabolism and Status During Pregnancy. In general, a lowered urinary riboflavin excretion during pregnancy is reported [71]. Whole blood or erythrocyte riboflavin content is also lowered during pregnancy [72, 73], or unaffected [19]. Higher levels are found in cord blood [19, 54, 74] although the difference between paired cord and maternal samples was reported to be insignificant when riboflavin content was expressed as the mean corpuscular riboflavin concentration (MCRC) [73].

Riboflavin (metabolites) readily crosses the placenta [75]. Placental conversion of flavin adenine dinucleotide (FAD), the main circulating form in maternal blood, to free riboflavin, and a different transplacental transport of these molecules has been suggested to explain the higher cord blood levels [76, 77]. Contrary to various pregnant animals, no specific high-affinity riboflavin-binding protein has been identified in the plasma of pregnant women [78].

With the EGR stimulation test a relatively high incidence of too high stimulation ratios (>1.30) was found in some, but not in all studies [19, 32, 63, 67, 79, 80]. The erythrocyte glutathione reductase (EGR) apoenzyme content generally does not show a significant trend [66]. In cord blood a significantly higher EGR activity and a lower EGR stimulation ratio is generally found as compared with the corresponding maternal values [19, 32, 63, 67, 80]. A modulating effect of the iron status on the riboflavin status has been reported [81]. Decker et al. [82] observed a coincidence between low haemoglobin levels and increased EGR stimulation.

Riboflavin-Related Pathology in Pregnancy. An increased incidence of hyperemesis gravidarum and prematurity was reported in some older studies [71]. In more recent studies in developed countries no relationship between (biochemical) riboflavin deficiency and pregnancy-induced pathology was found [79]. Clinical signs of riboflavin deficiency, like glossitis and angular stomatitis, have been observed in pregnancy in undernourished populations [10, 83].

Requirements. NAS/NRC [4] recommends an additional 0.3 mg/day to compensate for the increased requirements, as evidenced by the changes in biochemical indices of the riboflavin status. As for thiamine, WHO [3] does not differentiate between pregnant and non-pregnant women and recommends 0.55 mg/1,000 kcal for both groups. An increase in energy intake with about 300 kcal/day may result in an extra daily riboflavin intake of about 0.2 mg. It should be noted that in some studies a relatively high incidence of biochemical abnormality, especially with the EGR stimulation test, is found in spite of an apparently adequate riboflavin intake [10, 19].

Vitamin B_6

Vitamin B_6 Metabolism and Status During Pregnancy. In general, biochemical indices of the maternal vitamin B_6 status indicate a negative vitamin B_6 balance during pregnancy. Plasma pyridoxal 5′-phosphate (PLP) content decreases dramatically [19, 84], even during (oral) supplementation with pyridoxine in amounts up to 10 mg/day [85–87]. We [19] found a spontaneous reversal (i.e. without supplementation) of the pregnancy-induced changes after delivery (table III), although 6 months after delivery about a quarter of the population studied showed plasma PLP levels still below the lower limit of the reference range (15 nmol/l).

A relatively high incidence of abnormal values, indicative of a vitamin B_6 deficiency, has been reported for the tryptophan load test [88]. However, the validity of this test as an index of vitamin B_6 status is doubtful, as the alterations in tryptophan metabolism seem to be primarily caused by the changing hormonal environment rather than by vitamin B_6 deficiency [89, 90]. During pregnancy, urinary 4-pyridoxic acid excretion is lowered or unaffected [91]. With the transaminase stimulation tests as (functional) indices of the vitamin B_6 status, a percentage of abnormal stimulation ratios between 30 and 60% is reported [19, 22, 32, 63, 92]. The sensitivity and reproducibility of this test has, however, been questioned [84, 87]. Erythrocyte glutamate oxaloacetate transaminase (EGOT) apo-enzyme turnover is affected by both nutritional [87] and non-nutritional factors [93]. We [19] observed a different time trend in the course of pregnancy between plasma PLP and the EGOT stimulation test. Plasma PLP decreases already in early pregnancy, while the incidence of abnormal EGOT stimulation ratios increases when pregnancy progressed (table III).

Low diamine oxidase (DAO) activity in plasma and in the placenta has been associated with vitamin B_6 deficiency [68, 94]. DAO is a PLP-dependent enzyme, produced by the placental decidua [95].

The foetus is able to synthesize PLP, but evidence has been presented that PLP in the foetal circulation is mainly derived from the maternal circulation [86, 96]. The PLP concentration in cord blood is on average 3–5 times higher than in the maternal circulation [19, 67, 87]. In nearly all studies a higher basal EGOT (EGPT) activity and a lower stimulation ratio is reported in cord as compared with maternal erythrocytes. Also the placenta contains PLP, but to a much lesser extent than in animal species, e.g. the rat [97].

Vitamin B_6-Related Pathology in Pregnancy. Toxaemia [97–99], hyperemesis gravidarum [100, 101], depressive syndromes [102] and impaired glucose tolerance [103] have all been related with a disturbance in vitamin B_6 metabolism or with a marginal or deficient vitamin B_6 status in pregnancy. Low plasma DAO activity (induced by vitamin B_6 deficiency?) has been associated with pregnancy wastage, stillbirth and spontaneous abortion [104]. However, data are as yet inconclusive and await further confirmation. Recently, Schuster et al. [163] found no difference in vitamin B_6 status between pregnant women experiencing morning sickness and women who did not.

In some studies a relationship between vitamin B_6 status and birth weight was reported [32, 105, 106]. However, such a relationship was not found by others, like Heller et al. [92] and Vir et al. [22]. Also, Roepke and Kirksey [108] could not demonstrate such an effect, but reported lower Apgar scores in new-borns of mothers who were vitamin B_6-deficient, while Schuster et al. [109] reported a positive effect of maternal vitamin B_6 supplementation on the Apgar scores. Other vitamin supplementation studies have failed to show a positive effect on the incidence of specific pathology, except for a lower incidence of dental caries in women who were supplemented with 20 mg/day vitamin B_6 [110, 111].

Requirements. Although numerous studies indicate a negative vitamin B_6 balance, based on the changes in biochemical indices of the maternal vitamin B_6 status, the question how much extra vitamin B_6 is actually needed is still unanswered. Rather high supplementary doses are needed (5–10 mg/day) to maintain the biochemical parameters within the non-pregnant range [85–87]. Clinical evidence for an increased requirement is limited (see above). The only functional impairment may be on the level of foetal development [107–109]. NAS/NRC [4] recommends therefore 'only' an additional allowance of 0.6 mg/day above the 2.0 mg/day accepted for non-pregnant females (0.02 mg/g protein, with an estimated protein intake of 100 g/day), to compensate for the additional protein allowance.

Vitamin B_{12}

Vitamin B_{12} Metabolism and Status During Pregnancy. Serum vitamin B_{12} levels fall progressively during pregnancy [19, 112, 113, 159]. This pattern was reported to be unchanged even after vitamin B_{12} supplementation [114]. This decrease should be interpreted as 'normal physiology of pregnancy', as Kalamegham and Krishnaswamy [115] measured no increase in methylmalonic acid excretion after an oral valine load, even when serum vitamin B_{12} was below 100 pg/ml (75 pmol/l). In the postpartum period we [19] observed also for this vitamin a spontaneous rise towards the pre-pregnant range (table III). The transcobalamins, the vitamin B_{12} carrier proteins, show complex changes during pregnancy and are unlikely to be related with the changes occurring in maternal serum vitamin B_{12} content [116].

Vitamin B_{12} is readily transported across the placenta [75, 117]. Cord serum vitamin B_{12} levels are generally two times as high as in the corresponding maternal serum [19, 67]. The placenta can accumulate high concentrations of vitamin B_{12} in the intervillous space [118].

Vitamin B_{12}-Related Pathology in Pregnancy. The incidence of pernicious anaemia during pregnancy is negligible [113]. No evidence is available for specific pathology related with vitamin B_{12} in pregnancy. In one study low serum vitamin B_{12} levels were reported in women who gave birth to children with neural tube defects [119].

Requirements. Compared with maternal stores the amount of vitamin B_{12} accumulating in the foetus is relatively small (± 50 μg), i.e. about 1–2% of the total maternal store [113]. To compensate for this (average) foetal sequestration of 0.2–0.3 μg/day, both WHO [3] and NAS/NRC [4] recommend an additional daily allowance of 1.0 μg/day above 2.0 and 3.0 μg/day, respectively, for non-pregnant adults. Vegan women may have low vitamin B_{12} stores. This seems not to involve complications during pregnancy, but may cause serious problems during lactation [120].

Folacin

Folacin Metabolism and Status During Pregnancy. A progressive decline of serum and red cell folacin content has been reported [19, 157; for review of the (older) literature see ref. 121, 132]. This decrease is thought to reflect depletion of maternal stores caused by increasing foetal demands, blood volume expansion [122] and increased urinary excretion [123]. In our study on healthy pregnant women with uncomplicated pregnancies and delivery of a healthy baby, we observed significantly lower serum folacin levels at 6 months postpartum than measured at the 16th week of pregnancy, indicating that a normal pregnancy indeed 'costs' folacin. The decrease during pregnancy could not be explained by haemodilution [124]. Folacin plasma clearance is increased independent of creatinine clearance, and significantly correlated with the serum folacin level [123]. Folacin absorption, mainly in the upper part (jejunum) of the gastro-intestinal tract, seems unchanged during pregnancy [125]. Folacin deficiency in pregnancy has in one study been explained by increased enzymatic degradation [126].

Like the transcobalamins, folacin-binding proteins (FBP) in maternal blood show complex changes [127]. An unspecific FBP (low affinity, high capacity) in maternal serum has been reported to be involved in supplying folacin to the foetus. The FBP levels seem to be hormone-regulated [128].

Folacin levels in cord serum and red cells are invariably higher than corresponding maternal levels [19, 54, 67]. Placental transfer seems to be an efficient process [75, 77]. A specific FBP has been identified in cord serum [129]. An earlier study suggested that formyl folacin derivatives form an important constituent of foetal blood [130]. Foetal hepatic folacin stores were found to be related with foetal weight. At term the foetal liver contains about 300 μg [131].

Folacin-Related Pathology During Pregnancy. Megaloblastic anaemia due to folacin deficiency has a relatively high incidence during pregnancy. In industrialized societies rates between 1 and 5%, in developing countries rates up to 50% have been reported [121, 132]. Pre-anaemic bone marrow changes may have an even higher incidence. Toxaemia, abruptio placentae, abortion and stillbirth have all been associated with folacin deficiency, but a causal relationship is unlikely [111, 121]. In various studies a significant, positive relationship between birth weight and maternal folacin status, and/or a positive effect of folacin supplementation was reported [133, 134]. There is growing evidence that folacin deficiency is related with congenital malformations in the central nervous system [135]. Prospective studies from Smithells et al. [136, 137] and Laurence et al. [138] indicate a beneficial effect of (dietary) folacin treatment before conception and in early pregnancy on the recurrence risk for foetal neural tube defects. Maternal folacin deficiency may enhance the maternal immunosuppression that occurs in pregnancy as well as in malaria infection, diminishing passive immunity acquired by the foetus [139, 157].

Requirements. During pregnancy folacin requirements are increased as a consequence of rapid cell growth and cell differentiation, increased urinary losses (about 15 μg/day), and possibly increased folacin turnover. Supplementary folacin up to 300 μg/day seems required to maintain the whole blood folacin level. An extensive review of these studies on folacin requirements by Rodriguez [121] is available. However, there are still many unanswered questions, like the availability of food folacin and the variability in folacin stores and requirements between persons. At present WHO [3] and NAS/NRC [4] both recommend intakes of 800 μg total folacin (i.e. 400 μg 'free' folacin) a day for pregnant women, which is twice the amount for non-pregnant adults.

Vitamin C

Vitamin C Metabolism and Status During Pregnancy. The plasma as well as the leucocyte vitamin C content declines during pregnancy [140–142]. Urinary excretion of a test dose of ascorbic acid is reduced [143]. An extensive review of the literature on vitamin C metabolism and requirements during pregnancy has been compiled by Irwin and Hutchins [144]. Vitamin C levels in cord blood are about twice as high as the corresponding maternal levels [54, 67]. Ascorbic acid and dehydroascorbic acid are taken up from maternal blood by the placenta. Although dehydroascorbic acid seems the predominant form in the foetal tissues both forms are transported by the placenta across the cell membrane at the same rate [145].

Vitamin-C-Related Pathology During Pregnancy. It has been suggested that decreased ascorbic acid levels are associated with stillbirth and increased neonatal mortality, but this was not confirmed in other, more recent studies [141, 142]. In the study by Schorah et al. [142], a higher prevalence of low ascorbic acid levels was observed in mothers delivering babies with lower birth weights. However, an interfering effect of smoking could not be excluded. Sharma et al. [158] reported lower vitamin C blood levels in abruptio placentae patients, but it remains to be established whether these lower levels are causative, or result from a common aetiologic factor.

Requirements. Vitamin C requirements are thought to be greater in pregnant women than in non-pregnant women [144]. Smoking during pregnancy may even further increase vitamin C requirements. To cover the increasing foetal needs NAS/NRC [4] recommends an extra daily allowance of 20 mg above the 60 mg recommended for non-pregnant adults. Also, WHO [3] assumes an increased requirement and recommends an additional 20 mg/day making a total of 50 mg/day.

Other Vitamins

For the other vitamins like niacin, pantothenic acid and biotin, data on requirements during pregnancy are limited. There is some earlier evidence that pregnant women can convert tryptophan into niacin more efficiently than non-pregnant women [161]. There is no evidence for any relationship between niacin deficiency and specific pathology in pregnancy. Based on the recommended increase in energy intake of 300 kcal daily the allowance set by NAS/NRC [4] for pregnant women is increased with 2–15 niacin equivalents per day. WHO [3] recommends 6.6 niacin equivalents per 1,000 kcal for both pregnant and non-pregnant women.

Data on the changes in blood pantothenic acid content are inconsistent [146–148]. The higher cord blood levels reported indicate an active transport across the placenta. Although there is no 'official' RDA, the NAS/NRC [4] considers a pantothenic acid intake between 4 and 7 mg/day as 'safe and adequate'.

A progressive decline in biotin blood levels in the course of pregnancy was reported by Bhagavan [149], although there are large intra- and inter-individual variations [150]. Cord blood levels are 1.5–2 times as high as corresponding maternal levels [54, 67]. In one study a low biotin content was reported in the livers of babies having died from sudden infant death syndrome (SIDS) [151]. NAS/NRC [4] considers an intake of 100–200 μg/day as safe and adequate.

Vitamin Supplementation; Toxicity

As already indicated on page 99, a useful approach to the estimation of vitamin requirements is controlled supplementation. A number of supplementation studies have already been mentioned in the previous paragraphs. Hemminki and Starfield [111] reviewed a number of controlled clinical trials on the effect of routine administration of vitamins (and iron) on birth weight, length of gestation as well as on maternal and neonatal morbidity and mortality. In one trial a positive effect of vitamin B_6 on the incidence of dental caries was found, while in two other studies a positive effect of multivitamin supplementation on the incidence of pre-eclampsia was reported. Intervention trials with folacin supplements have recently been reviewed by Kristoffersen and Rolschau [135]. A positive effect on birth weight is reported in the results of some, but not of all, studies. The effect on early abortion and on congenital malformations, i.e. the recurrence risk for neural tube defects, is still under study (see page 111).

In The Gambia [154] riboflavin supplementation studies were carried out to assess riboflavin requirements during pregnancy and lactation. Supplementation with 2 mg/day was needed to achieve biochemical normality. The NAS/NRC [4] recommendation is slightly lower (1.5 mg).

In general, the use of supplements containing pharmacological doses of vitamins is controversial or even contra-indicated, especially during pregnancy. As demonstrated for most water-soluble vitamins the placenta is able to transfer vitamins to the foetal compartment against a concentration gradient [75]. Although no specific complications of foetal hypervitaminosis are known, adverse effects cannot be excluded as high levels of coenzyme may affect (foetal) enzyme turnover and induce a state of increased vitamin requirements after birth.

Recently, a case of retinoic acid embryopathy was reported [152]; also, for some other vitamins, toxic effects are known [153]. In general, vitamin supplementation during normal pregnancy, e.g. to supply or protect maternal stores, should not exceed two times the RDA.

General Discussion

There can be no doubt that (absolute) vitamin requirements during pregnancy are higher as compared with the non-pregnant state. The only question is: To what extent? The factorial approach to estimate the 'extra' needs gives, as indicated, no satisfactory answer, because accurate knowledge on vitamin contents of the foetal and placental tissues is lacking. As far as data are available, like for folacin, vitamin A and vitamin B_{12}, it seems, however, that foetal stores are relatively small as compared with maternal stores.

The supply of vitamins to the foetus seems well protected by the placenta, although the early phase of pregnancy when the placenta is not yet fully developed may be critical. This can be concluded from the detrimental effects of inadequate vitamin supply in embryonic development, demonstrated in various animal models [35], and the effect of folacin supplementation on the recurrence risk of a neural tube defect. Placental vitamin transfer and foetal storage capacity seem to increase as pregnancy progresses.

Evidence for maternal, vitamin-related pathology pregnancy is also limited. The only well-established relationship between maternal vitamin deficiency and pregnancy-related pathology is that between folacin deficiency and megaloblastic anaemia. Other reported associations, including the effect of vitamin supplements on birth weight, need further confirmation in well-controlled studies to ascertain whether these relationships are causal or just incidental.

Actually, the higher RDA for vitamins during pregnancy are in many cases based on data on biochemical indices of the vitamin status obtained at the various stages of pregnancy, i.e. on the amount of vitamin required to maintain 'biochemical normality'. However, also this criterion can be challenged. Adaptation of maternal physiology to the pregnant state, i.e. the so-called physiological adjustment of pregnancy, may secondarily affect biochemical indices of the vitamin nutritional status. In our study we could not demonstrate a significant relationship between the fall in vitamin blood levels and dietary vitamin intake [19]. We used the 'recovery' of the pregnancy-induced changes in some vitamin status parameters during the postpartum period as a criterion to evaluate the 'vitamin cost of pregnancy'. For all parameters measured such a spontaneous recovery was observed, i.e. the mean values at 6 weeks postpartum were at the same level (or better) than those at the 16th week of pregnancy, the first time of measurement, except for folacin (table III). It should be mentioned that the majority of women in our study have bottle-fed their babies, so that there was no further drain on maternal stores due to lactation. Dietary vitamin intakes in our population met NAS/NRC standards, i.e. the mean intake was equal to, or greater than, the RDA, except for vitamin B_6

(mean intake ca 55% of RDA) and vitamin D (mean intake ca 30% of RDA) (table II). Unfortunately, we were not able to calculate folacin intakes from the dietary histories, but in comparable studies folacin intake is regularly found to be below recommendations (see page 99). Although the mean plasma PLP level at 6 weeks postpartum was slightly higher than that at week 16 of pregnancy, the relatively high incidence of abnormal values (25%) after delivery might indicate that for a considerable number of women vitamin B_6 stores were marginal, and that, on the average, a dietary intake of 1.4 mg/day is at least insufficient to replenish maternal stores. The existence of marginal stores before conception cannot be excluded and may have augmented the pregnancy-induced changes. Long-term use of hormonal contraceptives before conception has been reported to affect vitamin B_6 and folacin blood levels during pregnancy [108, 155].

Although the vitamin absorption from the diet of pregnant and non-pregnant women does not seem to differ, the urinary vitamin B excretion is generally lower during pregnancy, except for folacin (page 111). This increase in vitamin retention occurs already early in pregnancy when foetal needs are relatively small.

Based on experimental studies in energy and protein metabolism, Naismith [156] developed the concept of an anabolic and catabolic phase in maternal metabolism. During the first half of pregnancy, the anabolic phase, 'extra' energy and protein is stored, which is again mobilized during the second half (and during lactation), the catabolic phase. The change-over from an anabolic to a catabolic state is under hormonal control. The question is whether this concept has relevance to vitamin metabolism and requirements. The role of the placenta and the extravascular compartment as a temporary vitamin depot deserves further consideration. The different trends between vitamin serum/plasma levels and parameters reflecting vitamin tissue stores may indicate a redistribution between the cellular and extracellular compartments during pregnancy.

Recommendations aiming at biochemical normality for nearly all members of the pregnant population as the ultimate goal are therefore questionable, and probably too high, at least higher than those aiming at the prevention of specific pathology.

The most desirable approach would be relating vitamin requirements to functional criteria of both foetal and maternal health [2]. However, there are as yet no, or hardly any, validated functional criteria available to evaluate the vitamin status.

For the time being it seems that WHO and/or NAS/NRC recommendations, if applied in the right way, and keeping in mind the limitations of the RDA concept, are the 'best guess' considering the available knowledge.

References

1 Sandstead, H.H.: Methods for determining nutrient requirements in pregnancy. Am. J. clin. Nutr. *34:* 697–704 (1981).

2 Beaton, G.H.: Nutritional needs of the pregnant and lactating mother; in Hambraeus, Sjölin, The mother/child dyad-nutritional aspects. Symp. Swedish Nutrition Foundation XIV, pp. 26–34 (Almqvist & Wiksell, Stockholm 1979).

3 WHO: Handbook on human nutritional requirements. Monogr. Ser., No. 61 (WHO, Genève 1974).

4 National Academy of Sciences – National Research Council: Committee on Dietary Allowances of the Food and Nutrition Board; 9th rev. ed. (National Academy of Sciences, Washington 1980).

5 Department of Health and Social Security: Recommended daily intakes of energy and nutrients for the UK Rep. Publ. Hlth Med., No. 120 (DHSS, London 1969).

6 Rosso, P.; Cramoy, C.: Nutrition and pregnancy; in Alfin-Slater, Kritchevsky, Human nutrition. A comprehensive treatise. I. Nutrition, pre- and postnatal development, pp. 133–227 (Plenum Press, New York 1980).

7 Hytten, F.E.; Leitch, J.: The physiology of human pregnancy (Blackwell, Oxford 1971).

8 Hegsted, D.M.: Balance studies. J. Nutr. *106:* 307–311 (1976).

9 Dempsey, W.B.: Vitamin B_6 and pregnancy; in Human vitamin B_6 requirements, pp. 202–209 (Natn. Academy of Science, Washington 1978).

10 Bates, C.J.; Prentice, A.M.; Paul, A.A.; Sutcliffe, B.A.; Watkinson, M.; Whitehead, R.G.: Riboflavin status in Gambian pregnant and lactating women and its implications for recommended dietary allowances. Am. J. clin. Nutr. *34:* 928–935 (1981).

11 Bates, C.J.; Prentice, A.M.; Prentice, A.; Lamb, W.H.; Whitehead, R.G.: The effect of vitamin C supplementation on lactating women in Keneba, a West African rural community. Int. J. Vitam. Nutr. Res. *53:* 68–76 (1983).

12 Report by Committee 1/5 of the International Union of Nutritional Sciences (IUNS): Recommended dietary intakes around the world. Nutr. Abstr. Rev. *53:* 940–1015 (1983).

13 Gräfe, H.K.: Aktueller Beitrag zur Schwangeren-Ernährung. 1. Bericht über die Ernährungsbefunde von 89 Frauen im 5. Monat der Schwangerschaft. 2. Bericht über die Ernährungsbefunde von 89 Frauen im 8. Monat der Schwangerschaft. Dt. GesundhWes. *16:* 461–468, 813–821, 845–850 (1961).

14 Lunell, N.O.; Persson, B.; Sterky, G.: Dietary habits during pregnancy. Acta obstet. gynec. scand. *48:* 187–194 (1969).

15 Smithells, R.W.; Ankers, C.; Carver, M.E.; Lennon, D.; Schorah, C.J.; Sheppard, S.: Maternal nutrition in early pregnancy. Br. J. Nutr. *38:* 497–506 (1977).

16 Darke, S.J.; Disselduff, M.M.; Try, G.P.: Frequency distributions of mean daily

intakes of food energy and selected nutrients obtained during nutrition surveys of different groups of people in Great Britain between 1968 and 1971. Br. J. Nutr. *44:* 243–252 (1980).
17 Doyle, W.; Crawford, M.A.; Laurance, B.M.; Drury, P.: Dietary survey during pregnancy in a low socio-economic group. Human Nutr. appl. Nutr. *36A:* 95–106 (1982).
18 Papoz, L.; Eschwege, E.; Pequignot, G.; Barnat, J.: Dietary behaviour during pregnancy; in Dobbing, Maternal nutrition during pregnancy, pp. 41–69 (Academic Press, London 1981).
19 Van den Berg, H.; Bruinse, H.W.: On the role of nutrition in normal human pregnancy; thesis, Utrecht (1983).
20 Bates, C.J.; Phillipsen, D.R.: Folic acid – established facts and new horizons. BNF Nutr. Bull. *38:* 81–92 (1983).
21 Elsborg, L.; Rosenquist, A.: Folate intake by teenage girls and by pregnant women. Int. J. Vitam. Nutr. Res. *49:* 70–76 (1979).
22 Vir, S.C.; Love, A.H.G.; Thompson, W.: Vitamin B_6 status during pregnancy. Int. J. Vitam. Nutr. Res. *50:* 403–411 (1980).
23 Fraser, D.R.: The physiological economy of vitamin D. Lancet *i:* 969–972 (1983).
24 Takahashi, Y.I.; Smith, J.E.; Goodman, D.S.: Vitamin A and retinol binding protein metabolism during fetal development in the rat. Am. J. Physiol. *233:* 63–72 (1977).
25 Montreewasuwat, N.; Olson, J.A.: Serum and liver concentrations of vitamin A in Thai fetuses as a function of gestational age. Am. J. clin. Nutr. *32:* 601–606 (1979).
26 Iyenger, L.; Apte, S.V.: Nutrient stores in human foetal livers. Br. J. Nutr. *27:* 313–317 (1973).
27 Gal, I.; Sharman, I.; Pryse-Davies, J.: Vitamin A in relation to human congenital malformations. Adv. Teratol. *5:* 143 (1972).
28 Rutishauser, I.H.E.: Vitamin A. J. Food Nutr. *42:* 2 (1986).
29 Rodriguez, M.S.; Irwin, M.I.: A conspectus of research on vitamin A requirements of man. J. Nutr. *102:* 909–968 (1972).
30 Underwood, B.A.; Loerch, J.D.; Lewis, K.C.: Effects of dietary vitamin A deficiency; retinoic acid and protein quantity and quality on serially obtained plasma and liver levels of vitamin A in rats. J. Nutr. *109:* 796–806 (1979).
31 Gal, I.; Parkinson, C.E.: Effects of nutrition and other factors on pregnant women's serum vitamin A levels. Am. J. clin. Nutr. *27:* 688–695 (1974).
32 Kübler, W.; Moch, K.J.: Zur Deckung des Vitaminbedarfs in der Schwangerschaft; in Brubacher, Ritzel, Zur Ernährungssituation der Schweizerischen Bevölkerung, pp. 233–241 (Huber, Bern 1975).
33 Metcoff, J.: Association of fetal growth with maternal nutrition; in Falkner, Tanner, Human growth, vol. 1, pp. 415–460 (Plenum Press, New York 1978).
34 Ismadi, S.D.; Olson, J.A.: Vitamin A transport in human fetal blood. Am. J. clin. Nutr. *28:* 967–972 (1975).
35 Weiner, M.: The significance of marginal nutritional deficiency during pregnancy. Nutr. Rep. int. *21:* 653–658 (1980).
36 Basu, S.H.J.; Arulanantham, R.: A study of serum protein and retinol levels in pregnancy and toxaemia of pregnancy in women of low socio-economic status. Indian J. med. Res. *61:* 589–595 (1973).

37 Sharma, S.C.; Bonnar, J.; Dostalova, L.: Comparison of blood levels of vitamin A, β-carotene and vitamin E in abruptio placentae with normal pregnancy. Int. J. Vitam. Nutr. Res. *56:* 3–9 (1986).
38 Bates, C.J.: Vitamin A in pregnancy and lactation. Proc. Nutr. Soc. *42:* 65 (1983).
39 Bouillon, R.; Van Assche, F.A.: Perinatal vitamin D metabolism. Dev. Pharmacol. Ther. *4:* suppl. 1, pp. 38–44 (1982).
40 Weisman, Y.; Harell, A.; Edelstein, S.; David, M.; Spirer, Z.; Colander, A.: 1α,25-Dihydroxyvitamin D_3 and 24,25-dihydroxyvitamin D_3 in vitro synthesis by human decidua and placenta. Nature *282:* 317–319 (1979).
41 Sunaga, S.; Horiuchi, N.; Takchashi, N.; Okuyama, K.; Suda, T.: The site of 1α,25-dihydroxyvitamin D_3 reduction in pregnancy. Biochem. biophys. Res. Commun. *90:* 948–955 (1979).
42 Van den Berg, H.; Boshuis, P.G.; Bruinse, H.W.: Seasonal variation in 25-hydroxy vitamin D serum content during pregnancy. J. Steroid Biochem. *17:* 53 (1982).
43 Reiter, E.O.; Braunstein, G.D.; Vargas, A.; Root, A.W.: Changes in 25-hydroxyvitamin D and 24,25-dihydroxyvitamin D during pregnancy. Am. J. Obstet. Gynec. *135:* 227–229 (1979).
44 Satyanarayana Reddy, G.; Norman, A.W.; Willis, D.M.; Goltzman, D.; Guyda, H.; Solomon, S.; Philips, D.R.; Bishop, J.E.; Mayer, E.M.: Regulation of vitamin D metabolism in normal human pregnancy. J. clin. Endocr. Metab. *56:* 363–370 (1983).
45 Barragry, I.M.; Corless, D.; Auton, J.F.; Carter, N.D.; Long, R.G.; Maxwell, I.D.; Switala, S.: Plasma vitamin-D-binding globulin in vitamin D deficiency, pregnancy and chronic liver disease. Clinica chim. Acta *87:* 359–365 (1978).
46 Hillman, L.; Haddad, J.G.: Human perinatal vitamin D metabolism 1:25-hydroxyvitamin D in maternal and cord blood. J. Pediat. *84:* 742–749 (1974).
47 Bouillon, R.; Van Assche, F.A.; Van Baelen, H.; Heyns, W.; De Moor, P.: Influence of the vitamin-D-binding protein on the serum concentration of 1,25-dihydroxyvitamin D: significance of the free 1,25-dihydroxyvitamin D_3 concentration. J. clin. Invest. *67:* 589–596 (1981).
48 Wieland, P.; Fischer, J.A.; Treeksel, U.; et al.: Perinatal parathyroid hormone, vitamin D metabolites and calcitonin in man. Am. J. Physiol. *239:* E385–E390 (1980).
49 Markestad, T.; Aksnes, L.; Ulstein, M.; Aarskog, D.: 25-Hydroxyvitamin D and 1,25-dihydroxyvitamin D of D_2 and D_3 origin in maternal and umbilical cord serum after vitamin D_2 supplementation in human pregnancy. Am. J. clin. Nutr. *40:* 1057–1063 (1984).
50 Purvis, R.J.; MacKay, G.S.; Cockburn, F.; Barry, W.J.; Forfer, J.O.: Enamel hypoplasia of the teeth associated with neonatal tetany. A manifestation of maternal vitamin D deficiency. Lancet *ii:* 811–814 (1973).
51 Rosen, J.; Roginsky, M.; Nathenson, G.; Finberg, L.: 25-Hydroxyvitamin D. Plasma levels in mothers and their premature infants with neonatal hypocalcemia. Am. J. Dis. Child. *127:* 220 (1974).
52 Takahashi, Y.; Shitara, H.; Uruno, K.; Kimura, S.: Vitamin E and lipoprotein levels in the sera of pregnant women. J. Nutr. Sci. Vitam. *24:* 471–476 (1978).
53 Jagadeesan, V.; Prema, K.: Plasma tocopherol and lipid levels in pregnancy and oral contraceptive users. Br. J. Obstet. Gynaec. *87:* 903–907 (1980).

54 Baker, H.; Frank, O.; Thompson, A.D.; Langer, A.; Munves, A.D.; Angelis, B. de; Kaminetzky, H.A.: Vitamin profile of 174 mothers and newborns at parturition. Am. J. clin. Nutr. *28:* 59–65 (1975).
55 Horwitt, M.K.; Harvey, C.C.; Dahm, C.H.; Searcy, M.T.: Relationship between tocopherol and serum lipid levels for determination of nutritional adequacy. Ann. N.Y. Acad. Sci. *203:* 223–236 (1972).
56 Haga, P.; Lunde, G.: Selenium and vitamin E in cord blood from preterm and full-term infants. Acta paediat. scand. *67:* 735–739 (1978).
57 Jagadeesan, V.; Prema, K.: Plasma tocopherol and lipid levels in mother and umbilical cord; influence on birth weight. Br. J. Obstet. Gynaec. *87:* 908–910 (1980).
58 Vobecky, J.S.; Vobecky, J.; Shapcott, D.; Blanchard, R.; La Fond, R.; Cloutier, D.; Munnan, L.: Serum α-tocopherol in pregnancies with normal or pathological outcomes. Can. J. Physiol. Pharmacol. *52:* 384–388 (1974).
59 Fomon, S.J.: Vitamin K deficiency in infancy. Proc. Int. Symp. on Vitamins and Minerals in Pregnancy and Lactation, Innsbruck 1986. Nestlé Nutrition Workshop Ser. (in press).
60 Kries, R. van; Maase, B.; Becker, A.; Göbel, U.: Latent vitamin K deficiency in healthy infants? Lancet *ii:* 1421–1422 (1985).
61 Shearer, M.J.; Barkhan, P.; Rahim, S.; Stimmler, L.: Plasma vitamin K_1 in mothers and their newborn babies. Lancet *ii:* 460–463 (1982).
62 Darby, W.J.; McGanity, W.J.; Martin, M.P.; et al.: The Vanderbilt cooperative study of maternal and infant nutrition. IV. Dietary, laboratory and physical findings in 2,129 delivered pregnancies. J. Nutr. *51:* 565–597 (1953).
63 Van den Berg, H.; Schreurs, W.H.P.; Joosten, G.P.A.: Evaluation of the vitamin status in pregnancy. Int. J. Vitam. Nutr. Res. *48:* 12–21 (1978).
64 Heller, S.; Salkeld, R.M.; Körner, W.F.: Vitamin B_1 status in pregnancy. Am. J. clin. Nutr. *27:* 1221–1224 (1974).
65 Vir, S.C.; Love, A.H.G.; Thompson, W.: Thiamin status during pregnancy. Int. J. Vitam. Nutr. Res. *50:* 131–140 (1980).
66 Dirige, O.V.; Jacob, M.; Ostergard, N.; Hunt, J.: Apoenzyme activities of erythrocyte transketolase, glutathione reductase, and glutamic-pyruvic transaminase during pregnancy. Am. J. clin. Nutr. *31:* 202–205 (1978).
67 Dostalova, D.: Correlation of the vitamin status between mother and newborn during delivery. Dev. Pharmacol. Ther. *4:* suppl. 1, pp. 45–57 (1982).
68 Ramsay, V.P.; Neumann, C.; Clark, V.; Swenseid, M.E.: Vitamin cofactor saturation indices for riboflavin, thiamin, and pyridoxine in placental tissue of Kenyan women. Am. J. clin. Nutr. *37:* 969–973 (1983).
69 Endtz, J.: Hyperemesis gravidarum: Een ziektebeeld met complicaties. Ned. Tijdschr. Geneesk. *114:* 890–891 (1970).
70 Chaudhuri, S.K.: Nutrition and toxemia of pregnancy. Am. J. Obstet. Gynec. *110:* 46–48 (1971).
71 Brzezinsky, A.; Bromberg, Y.M.; Braun, K.: Riboflavin excretion during pregnancy and early lactation. J. Lab. clin. Med. *39:* 84–90 (1952).
72 Clarke, H.C.: Relationship between whole blood riboflavin levels and results of riboflavin stimulation tests in normal and pathological conditions in man. Int. J. Vitam. Nutr. Res. *39:* 238–245 (1969).
73 Knobloch, E.; Hodr, R.; Janda, J.; Herzmann, J.; Houdkova, V.: Spectrofluorimetric

micromethod for determining riboflavin in the blood of newborn babies and their mothers. Int. J. Vitam. Nutr. Res. *49:* 144–151 (1979).
74 Clarke, H.C.: Relationship between whole blood riboflavin levels in the mother and in the prenate. Am. J. Obstet. Gynec. *111:* 43–46 (1971).
75 Munro, H.N.: The placenta in nutrition. Annu. Rev. Nutr. *3:* 97–124 (1983).
76 Lust, J.E.; Hagerman, D.D.; Villee, C.A.: The transport of riboflavin by human placenta. J. clin. Invest. *33:* 38–40 (1954).
77 Kaminetzky, H.A.; Baker, H.; Frank, O.; Langer, A.: The effect of intravenously administered water-soluble vitamins during labor in normovitaminemic and hypovitaminemic gravidas on maternal and neonatal blood vitamin levels at delivery. Am. J. Obstet. Gynec. *120:* 697–703 (1974).
78 Merrill, A.H.; Froehlich, J.A.; McCormick, D.B.: Purification of riboflavin-binding proteins from bovine plasma and discovery of a pregnancy-specific riboflavin binding protein. J. biol. Chem. *254:* 9362–9364 (1979).
79 Heller, S.; Salkeld, R.M.; Körner, W.F.: Riboflavin status in pregnancy. Am. J. clin. Nutr. *27:* 1225–1230 (1974).
80 Vir, S.C.; Love, A.H.G.; Thompson, W.: Riboflavin status during pregnancy. Am. J. clin. Nutr. *34:* 2699–2705 (1981).
81 Ramachandran, M.; Iyer, G.Y.N.: Erythrocyte glutathione reductase in iron deficiency anaemia. Clinica Chim. Acta. *52:* 225–229 (1974).
82 Decker, K.; Dotis, B.; Glatzle, D.; Hinselmann, M.: Riboflavin status and anaemia in pregnant women. Nutr. Metab. *21:* suppl. 1, pp. 17–19 (1977).
83 Bamji, M.S.: Enzymic evaluation of thiamin, riboflavin and pyridoxine status of parturient women and their newborn infants. Br. J. Nutr. *35:* 259–265 (1976).
84 Shane, B.; Contracter, S.F.: Assessment of vitamin B_6 status. Studies on pregnant women and oral contraceptive users. Am. J. clin. Nutr. *28:* 739–747 (1975).
85 Hamfelt, A.; Tuvemo, T.: Pyridoxal phosphate and folic acid concentration in blood and erythrocyte aspartate amino-transferase activity during pregnancy. Clinica chim. Acta *41:* 287–298 (1972).
86 Cleary, R.E.; Lumeng, L.; Li, T.K.: Maternal and fetal plasma levels of pyridoxal phosphate at term: adequacy of vitamin B_6 supplementation during pregnancy. Am. J. Obstet. Gynec. *121:* 25–28 (1975).
87 Lumeng, L.; Cleary, R.E.; Wagner, R.; Yu, P.L.; Li, T.K.: Adequacy of vitamin B_6 supplementation during pregnancy: a prospective study. Am. J. clin. Nutr. *29:* 1376–1383 (1976).
88 Wachstein, M.: Evidence for a relative vitamin B_6 deficiency in pregnancy and some disease states. Vitams Horm. *22:* 705–719 (1964).
89 Leklem, J.E.; Rose, D.P.; Linksweiler, H.N.: Vitamin B_6 requirements of women using oral contraceptives. Am. J. clin. Nutr. *28:* 535–541 (1975).
90 Bender, D.A.; Wynick, D.: Inhibition of kynureninase by oestrone sulphate: an alternative explanation for abnormal results of tryptophan load tests in women receiving oestrogenic steroids. Br. J. Nutr. *45:* 269–275 (1981).
91 Contractor, S.F.; Shane, B.: Blood and urine levels of vitamin B_6 in the mother and fetus before and after loading of the mother with vitamin B_6. Am. J. Obstet. Gynec. *107:* 635–640 (1970).
92 Heller, S.; Salkeld, R.M.; Körner, W.F.: Vitamin B_6 status in pregnancy. Am. J. clin. Nutr. *26:* 1339–1348 (1973).

93 Rose, D.P.: Oral contraceptives and vitamin B_6; in Human vitamin B_6 requirements, pp. 193–201 (Natn. Academy of Science, Washington 1978).
94 Martner-Hewes, P.M.; Hunt, I.F.; Murphy, N.J.; Swendseid, M.E.; Settlage, R.H.: Vitamin B_6 nutriture and plasma diamine oxidase activity in pregnant Hispanic teenagers. Am. J. clin. Nutr. *44:* 907–913 (1986).
95 Southern, A.L.; Kobayashi, A.L.; Weingold, A.B.; Carmody, N.C.: Serial plasma diamine oxidase (DAO) assays in first- and second trimester complications of pregnancy. Am. J. Obstet Gynec. *96:* 502–510 (1968).
96 Shane, B.; Contractor, S.F.: Vitamin B_6 status and metabolism in pregnancy; in Tryfiates, Vitamin B_6 metabolism and role in growth, pp. 137–171 (Food & Nutrition Press, Westport 1980).
97 Klieger, J.A.; Altshuler, C.H.; Krakow, G.; Hollister, C.: Abnormal pyridoxine metabolism in toxemia of pregnancy. Ann. N.Y. Acad. Sci. *166:* 288–296 (1969).
98 Brophy, M.H.; Siiteri, P.K.: Pyridoxal phosphate and hypertensive disorders of pregnancy. Am. J. Obstet. Gynec. *121:* 1075–1079 (1975).
99 Gaynor, R.; Dempsey, W.B.: Vitamin B_6 enzymes in normal and preeclamptic human placentae. Clinica chim. Acta *37:* 411–416 (1972).
100 Willis, R.S.; Winn, W.W.; Morris, A.T.; Newson, A.A.; Massay, W.E.: Clinical observations in treatment of nausea and vomiting in pregnancy with vitamin B and B_6. Am. J. Obstet. Gynec. *44:* 265–271 (1942).
101 Reinken, L.; Gant, H.: Vitamin B_6 nutrition in women with hyperemesis gravidarum during the first trimester of pregnancy. Clinica chim. Acta *55:* 101–102 (1974).
102 Pulkkinen, M.O.; Salminen, J.; Virtanen, S.: Serum vitamin B_6 in pure pregnancy depression. Acta obstet. gynec. scand. *57:* 471–472 (1978).
103 Coelingh Bennink, H.J.T.; Schreurs, W.H.P.: Improvement of oral glucose tolerance in gestational diabetes by pyridoxine. Br. med. J. *iii:* 13–15 (1975).
104 Gahl, W.A.; Raubertas, F.; Vale, A.M.; Golubjatnikow, R.: Maternal serum diamine oxidase in fetal death and low birth-weight infants. Br. J. Obstet. Gynaec. *89:* 202–207 (1982).
105 Baker, H.; Thind, I.S.; Frank, O.; Angelis, B. de; Caterini, H.; Louria, D.B.: Vitamin levels in low-birth weight newborn infants and their mothers. Am. J. Obstet. Gynec. *129:* 521–524 (1977).
106 Reinken, L.; Dapunt, O.: Vitamin B_6 nutrition during pregnancy. Int. J. Vitam. Nutr. Res. *48:* 341–347 (1978).
107 Roepke, J.L.B.; Kirksey, A.: Vitamin B_6 nutriture during pregnancy and lactation. I. Vitamin B_6 intake, levels of the vitamin in biological fluids and condition of the infant at birth. Am. J. clin. Nutr. *32:* 2249–2256 (1979).
108 Roepke, J.L.B.; Kirksey, A.: Vitamin B_6 nutriture during pregnancy and lactation. II. The effect of long-term use of oral contraceptives. Am. J. clin. Nutr. *32:* 2257–2264 (1979).
109 Schuster, K.; Bailey, L.B.; Mahan, C.S.: Effect of maternal pyridoxine HCL supplementation on the vitamin B_6 status of mother and infant and on pregnancy outcome. J. Nutr. *114:* 977–988 (1984).
110 Hillmann, R.W.; Cabard, P.G.; Nilsson, D.E.; Arpin, P.D.; Tufano, R.J.: Pyridoxine supplementation during pregnancy: clinical and laboratory observations. Am. J. clin. Nutr. *12:* 427–430 (1963).

111 Hemminki, E.; Starfield, B.: Routine administration of iron and vitamines during pregnancy: review of controlled clinical trials. Br. J. Obstet. Gynaec. *85:* 404–410 (1978).
112 Okuda, K.; Helliger, A.E.; Chow, B.P.: Vitamin B_{12} serum level and pregnancy. Am. J. clin. Nutr. *4:* 441–443 (1956).
113 Chanarin, I.: The megaloblastic anemias (Blackwell, Oxford 1969).
114 Metz, J.; Festenstein, H.; Welch, P.: Effect of folic acid and vitamin B_{12} supplementation on tests of folate and vitamin B_{12} nutrition in pregnancy. Am. J. clin. Nutr. *16:* 472–479 (1965).
115 Kalameghan, R.; Krishnswamy, K.: Functional significance of low serum vitamin B_{12} levels in pregnancy. Int. J. Vitam. Nutr. Res. *47:* 52–69 (1977).
116 Fernandez-Costa, F.; Metz, J.: Levels of transcobalamins I, II and III during pregnancy and in cord blood. Am. J. clin. Nutr. *35:* 87–94 (1982).
117 Luhbi, A.L.; Cooperman, J.M.; Stone, M.L.; Slobody, B.: Physiology of vitamin B_{12} in pregnancy, the placenta and the newborn. Am. J. Dis. Child. *102:* 753–754 (1961).
118 Giugliani, E.R.J.; Jorge, S.M.; Gonçalves, A.L.: Serum vitamin B_{12} levels in parturients, in the intervillous space of the placenta and in full-term newborns and their interrelationships with folate levels. Am. J. clin. Nutr. *41:* 330–335 (1985).
119 Schorah, C.J.; Smithells, R.W.; Scott, J.: Vitamin B_{12} and anencephaly. Lancet *i:* 880 (1980).
120 Higginbottom, M.C.; Sweetman, L.; Nyhan, W.L.: A syndrome of methylmalonic aciduria, homocystinuria, megaloblastic anemia and neurologic abnormalities in a vitamin B_{12}-deficient breast-fed infant of a strict vegetarian. New Engl. J. Med. *299:* 317–323 (1978).
121 Rodriguez, M.S.: A conspectus of research on folacin requirements of man. J. Nutr. *108:* 1983–2103 (1978).
122 Hall, M.H.; Pirani, B.B.K.; Campbell, D.: The cause of the fall in serum folate in normal pregnancy. Br. J. Obstet. Gynaec. *83:* 132–136 (1976).
123 Fleming, A.F.: Urinary excretion of folate in pregnancy. J. Obstet. Gynaec. Br. Commonw. *79:* 916–928 (1972).
124 Bruinse, H.W.; Berg, H. van den; Haspels, A.A.: Maternal serum folacin levels during and after normal pregnancy. Eur. J. Obstet. Gynec. Reprod. Biol. *20:* 153–158 (1985).
125 Landon, M.J.; Hytten, F.E.: Plasma folate levels following an oral load of folic acid during pregnancy. J. Obstet. Gynaec. Br. Commonw. *79:* 577–583 (1972).
126 Davis, M.; Simmons, C.J.; Dordoni, B.; Maxwell, J.D.: Induction of hepatic enzymes during normal human pregnancy. J. Obstet. Gynaec. Br. Commonw. *82:* 374–381 (1975).
127 Da Costa, M.; Rothenberg, S.P.: Appearance of a folate binder in leucocytes and serum of women who are pregnant or taking oral contraceptives. J. Lab. clin. Med. *83:* 207–214 (1974).
128 Markkanen, T.; Virtanen, S.; Pajula, R.L.; Himanen, P.: Hormonal dependence of folic acid protein binding in human serum. Int. J. Vitam. Nutr. Res. *44:* 81–94 (1974).
129 Kamen, B.A.; Caston, J.D.: Purification of folate binding factor in normal umibilical cord serum. Proc. natn. Acad. Sci. USA *72:* 4261–4264 (1979).

130 Grossowitz, N.; Izak, G.; Rachmilewitz, M.: Effect of anaemia on the concentration of folate derivatives in paired fetal-maternal blood. Israel J. med. Scis *2:* 510–512 (1966).
131 Vaz Pinto, A.; Torras, V.; Sandoval, J.F.F.: Folic acid and vitamin B_{12} determination in fetal liver. Am. J. clin. Nutr. *28:* 1085–1086 (1975).
132 Rothman, D.: Folic acid in pregnancy. Am. J. Obstet. Gynec. *108:* 149–175 (1970).
133 Gandy, G.; Jacobson, W.: Influence of folic acid on birth weight and growth of the eryblastotic infant I. Birth weight. Archs Dis. Childh. *52:* 1–6 (1977).
134 Rolschau, J.; Date, J.; Kristoffersen, K.: Folic acid supplement and intrauterine growth. Acta obstet. gynec. scand. *58:* 343–346 (1979).
135 Kristoffersen, K.; Rolschau, J.: Vitamin supplements and intrauterine growth; in Briggs, Recent vitamin research, pp. 84–101 (CRC Press, Boca Raton 1984).
136 Smithells, R.W.; Sheppard, S.; Schorah, C.J.: Vitamin deficiencies and neural tube defects. Archs Dis. Childh. *51:* 944–950 (1976).
137 Smithells, R.W.; Sheppard, S.; Schorah, C.J.: Possible prevention of neural tube defects by preconceptional vitamin supplementation. Lancet *i:* 339–340 (1980).
138 Laurence, K.M.; James, N.; Miller, M.H.J.; Tennant, G.B.; Campbell, H.: Double-blind randomised controlled trial of folate treatment before conception to prevent recurrence of neural-tube defects. Br. med. J. *282:* 1509–1511 (1981).
139 Brabin, B.J.: Hypothesis: the importance of folacin in influencing susceptibility to malaria infection in infants. Am. J. clin. Nutr. *35:* 146–151 (1982).
140 Mason, M.; Rivers, J.M.: Plasma ascorbic acid levels in pregnancy. Am. J. Obstet. Gynec. *1971:* 960–961.
141 Vobecky, J.S.; Vobecky, J.; Shapcott, D.; Munnan, L.: Vitamin C and outcome of pregnancy. Lancet *i:* 630 (1974).
142 Schorah, C.J.; Zemroch, P.J.; Sheppard, S.; Smithells, R.W.: Leucocyte ascorbic acid and pregnancy. Br. J. Nutr. *39:* 139–149 (1978).
143 Toverud, K.U.: The vitamin C need in pregnant and lactating women. Acta paediat. *24:* 332–340 (1939).
144 Irwin, M.J.; Hutchins, B.K.: A conspectus of research on vitamin C requirements of man. J. Nutr. *106:* 821–897 (1976).
145 Streeter, M.L.; Rosso, P.: Transport mechanism for ascorbic acid in the human placenta. Am. J. clin. Nutr. *34:* 1706–1711 (1981).
146 Cohenour, S.H.; Calloway, D.H.: Blood, urine and dietary pantothenic acid levels of pregnant teenagers. Am. J. clin. Nutr. *25:* 512–517 (1972).
147 Srinivasan, V.; Belavady, B.: Nutritional status of pantothenic acid in Indian pregnant and nursing women. Int. J. Vitam. Nutr. Res. *46:* 433–438 (1976).
148 Song, W.O.; Wyse, B.W.; Hansen, R.G.: Pantothenic acid status of pregnant and lactating women. J. Am. diet. Ass. *85:* 192–198 (1985).
149 Bhagavan, H.N.: Biotin content of blood during gestation. Int. J. Vitam. Nutr. Res. *39:* 235–237 (1969).
150 Salmenpera, L.; Perheentupa, J.; Pispa, J.P.; Siimes, M.A.: Biotin concentrations in maternal plasma and milk during prolonged lactation. Int. J. Vitam. Nutr. Res. *55:* 281–285 (1985).
151 Johnson, A.R.; Hood, R.L.; Emery, J.L.: Biotin and the sudden infant death syndrome. Nature *285:* 159–160 (1980).

152 Lammer, E.J.; Chen, D.T.; Hoar, R.M.; et al.: Retinoic acid embryopathy. New Engl. J. Med. *313:* 837–841 (1985).
153 Marks, J.: Vitamin safety. Vitamin information; 3rd rev. ed. Roche (Hoffmann-La Roche, Basel 1986).
154 Bates, C.J.; Prentice, A.M.; Watkinson, M.; Morrell, M.; Foord, F.A.; Watkinson, A.; Cole, T.J.; Whitehead, R.G.: Efficacy of a food supplement in correcting riboflavin deficiency in pregnant Gambian women. Hum. Nutr. Clin. Nutr. *38C:* 363–374 (1984).
155 Martinez, O.; Roe, DA.: Effect of oral contraceptives on blood folate levels in pregnancy. Am. J. Obstet. Gynec. *128:* 255–261 (1977).
156 Naismith, D.J.: Maternal nutrition and the outcome of pregnancy – a critical appraisal. Proc. Nutr. Soc. *39:* 1–11 (1980).
157 Brabin, B.J.; Van den Berg, H.; Nijmeijer, F.: Folacin, cobalamin, and hematological status during pregnancy in rural Kenya: the influence of parity, gestation, and *Plasmodium falciparum* malaria. Am. J. clin. Nutr. *43:* 803–815 (1986).
158 Sharma, S.C.; Walzman, M.; Bonnar, J.; Molloy, A.: Blood ascorbic acid and histamine in patients with placental bleeding. Hum. Nutr. Clin. Nutr. *39C:* 233–238 (1985).
159 Löwenstein, L.; Lalonde, M.; Deschenes, E.B.; Shapiro, L.: Vitamin B_{12} in pregnancy and the puerperium. Am. J. clin. Nutr. *8:* 265–275 (1960).
160 Mino, M.; Hishino, H.: Fetal and maternal relationship in serum vitamin E level. J. Nutr. Sci. Vitaminol. *19:* 475–482 (1973).
161 Wertz, A.W.; Loikin, M.E.; Bouchard, B.S.; Derby, M.B.: Tryptophan-niacin relationships in pregnancy. J. Nutr. *64:* 339–353 (1958).
162 Van den Berg, H.; Van de Zedde, A.; Bruinse, H.W.; Mommersteeg-Flipse, E.: Voeding en zwangerschap: gegevens over de voedselconsumptie van een groep Nederlandse vrouwen tijdens en na de zwangerschap. Voeding *45:* 285–291 (1984).
163 Schuster, K.; Bailey, L.B.; Dimperio, D.; Mahan, C.S.: Morning sickness and vitamin B_6 status of pregnant women. Hum. Nutr. Clin. Nutr. *39C:* 75–79 (1985).

H. van den Berg, MD, TNO-CIVO Toxicology and Nutrition Institute,
P.O. Box 360, 3700 AJ Zeist (The Netherlands)

Wld Rev. Nutr. Diet., vol. 57, pp. 126–213 (Karger, Basel 1988)

Is Our Knowledge of Human Nutrition Soundly Based?

F.B. Shorland[1]

Department of Biochemistry, Victoria University of Wellington, Wellington, New Zealand

Contents

[1] The author would like to acknowledge statistical help by Dr. S.F.L. Gallot of the DSIR Applied Mathematics Division, Wellington, New Zealand.

I. Introduction

In this review 'our knowledge' is taken to mean the information that is available in the scientific literature on human nutrition. To indicate how far that knowledge is soundly based the author has selected a few examples taken from areas with which he is familiar.

It is recognised that our knowledge of human nutrition is limited by the extent to which the human may be subjected to the extremes of dietary change used for animal nutrition experiments. Additionally, it will be shown using historical hindsight, that soundly based experiments on humans have been ignored even at the international level and that at times nutritional decisions have been made without asking for the experimental evidence.

Sources of our knowledge of human nutrition include also news media, lectures, books and popular beliefs. These sources often form a valuable line of communication with the public. They can unfortunately also promote nutritional misinformation. As an example, one may cite the popular books of the late Adelle Davis that rank highly amongst the sources of nutritional information as shown by the sale of more than 10,000,000 copies. Rynearson [1974], in a review entitled 'Americans Love Hogwash', notes that her book 'Get Well' lists 2,402 references to document 34 chapters. The references, she claims, are drawn mainly from studies conducted by doctors, 25% of whom are professors in medical schools. However, as revealed by Rynearson [1974], none of them had, in fact, corresponded with Miss Davis and less than 10% were professors. The references had misquotations and inaccuracies. An example is 'that autopsies reveal that 90% of persons dying with kwashiorkor have lung cancer'. The reference is to Prof. J.F. Bock of Capetown – the foremost worker on the subject. He replied 'I have never met her, nor have I seen her book. The statement is, of course, nonsense'.

It is of course of incidental interest that the above classical contribution by Emeritus Professor Rynearson of the Mayo Clinic and Foundation,

Rochester, Minn., is based on an address delivered at the Scientific Awards Dinner at the meeting of the American Medical Association, New York, on 26 June 1973. However, there is no record of either the author or the title to be found in Biological Abstracts, Chemical Abstracts, or Nutrition Abstracts and Reviews. The impact of misinformation may thus be much greater than that of a valuable contribution.

The scientific literature on human nutrition is made up of: (1) investigations using humans as experimental subjects; (2) experiments using animals as models for human nutrition, and (3) epidemiological investigations. Obviously, of the three methods listed the most soundly based would be those using humans but for a variety of reasons this may not be feasible. For ethical reasons, for example, the experiment must not endanger health. Thus, information relating to the effects of extreme deprivation has to be gleaned from wartime situations or other adverse circumstances as may occur in polar exploration. Nevertheless, there have been many useful experiments on humans but as will be described in section IV some of these have been ignored by present-day workers. On the other hand, other information for which there is no basis, such as Voit's contention during the previous century that the working man required 340 g beef daily to replace the protein lost during muscular exertion, has not been entirely discarded even to this day.

Concerning the use of animals, especially rats, as models for exploring human nutritional needs, there are indisputable advantages in terms of relatively rapid evaluation and the freedom to impose extreme conditions. As indicated in the section II, dealing with the evolution of human diets, McCarrison [1944] gained insights into the nutritional value of the national diets in India by means of rats which gave increased confidence that the marked differences between the performance, health and physical appearance of the different races were diet related. However, as described in section IV, Mendel's [1923] investigations showing that wheat protein would not support the growth of weanling rats has been interpreted by nutritionists wrongly as applying also to humans, despite the experimental evidence to the contrary. Textbooks on nutrition, such as Orten and Neuhaus [1975], continue to emphasise the need for first-class animal protein as distinct from second-class plant protein. There is therefore a need to realise that in using the rat as a model for human nutrition the response of the rat to a nutrient may differ qualitatively from that of the human, or as in the case of vitamin C the response may be absent.

Because of the incomplete answers to human nutrition offered in many instances, by the limitations of direct experimentation on humans and by the use of animal models, one may be forced to have recourse to epidemiology. Here one may take two populations with similar nutritional, environmental and genetic characteristics but which differ, for example, in one particular aspect, such as salt intake, which can then be related to a physiological difference, such as hypertension.

The epidemiological evidence can be suggestive rather than offering a final answer which may need to be sought by appropriately designed experiments. The build-up of evidence on the causation of coronary heart disease (CHD) is largely a case of an interweaving of epidemiology and experimentation.

Epidemiology has the advantage of providing long-term predictions from experimental work which, because of the 70-year life cycle of the human, would prove too costly to carry out for such a prolonged period.

In this review following the introduction (section I), the remaining sections (II–VII) have been assigned to evolution of the human diet and its implications, recommended daily dietary allowances, the protein requirement saga, CHD and nutrition, other nutritional considerations and concluding remarks.

It was felt that the evolution of the human diet and its implications, especially the fact that the composition of today's diets includes a wide range of food components, should be first considered. This range includes the diet of the Eskimos which in the natural state is made up almost entirely of animal protein and fat derived from the flesh of mammals and fish through to the almost completely vegetarian diets. Such diets may be largely based on rice or other cereals. In other cases, cereals are absent and the plant food may comprise largely sweet potatoes or other root crops. In some instances coconuts are the basis of mainly vegetarian diets. The fact that great variations in food composition provide the means of apparently adequate sustenance poses nutritional questions and provides a challenge alike to dietary theories, such as the dietary fibre theory of Burkitt and Trowell [1975], as well as to the dietary goals provided by many developed countries.

In the USA, the National Research Council's [1980] Recommended Dietary Allowances (RDA); have already come under scrutiny. It is now self-evident that our knowledge of human nutrition is not soundly enough based to meet the challenges of those who point out deficiencies of the RDA.

In the remaining sections, it is similarly shown that our knowledge of human nutrition will need to be expanded before it can be deemed to be soundly based. This assertion, however, does not detract from the advances made, often in the face of serious experimental odds, or that the problems now faced cannot be solved in the future. It is equally important that the knowledge so gained is applied. That this does not happen to the extent that is desired is obvious to all who study human nutrition. The national and international organisations dealing with food production are generally concerned with the sale and the short-term safety of their products rather than with the long-term health effects.

II. Evolution of the Human Diet and Its Implications

To understand the pattern of the human diet of today and the development of some of the distortions which some have related to the occurrence of the Western type diseases, it is necessary to consider, albeit briefly, the course of its evolution. For this purpose the author has drawn from *Food in History* by Tannahill [1975].

With this background the author has taken the FAO [1971] Food Balance Sheets to calculate the relative contributions of the food components expressed as a percentage intake of the total calories in selected countries. Such a procedure does not take into account individual variations but provides nonetheless an indication of the general levels of the food items consumed in today's diet.

The Prehistory Diet

It appears that in the course of transformation of ape to man the shortage of nestlings and fruit drove him from his habitat in the trees to forage on the grasslands for lizards, porcupines, tortoises, ground squirrels, moles, plump insects and grubs. The extent to which this theory was selectively applied to such apes is not explained.

During the next three million years he learnt how to kill larger animals. Speech developed. His forefeet became hands with which he made tools. About half a million years ago with the icy climatic conditions Australopithecus became *Homo erectus,* more man than ape. The cave evidence indicates from the bone remains that venison made up about 70% of his diet with the addition of tiger, buffalo, and the rhinoceros. After the disappearance of *Homo erectus* or Neanderthal man, about 30,000 BC there came a more advanced breed *Homo sapiens.* Bone and horn were used to make new lightweight hunting weapons, fishing hooks and needles to sew up fitted garments.

It is important to realise that in the course of domestication of animals for meat production the selection of pigs, sheep and cattle in recent times has involved breeding programmes to increase the rate of growth and with it the level of fat in the carcase. The composition of meat has been thus greatly modified: the fat in such animals exceeding several times that of the protein. Even the dissected muscle tissues from the leanest joints, such as a leg of lamb, contain 3.2–8.0% fat (average 5.7%) [Barnicoat and Shorland, 1952].

In contrast, animals in their natural state are relatively lean and therefore the meat is mainly protein. As described by Eaton and Connor [1985] in the hunting society of our palaeolithic ancestors, meat provided a large fraction of each day's food ensuring high iron and folate levels. At that stage aquatic food sources were little used as evidenced by the general absence of shells and fish bones. Protein contributed twice to nearly five times the proportion of total calories that it does for Americans today. Not only is there more fat in domesticated animals than in free-living herbivores, but its composition is different. Wild game fat contains over five times more polyunsaturated fatty acids (PUFA) than the fat of domestic livestock. Furthermore, the fat of wild animals contains approximately 4% of eicosapentaenoic acid currently under investigation because of its apparent anti-atherogenic properties. Domestic beef contains almost undetectable amounts of this nutrient [Crawford et al., 1969].

Compared with the recommendations of the US Select Senate Committee on Nutrition and Human Needs [Eckholm and Record, 1977] involving a reduction for fat consumption from 40 to 30% of the total calories, the palaeolithic human would have had much less fat. As stated above, such fat would have contained much more PUFA than would be the case in our meat of today. The fatty material of the meat of the palaeolithic human would have been made up largely of structural lipids, especially phospholipids, rich in polyunsaturated C_{20} and C_{22} acids with low levels of depot fat.

The extent to which fatty components of today's meat are responsible for the chronic diseases of our industrialised society is still open to debate, but medical research is beginning to define a generally preventive diet against conditions ranging from atherosclerosis to cancer.

About 11,000 BC the ice began to retreat and with the warm winds great fields of wild grain appeared in the Near East. There followed with the aid of irrigation the deliberate culture of plants and the domestication of animals, including sheep, cattle and pigs. Food had already played its part in making man, now it was to make history, and never more decisively than in the millenia between 10,000 and 3,000 BC. There appeared villages and then towns followed by cities made possible by the agricultural revolution.

The early grain cooking involved separation of seeds assisted by heating. This was followed by grinding between stones or in a mortar. The resulting unleavened flour was mixed with a little water, made into a paste and apparently cooked on a heated stone.

Food of Egypt, Greece and Rome

In Egypt knowledge of fermentation became available but the precise date and evidence is elusive. With this knowledge the production of beer and leavened bread occurred. However, the demanding process of making leavened bread required a particular type of grain which meant that such bread was not commonly available until many centuries later.

Bread, beer and onions formed the basic diet of the peasant in dynastic Egypt. By the 12th century BC there were bread stalls in the villages selling the commonist type of flat bread. However, the priests and nobles could choose as many as 40 types of breads and pastries. The available food is indicated from a tomb dated third millenium BC which contained dishes of barley porridge, cooked quail, kidneys, pigeon stew, fish, beef ribs, wheaten bread, cakes, stewed figs, fresh berries, cheese, wine and beer enough food to keep the deceased going until she reached the other world.

In classical Greece the peasant ate not only barley pastes but also barley gruel and barley bread with the addition of a handful of olives and a few figs or some goat's milk. Occasionally, there would be a salt fish as a relish. Meat was a rarity for the poor but accessible to the rich.

The basic diet of the Roman poor comprised grain pastes or coarse bread bristling with chaff and a polenta-like porridge made from millet. Sometimes the poor would buy a slice of roast pork or more often they ate olives, raw beans, figs or cheese. The food of the rich was very different; it could include ample meat made up from pork or kid with a variety of birds, fish, pickles from Spain, ham from Gaul, oysters from Britain and much else. The city of Rome had first call on wheat of Egypt, North Africa and Sicily. There was the policy of free grain for the poor which in the days of Augustus involved 320,000 people or one third of the population of Rome.

Food in Medieval Europe

The expansion of Europe prior to the Middle Ages was dependent on the mouldboard plough which took the heavy clay soil of the north in its stride. The alternation of crops and the laying aside of fallow land produced not only more but also better food. There followed also the development of the markets in the towns and cities. Nevertheless, the medieval table of Europe, especially in the north, had to cope with long periods when no fresh meat or fish were available. Winter fodder made up of beans, dried plant stems, chaff and straw was sufficient to keep alive only the young and the strong animals. At the end of the year, beef, pork, game and fresh-water fish were salted down. In the salt fish trade, herrings in the 14th and 15th centuries were the most important items. The second major process for preservation was drying; this was used more often in Europe for meat than for fish.

Medieval menus for the poor in Europe in the 14th century consisted of dark bread made from rye, barley or maslin – sometimes with pea or bean flour mixed in with some cheese or curds to round the meal off. As typical the meals of the rich were much more sumptuous as identified in a company dinner with large number of dishes placed on the table at the same time. The meals would contain meat and fish dishes in abundance not to mention frumenty derived from whole wheat soaked in warm water at the side of the fire. After some hours the preparation swells and gelatinises into a delicious kind of aspic.

The Expanding World

In the period of the expanding world (1490–1800), Venice alone brought back to Europe 2,500 tons of pepper and ginger a year and almost as much again of other spices. The discovery of the New World did not achieve, as expected, more of the traditional spices but instead a number of new foodstuffs of great importance were made available. Indian corn became the staple food of Northern Spain, Portugal and Italy and later the Balkans. Potatoes became a useful source of vitamin C to many peoples. Chocolate, peanuts, vanilla, the tomato, pineapple, French beans, runner beans, the scarlet runner, red peppers, green peppers, tapioca all widened the cuisine of Europe, Asia and Africa. Australasia benefited from all other parts of the world. Sugar and the slave trade became interdependent soon after the discovery of the New World.

The evolution of a greatly diversified diet was not accompanied by a corresponding understanding of even the rudiments of good nutrition. The need for food to support life would have been all too apparent but the understanding of the relationship between food and nutritional deficiencies was not developed. Nevertheless, the now well-known *Treatise on Scurvy* published by Lind in 1753 provided a beginning in this direction. In addition, based on Biblical considerations gluttony was recognised as a sin whereas abstemious living as practised by Conaro, the Venetian, who lived to be 103 years was regarded as desirable [Walford, 1983].

The industrial revolution and the increasing population with the growth of new towns and cities thrown up to accommodate factories and associated services was accompanied by malnutrition, associated with scurvy and rickets. In the 1830s and 1840s the worker in Britain might earn anything from 25p to £2 a week. Twenty five pence would buy six four-pound loaves – just enough to feed two adults and three children. The weekly budget would include potatoes along with bread and a little meat as a poverty line diet with tea. The food of the rich remained as good if not better than before being based on access to the markets of the world.

Contemporary Patterns of Food Consumption

The dietary patterns of today's industrialised world evolved mainly during the present century. Wheat, formerly the basis of the nation's food supply diminished in significance. As reviewed by Hollingsworth [1974] during 1880–1972 grain diminished in Britain from 49 to 22% of the total calories with a temporary rise to 37% during World War II. Over the same period dairy products, excluding butter, rose from 8 to 12%, meats 13 to 17%, oils and fats 7 to 18%, sugar 11 to 18%, whereas potato consumption fell from 8 to 5%. Dupin et al. [1984] record that in France the daily bread consumption per person dropped from 600 g in 1880 to 500 g in 1910 declining progressively to 172 g in 1980. From 1925 to 1980 the annual consumption of potatoes per person fell from 178 to 84.5 kg. Similar changes occurred in other industrialised countries in Europe associated with increased consumption of meat, milk products, sugar, oils and fats. In USA wheat and potato consumption per person was in 1909–1913 130 and 93 kg, respectively. But this fell to half by 1965 their place being taken by meat, milk, sugar, oils and fats [Friend, 1967; Leveille, 1975a, b].

The dietary patterns mentioned above are now embodied in many industrialised Western countries (tables I, II). In other countries the displacement of wheat by meat, milk products, oils and fats, and sugar is continuing (tables III, IV). The rate of change thus varies. One of the earliest examples is New Zealand which became a major exporter of meat and milk products at the turn of the century. Parowski and Pachett [1970] assessed the per capita annual intake of wheat and potatoes in New Zealand in 1886–1890 at 163 and 161 kg compared with 97.5 and 54.9 kg, respectively, in 1967–1968. However, the evidence including dietary surveys since 1928 [Davidson and Gilmour, 1969] and FAO Food Balance Sheets shows a virtually unchanged meat, milk dietary pattern suggesting that the change occurred well before 1928.

The changed dietary patterns seem unconnected with any conscious effort to supply nutrients at such levels as to ensure a healthy and active existence over a maximum life span. Nevertheless, now the requirements of vitamins and minerals are known with sufficient accuracy to prevent overt deficiencies. Diets seen as deficient in nutrient levels have been corrected in some instances. Salt has been iodised to combat goitre in deficient areas, and to reduce dental decay in fluoride-deficient areas fluoridation of the water supplies has taken place. The widespread fortification of nutrients in foods, as notably in USA, has mitigated against the occurrence of deficiency diseases. In developed countries considerable progress has also been made in the control of infectious diseases. We are now largely left with the non-infectious Western type diseases including CHD, cancer and stroke as the main causes of death.

It is now widely believed that the Western type diseases are of environmental origin and that nutrition plays a part. Nations accordingly are attempting to provide dietary guidelines. Following the Medical Guidelines on Peoples' Food in the Scandinavian Countries in 1968, policies on national diets have been announced in Canada, FRG, the Netherlands, UK, and Belgium [Clements and Rogers, 1983]. The most discussed of all were the Dietary Goals for the United States [1977] as the culmination of 10 year's work by the US Senate Select Committee on Nutrition and Human Needs [Eckholm and Record, 1977]. This committee recommended a reduction in fat consumption from 40 to 30% of the total calories, decreasing the intake of saturated fats particularly, with increased consumption of fresh fruits, vegetables and whole grain products while reducing the amount of sugar and salt in the diet. The ideas upon which the recommendations are based are in keeping with recent knowledge concern-

Table I. Food supply patterns of various countries. Component food items expressed as a percentage of the total calories. Derived from FAO [1971] Food Balance Sheets 1964–1966 Averages. Countries with meat, milk diets and high female life expectancy at birth [Keyfitz and Flieger, 1971]

	Life expectancy at birth (years)	kcal per day	Meat Milk[1]	Cereals Starchy[2] roots	Sugar Oils and fats	Eggs Fish	Vege-tables Fruit	Pulses[3] Butter[4]	Total meat, milk	Total sugar, oils and fats
Norway	F 76.9	2,963	8.7	24.2	15.6	1.2	0.6	1.7	25.7	34.8
	M 71.4		17.0	6.5	19.2	2.3	2.9	2.8		
Iceland	F 76.6	2,899	14.8	19.7	20.0	0.4	0.2	Tr	31.3	40.5
	M 71.4		16.5	2.3	20.5	4.0	1.5	6.3		
Netherlands	F 76.6	3,190	11.0	21.6	16.4	1.5	1.2	1.9	23.4	41.5
	M 71.2		12.4	5.5	25.1	0.6	2.8	2.6		
Sweden	F 76.6	2,907	12.4	22.0	15.4	1.5	0.8	1.5	27.9	33.7
	M 71.9		15.5	6.2	18.3	2.5	3.8	5.9		
UK	F 76.0	3,233	16.3	23.8	16.4	1.9	1.4	2.1	28.0	33.4
	M 69.6		11.7	6.1	17.0	0.9	2.4	5.4		
Switzerland	F 75.9	3,162	13.0	26.3	14.8	1.3	1.3	3.7	26.9	30.8
	M 69.7		13.9	3.6	16.0	0.8	5.2	4.1		
Canada	F 75.5	3,142	19.7	21.2	16.9	1.8	2.0	2.3	31.7	32.2
	M 68.9		12.0	4.9	15.3	0.7	3.2	5.2		
France	F 75.5	3,108	15.5	27.3	11.4	1.4	2.8	2.0	26.0	29.8
	M 68.0		10.5	6.3	18.4	1.4	3.1	5.7		
Denmark	F 75.4	3,220	14.2	21.7	15.9	1.5	1.1	1.0	26.2	37.3
	M 70.7		12.0	6.2	21.4	2.3	2.7	6.3		
Means with standard deviations in parentheses		3,092 (133)	14.0 (3.4)	23.1 (2.5)	15.9 (2.0)	1.4 (0.4)	1.3 (1.8)	1.8 (1.0)	27.5 (2.7)	34.9 (4.1)
			13.5 (2.3)	5.3 (1.4)	19.0 (2.9)	1.7 (1.3)	3.0 (1.0)	4.9 (1.0)		

F = Females, M = males.

[1] Includes all milk products except butter.

[2] Starchy roots here means potatoes.

[3] Pulses includes also nuts and oil seeds.

[4] Butter is included also in the oils and fats component.

Table II. Food sully patterns of various countries. Intakes of food items expressed as a percentage of the total calories. Derived from FAO [1984] Food Balance Sheets 1979–1981 Averages. Countries with meat, milk diets and high female life expectancy at birth. World Statistics in brief. United Nations [1985]. Data for 1983. For footnotes see table I.

	Life expectancy (years) at birth	kcal per day	Meat Milk[1]	Cereals Starchy roots[2]	Sugar Oils and fats	Eggs Fish	Vege-tables Fruit	Pulses[3] Butter[4]	Total meat, milk	Total sugar, oils and fats
Norway	F 79	3,391	12.1	25.9	14.0	1.3	1.0	1.0	27.8	32.4
	M 73		15.7	5.1	18.4	2.5	3.0	3.2		
Iceland	F 80	3,087	17.5	20.7	18.3	1.6	0.6	0.6	36.6	28.8
	M 74		19.1	4.3	10.5	6.4	0.4	3.3		
Netherlands	F 79	3,617	18.2	18.7	14.1	1.5	1.1	1.5	31.2	37.4
	M 73		13.0	5.0	23.3	0.5	3.1	2.0		
Sweden	F 79	3,146	18.0	21.3	14.9	1.6	1.1	0.9	32.2	32.6
	M 73		14.2	5.0	17.7	2.3	3.0	3.8		
UK	F 77	3,249	17.1	22.7	14.5	1.6	1.7	2.2	28.3	33.9
	M 71		11.2	6.8	19.4	0.8	2.0	4.0		
Switzerland	F 79	3,455	20.0	22.5	14.6	1.4	1.5	1.7	33.2	31.7
	M 73		13.2	2.9	17.0	0.5	4.6	4.5		
Canada	F 79	3,340	20.7	20.5	14.2	1.5	2.0	3.2	31.1	32.2
	M 71		10.4	4.7	18.0	1.0	3.8	2.7		
France	F 79	3,529	19.3	24.2	12.7	1.7	2.3	1.2	29.6	32.7
	M 71		10.3	4.8	20.0	1.1	2.4	4.7		
Denmark	F 78	3,548	21.3	20.2	13.8	1.6	1.0	0.6	32.0	34.4
	M 72		10.7	4.7	20.6	3.2	2.3	5.0		
Means with standard deviation in parentheses		3,374 (183)	18.3 (2.5)	21.9 (2.2)	14.6 (0.7)	1.5 (0.1)	1.4 (1.6)	1.4 (0.8)	31.4 (3.0)	32.9 (2.4)
			13.1 (3.0)	4.8 (1.1)	18.3 (3.5)	2.0 (1.9)	2.8 (0.9)	3.7 (2.8)		

Table III. Food supply patterns of various countries. Intakes of food items expressed as a percentage of total calories. Derived from FAO [1971] Food Balance Sheets 1964–1966 Averages. Countries with high-calorie wheat-based diets and moderate life expectancy at birth [Keyfitz and Flieger, 1971]. For footnotes see table I

	Life expectancy at birth (years)	kcal per day	Meat Milk[1]	Cereals Starchy[2] roots	Sugar Oils and fats	Eggs Fish	Vege-tables Fruit	Pulses[3] Butter[4]	Total meat, milk	Total sugar, oils and fats
Greece	F 74.5	2,901	5.2	44.5	6.6	1.2	3.0	5.1	14.5	22.2
	M 70.7		9.3	3.1	15.6	1.4	5.0	0.8		
Italy	F 74.2	2,818	6.1	45.4	9.6	1.3	3.3	3.2	13.6	24.9
	M 68.4		7.5	3.0	15.3	0.3	5.0	1.2		
Bulgaria	F 72.9	3,074	7.0	63.3	8.1	0.7	1.7	1.9	10.3	18.3
	M 68.9		3.3	1.4	10.2	0.2	2.2	0.7		
Yugoslavia	F 70.2	3,154	5.8	60.6	7.5	0.5	1.2	3.1	10.1	18.1
	M 66.1		4.3	3.9	10.6	0.1	2.4	0.5		
Rumania	F 73.5	3,012	9.5	60.3	6.2	0.7	1.2	2.9	15.2	13.7
	M 71.3		5.7	4.3	7.5	0.2	1.5	0.6		
Means with standard deviations in parentheses		2,990	6.7	54.7	7.6	0.9	2.1	3.3	12.7	19.4
		(132)	(1.7)	(9.1)	(2.6)	(0.8)	(1.0)	(1.2)	(2.4)	(4.2)
			6.0	3.2	11.8	0.5	3.2	0.8		
			(2.6)	(1.1)	(3.8)	(0.5)	(1.7)	(0.3)		

Table IV. Food supply patterns of various countries. Intakes of food items expressed as a percentage of the total calories. Derived from FAO [1984] Food Balance Sheets 1979–1981 Averages. Countries with high-calorie wheat-based diets and moderate life expectancy at birth. World Statistics in brief. United Nations [1985]. Data for 1983. For footnotes see table I

	Life expectancy at birth (years)	kcal per day	Meat Milk[1]	Cereals Starchy roots[2]	Sugars Oils and fats	Eggs Fish	Vege-tables Fruit	Pulses[3] Butter[4]	Total meat, milk	Total sugar, oils and fats
Greece	F 76 M 72	3,668	11.3 8.6	33.3 3.7	10.5 18.5	1.3 0.8	3.0 5.1	3.9 0.5	19.9	29.0
Italy	F 78 M 71	3,688	12.1 8.1	37.6 2.5	9.9 18.4	1.3 0.8	2.8 4.2	2.3 1.2	20.2	28.3
Bulgaria	F 75 M 70	3,619	9.6 6.9	46.6 1.7	10.7 14.7	1.7 0.3	1.7 3.9	2.2 1.3	16.5	25.4
Yugoslavia	F 74 M 69	3,550	7.7 7.1	48.9 3.3	9.6 14.7	1.0 0.2	1.7 2.6	3.2 0.4	14.8	24.3
Rumania	F 74 M 69	3,346	9.5 9.1	46.2 4.5	9.1 12.9	1.5 0.5	2.6 2.4	1.7 0.8	18.6	22.0
Means with standard deviations in parentheses		3,574 (140)	10.0 (1.7) 8.0 (1.0)	42.5 (6.6) 3.1 (0.8)	10.0 (0.6) 15.8 (2.2)	1.4 (0.3) 0.5 (0.3)	2.3 (0.6) 3.7 (1.1)	2.7 (1.0) 0.8 (0.4)	18.0 (2.3)	25.8 (2.9)

ing the cause of chronic diseases, especially CHD. This knowledge, however, may not be soundly based. It leaves unexplained such anomalies as the diets of Eskimos in their native state. Such diets despite their high fat content and lack of dietary fibre do not appear to be conducive to the Western type diseases as could be anticipated from the theory of Burkitt and Trowell [1975]. Similar considerations seem to apply to Pacific atoll populations living on coconuts which are rich in saturated fatty acids, particularly lauric acid, in contrast to palmitic acid characteristic of Western diets. There is little reason to suppose that a reduction in the high fat levels of the Eskimo diet would be beneficial. To reconcile the differences between the areas just mentioned and those of the West one needs to offer the hypothesis that the composition of the fat as well as the level of dietary intake has a bearing on the occurrence of the Western type diseases.

The existence of nutritional guidelines has some influence on the dietary patterns of today but it is believed that, even in the developed countries, as in the past, the factors of customs, acceptability, availability, economics and propaganda are influential in determining what the individual eats. Because of surveys made by FAO, incorporated in Food Balance Sheets [FAO, 1971, 1984], it is now possible to describe diets on a national basis recognising that there exist many groups whose dietary habits deviate from the mean values given by the whole population. Some are vegetarians, some do not eat fish and so on. Nevertheless, the mean intakes per capita give some insights into the differences in food consumption in different countries. It will be seen that many Western countries are characterised by high meat and dairy product consumption whereas many developing countries depend on cereals for their staple diet and to a large extent lack meat and dairy products which are too expensive to purchase.

The Food Balance Sheets [FAO, 1971, 1984], which are used here to describe the composition of today's diets, cover a wide range of dietary components. However, as will be later indicated, this range is considerably extended by inclusion of the diets of races living on their traditional food sources as is the case with the Eskimos and Pukapukans.

Dietary Patterns Derived from FAO [1971, 1984] Food Balance Sheets

In a previous investigation, Shorland [1978] used FAO [1971] Food Balance Sheets in association with the life expectancy data of Keyfitz and Flieger [1971] to determine the relationship between diet and life expectancy. It was suggested that with the decreased importance of infectious diseases and dietary deficiencies as a cause of death, the residue of non-infectious diseases, including CHD, cancer and stroke, had become the main causes of death, particularly in Western countries. The incidence of these diseases appears to be of environmental origin and in part at least related to diet (tables I, II). Countries with their per capita intakes of various food items were therefore ranked in order of female life expectancy at birth as an index of health. Data from various sources suggested that the female was less prone to accidents and less affected by smoking and alcohol. For the present purpose the data mentioned above have been regrouped with a view to identifying some of the characteristic diets of the world. This led to a classification based on the main dietary components into five categories including meat, milk; high-calorie wheat; low-calorie wheat; maize and rice diets.

By means of such a classification, similar diets are grouped together facilitating comparisons between countries and the diagnosis of the extent to which the diets deviate or conform to current dietary guidelines. The variations in the diets are furthermore suggestive in terms of relationships to health and the necessity or otherwise of following a rigid dietary pattern. Knowledge of the effects of varying the patterns of food components can also be useful for economic reasons. If a food component becomes expensive, it may be important to have an acceptable and nutritionally equivalent alternative. Clearly the diets that are currently acceptable on a national basis in countries with a relatively low incidence of Western type diseases tend to be low in saturated fats compared with the diets of countries where the incidence is much higher. A more widespread knowledge of these differences would enable the public to alter their dietary patterns on a sound basis.

In the tables which follow, the calories of each food item have been calculated from the relevant FAO [1971, 1984] Food Balance Sheets as a percentage of the total food items shown. However, the item 'butter' has been included in the oils and fats category and is therefore not counted again in making up the total food items. In the Food Balance Sheets the calories for alcohol and spices have sometimes been included. To ensure comparability between countries, such items have here been omitted. Although comparisons between countries are here based on FAO [1971] data, tables using FAO [1984] data are included. In general the percentage calories of items shown did not change significantly over the period. However, where relevant such changes as did occur will be mentioned. In the

Table V. Food supply patterns of various countries. Intakes of food items expressed as a percentage of the total calories. Derived from FAO [1971] Food Balance Sheets 1964–1966 Averages. Countries with low-calorie wheat diets and relatively low female life expectancy at birth [Keyfitz and Flieger, 1971]. For footnotes see table I

	Life expectancy at birth (years)	kcal per day	Meat Milk[1]	Cereals Starchy roots[2]	Sugars Oils and fats	Eggs Fish	Vege-tables Fruit	Pulses[3] Butter[4]	Total meat, milk	Total sugar, oils and fats
Algeria	F 66.9	1,892	2.2	70.6	9.5	0.3	1.1	2.2	4.4	15.2
	M 63.0		2.2	1.6	5.7	0.2	4.3	–		
Chile	F 66.2	2,516	8.1	53.3	13.4	0.6	2.0	2.3	14.4	19.3
	M 59.2		6.3	5.2	5.9	1.0	1.9	–		
Tunisia	F 63.2	2,205	3.1	61.6	7.6	0.4	2.0	3.1	6.1	22.4
	M 55.7		3.0	1.0	14.8	0.5	2.9	–		
Means with standard deviation in parentheses		2,204 (312)	4.5 (3.2)	62.0 (8.6)	10.0 (3.0)	0.4 (0.2)	1.7 (0.5)	2.5 (0.5)	8.4 (5.3)	19.0 (3.6)
			3.9 (2.2)	2.6 (2.1)	8.8 (5.3)	0.6 (0.4)	3.0 (1.2)	–		

case of an individual country where a marked change has occurred, this will be assessed for significance on the assumption that the standard deviation for the group applies also to that country. To match the FAO [1984] Food Balance Sheets the United Nations [1985] publication *Statistics in Brief* has been used as a source of life expectancy data for 1983 (tables III, IV).

In tables I–IX the diets are arranged in descending order of their percentage contribution of meat, milk products to the total calories (shown in parentheses with standard deviations), thus: meat, milk, 27.5 ± 2.7; wheat, high calorie, 12.7 ± 2.4; wheat, low calorie, 8.4 ± 5.3; maize, 7.2 ± 1.5, and rice, 4.3 ± 2.1. In each case the table giving FAO [1971] data is followed by a corresponding table with FAO [1984] data.

Considering first life expectancy data it will be seen (table I) that the meat, milk group in general outranks all other groups with female life expectancy at birth extending from 75.4 years in Denmark to 76.9 years in Norway. Not included in the table are USA, Australia and New Zealand which were ranked as the highest consumers of meat, milk products with female life expectancies of 74.8, 74.5 and 74.3 years, respectively. The female life expectancy of the high-calorie wheat group (70.2–74.5 years) approaches that of the meat, milk group (table III), then follows the low-calorie wheat group (table V) with life expectancies ranging from 63.2 to 66.9 years. The maize and rice groups (tables VII, VIII) present a divergence of female life expectancies covering 50.9–67.9 and 50.9–73.7 years, respectively.

The uniformly high life expectancy of the meat, milk group is associated with relatively low infant mortality so that the life expectancy potential of other groups with higher infant mortality tends to be obscured. This is indicated by comparing life expectancies at different ages. As shown in figures 1 and 2 the life expectancy of the low-calorie wheat group at 20 years or more may exceed that of the meat, milk group by several years using London as the standard for the highest female life expectancy given by Keyfitz and Flieger [1971]. It may be similarly shown that male life expectancy in Nicaragua (maize diet) is in excess of that of the male Swede taken from Keyfitz and Flieger [1971] as the highest value for male life expectancy. At birth the Greek male (high-calorie wheat diet) has a life expectancy of 70.7 years but at 1 year the expectancy rises to 72.2 years compared with 71.9 years for the male Swede. Clearly infant mortality tends to obscure the use of life expectancy as an index of nutrition but as infant mortality becomes more uniformly low this index will become more effective.

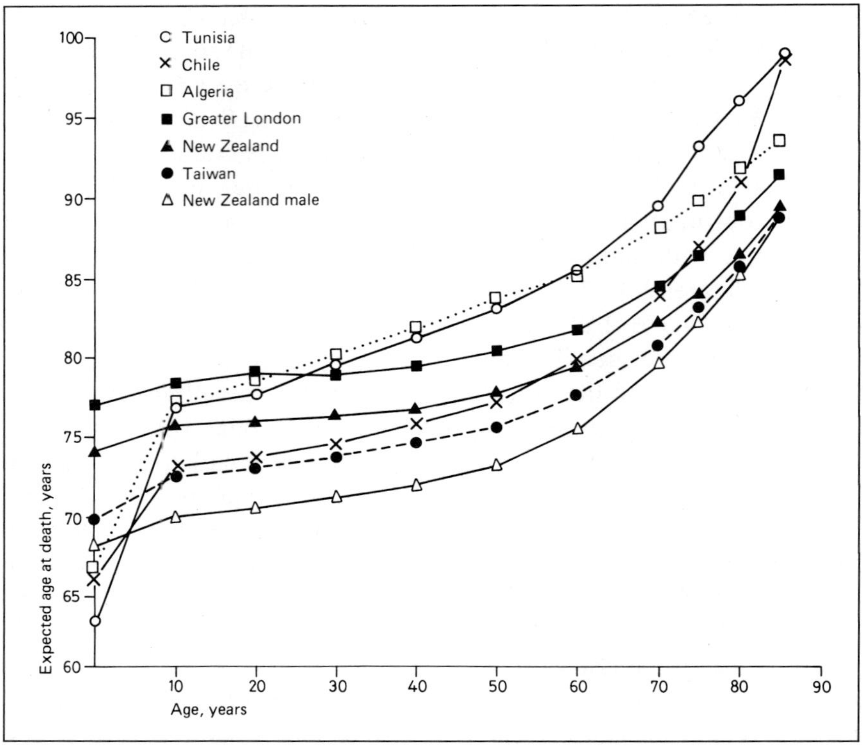

Fig. 1. Female life expectancy and diet. The London female is taken as the standard longevity. The diets involved are meat, milk (Greater London, New Zealand), low-calorie wheat (Algeria, Chile and Tunisia) and rice (Taiwan). See tables I, V, VIII [Shorland, 1978]. Life expectancy data taken from Keyfitz and Flieger [1971].

In figure 2 there has been added [Shorland, 1978] data for the US male which follow closely that of the New Zealand male, the life expectancies at birth being 67.6 and 68.2 years, respectively, compared with 71.9 years for the Swede male. However, in later life, differences in life expectancy converge. Males in USA, New Zealand and Sweden at 80 years have life expectancies of 7.36, 5.55 and 6.13 years, respectively (fig. 2). At 85+ years the corresponding values are 5.18, 4.11 and 4.49 years. Life expectancy data for Tunisian, Algerian and Nicaraguan males representing low-calorie wheat and maize diets also show convergence but at a higher level. At 80 years the life expectancies are 9.98, 10.88 and 11.76 years, respectively (fig. 2), the corresponding values for 85+ years being 9.25, 8.69 and 10.27

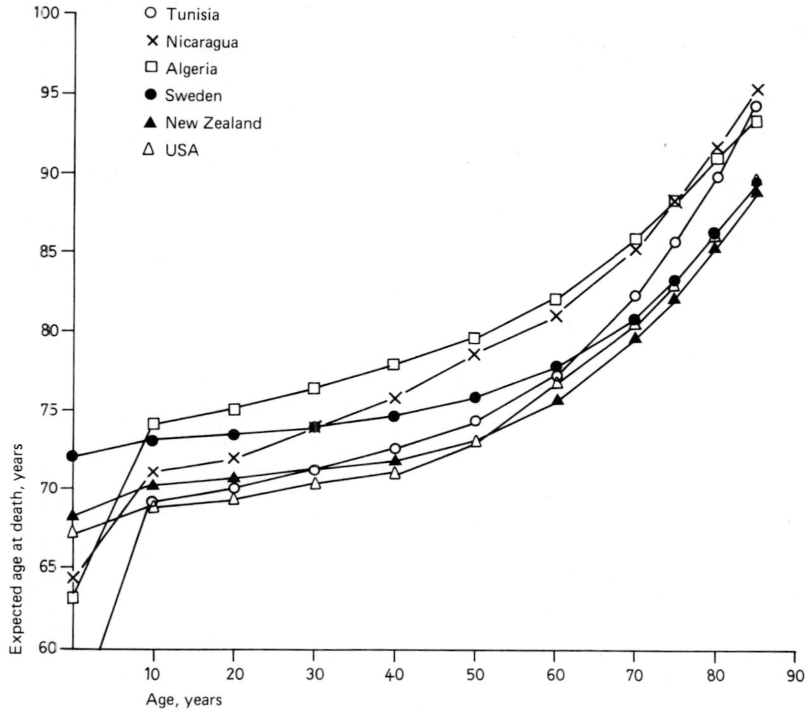

Fig. 2. Male life expectancy and diet. The Swedish male is taken as the standard for longevity. The diets involved are meat, milk (Sweden, New Zealand and USA), low-calorie wheat (Algeria, Tunisia) and maize (Nicaragua). See tables I, V, VII [Shorland, 1978]. Life expectancy data taken from Keyfitz and Flieger [1971].

years. This means that overall life expectancies at 80 and 85+ years in Tunisia, Algeria and Nicaragua are nearly double those found in USA, New Zealand and Sweden for males despite the considerable medical resources available in these latter countries. The results are consistent with those of the cereal based centenarian diets as reviewed by Shorland [1978].

Since 1971, there have been changes in life expectancy as shown by United Nations [1985] statistics. In the meat, milk countries the life expectancy of the female has risen by 2–3 years covering a range of 77–80 years with Iceland replacing Norway in showing greatest life expectancy (table II). The high-calorie wheat countries (table IV) and the rice countries (table

Table VI. Food supply patterns of various countries. Intakes of food items expressed as a percentage of the total calories. Derived from FAO [1984] Food Balance Sheets 1977–1979 Averages. Countries with low-calorie wheat diets and relatively low female life expectancy at birth. World Statistics in brief. United Nations [1985]. Data for 1983. For footnotes, see table I

	Life expectancy at birth (years)	kcal per day	Meat Milk[1]	Cereals Starchy roots[2]	Sugars Oils and fats	Eggs Fish	Vegetables Fruit	Pulses[3] Butter[4]	Total meat, milk	Total sugar, oils and fats
Algeria	F 59 M 57	2,586	2.0 6.0	57.3 2.2	11.8 13.2	0.4 0.2	1.0 3.6	2.2 1.5	8.0	25.0
Chile	F 70 M 64	2,759	7.0 6.1	51.1 3.6	14.4 8.4	0.7 1.5	2.4 2.6	2.2 0.7	13.1	22.8
Tunisia	F 61 M 60	2,763	2.7 3.8	56.5 1.3	9.4 14.9	0.6 0.5	2.9 3.1	4.3 1.6	6.5	24.3
Means with standard deviation in parentheses		2,703 (102)	3.9 (2.8) 5.3 (1.3)	55.0 (3.4) 2.4 (1.2)	11.8 (2.5) 12.2 (4.0)	0.5 (0.2) 0.7 (0.7)	2.1 (1.1) 3.1 (0.5)	2.9 (1.2)	9.2 (3.4)	24.0 (1.1)

IX) have similarly improved, whereas no such improvement is indicated in the low-calorie wheat countries. Data for the maize group are lacking except for Guatemala where there has been considerable improvement in life expectancy of some 10 years.

Perhaps the most outstanding change in life expectancy is shown by Japan which now ranks second in the developed countries. In 1964 life expectancies of the male and female at birth were 67.7 and 72.9 years, respectively. Over an 8-year period these expectancies rose to 70.5 and 75.9 years, now reaching as shown in table IX 74 and 79 years, respectively. According to Innami and Mickelsen [1969] the main changes during the previous 10 years expressed as a percentage of the 1956 values were as follows: eggs, 318; milk, 301; fats and oils, 230; fruits, 199 calories, 103, and protein, 106. There have also been increases in animal protein and fat of 123 and 177%, respectively. The calories from cereals decreased progressively from 70% in 1955 to 62% in 1966. With these changes there are associated increases in height and weight of the children. Cerebrovascular accidents account for 25.6%, cancer for 14.2% and CHD for about 10% of all deaths. With the change to more Westernised diets while maintaining high levels of fish intake, the disease pattern may continue to include a low proportion of deaths from CHD (tables V, VI). The increased levels of animal protein and fat in a diet previously low in these components have thus been associated with a marked increase in life expectancy, suggesting the possibility that the Japanese diet based on rice – a poor-quality protein low in thiamine – needs supplementation with small amounts of high-quality protein foods.

Before dealing with the patterns of the food components it is perhaps necessary to point out that the FAO Food Balance Sheets are based on consumption data derived from the disappearance of supplies. The per capita intakes thus calculated are in excess of those determined by dietary surveys. As shown previously [Shorland, 1978] a dietary survey [Davidson and Gilmour, 1969] indicated a daily per capita intake of 2,750 kcal for New Zealand compared with 3,454 kcal reported in the FAO [1971] Food Balance Sheets. However, food items expressed as a percentage of total calories derived from the two sets of data were in close agreement.

As seen from tables I and III, the intakes of meat, milk and high-calorie wheat groups approximate 3,000 kcal in the FAO [1971] survey whereas the remaining groups are shown to consume 2,500 kcal or less. Higher values for the FAO [1984] survey are unlikely to reflect higher intakes than for the FAO [1971] survey. As indicated by Call [1965] in

Table VII. Food supply patterns of various countries. Intakes of food items expressed as a percentage of the total calories. Derived from FAO [1971] Food Balance Sheets 1964–1966 Averages. Life expectancy data [Keyfitz and Flieger, 1971] and World Statistics in brief, United Nations [1985]. Data for 1983. Countries with maize diets and relatively low female life expectancy at birth. Data for Nicaragua and El Salvador were not included in the FAO [1984] Food Balance Sheets. However, the values for Guatemala were available in their publication and are included for convenience in this table. For footnotes see table I

		Life expectancy at birth (years)	kcal per day	Meat Milk[1]	Cereals Starchy roots[2]	Sugars Oils and fats	Eggs Fish	Vegetables Fruit	Pulses[3] Butter[4]	Total meat, milk	Total sugar, oils and fats
Nicaragua	F	67.9	2,253	0.9	50.7	12.9	0.9	0.4	9.3	7.7	22.4
	M	64.6		6.8	6.1	9.5	0.3	2.2	–		
El Salvador	F	60.7	1,877	2.1	56.1	15.0	1.1	0.9	5.1	7.9	22.8
	M	56.4		5.8	3.9	7.8	0.3	1.9	–		
Guatemala	F	50.9	1,952	2.2	64.8	13.0	1.0	0.9	5.2	5.2	18.7
	M	49.3		4.0	1.6	5.7	0.1	1.5	–		
Means with standard deviations in parentheses			2,027	1.7	57.2	13.6	1.0	0.7	6.5	7.2	21.3
			(199)	(0.7)	(7.1)	(1.2)	(0.1)	(0.3)	(3.4)	(1.5)	(2.3)
				5.5	3.9	7.7	0.2	1.9			
				(1.4)	(2.3)	(1.9)	(0.1)	(0.3)			
Guatemala FAO [1984]	F	60.0	2,138	3.6	59.0	16.0	0.9	0.7	5.5	7.3	22.9
	M	62.0		3.7	0.5	6.9	0.1	3.1	–		

USA the caloric intake determined from the disappearance of supplies is much greater than the needs of the basic unit of 2,900 kcal or the requirement of the young adult male.

Cereals, even in the meat, milk group, at 23.1 ± 2.5% remain the most important contributors of calories. In other groups, cereals contribute 40% or more of the total calories, the highest levels (68.3 ± 8.5%) being attained in the rice diets (tables I, III, V, VII and VIII).

Oils, fats and sugars together are large caloric contributors to the modern diet and are sometimes referred to as empty calories. As shown in tables I, III, V, VII and VIII they provide in the groups named the following percentage contributions to the total calories: meat, milk, 34.9 ± 4.1; high-calorie wheat, 19.4 ± 4.2; low-calorie wheat, 19.0 ± 3.6; maize, 21.3 ± 2.3; rice, 10.6 ± 5.6. The sugar contribution to the diets just mentioned expressed as a percentage of the total oils, fats and sugars is 46, 40, 53 and 70, respectively. In the rice group the contribution of the oils, fats and sugar components is very variable ranging from 1.4% in the Republic of Korea to 16.4% in Sri Lanka.

Of the major components just discussed the meat, milk group has significantly ($p < 0.05$) higher proportions of meat and milk products and of oils, fats and sugars but significantly ($p < 0.05$) lower proportions of cereals than the other dietary groups. These major components of the diet comprising meat and milk, oils, fats and sugars, and cereals make up in the diets named the following percentage contributions to the total calories: meat, milk, 85.5; high-calorie wheat, 86.8; low-calorie wheat, 89.4; maize, 85.7, and rice, 83.2.

The minor components of the diet include, starchy roots, eggs, fish, vegetables, fruit and pulses. In general the minor components provide individually less than 6% of the total calories. However, in some cases starchy roots provide up to 11% of the total calories. In Western countries starchy roots designates potatoes but in the rice countries starchy roots comprises sweet potatoes and in tropical countries cassava is included. In the item pulses here include also nuts and oil seeds which together generally make up less than 4% of the total calories. Sri Lanka provides an exception with 14.8% based on consumption of high levels of coconuts.

The respective contributions of the starchy roots as a percentage of total calories in the diets named (tables I, III, V, VII and VIII) are as follows: meat, milk, 5.3 ± 1.4; high-calorie wheat, 3.2 ± 1.1; maize, 3.9 ± 2.3; low-calorie wheat, 2.6 ± 2.1, and rice, 5.1 ± 3.9. Notably high values

Table VIII. Food supply patterns of various countries. Intakes of food items expressed as a percentage of total calories. Derived from FAO [1971] Food Balance Sheets Averages 1964–1966. Countries with rice diets and many with relatively low female life expectancy at birth [Keyfitz and Flieger, 1971]. For footnotes see table I

	Life expectancy at birth (years)	kcal per day	Meat Milk[1]	Cereals Starchy roots[2]	Sugars Oils and fats	Eggs Fish	Vege-tables Fruit	Pulses[3] Butter[4]	Total meat, milk	Total sugar, oils and fats
Japan	F 73.7	2,416	2.1	57.8	8.2	1.6	3.7	6.0	4.7	15.4
	M 68.5		2.6	5.5	7.2	3.5	1.7	1.4		
Taiwan	F 69.8	2,379	7.1	63.4	6.5	0.1	1.5	1.3	7.6	16.0
	M 65.2		0.5	6.1	9.5	2.1	1.8	–		
Sri Lanka	F 66.8	2,219	0.6	56.1	8.4	0.3	2.9	14.8	2.6	16.4
	M 65.1		2.0	4.5	8.0	1.7	0.7	–		
China	F 50.9	2,045	6.6	67.4	1.7	0.6	1.6	6.6	6.9	4.9
	M 57.0		0.3	11.0	3.2	0.7	0.3	–		
Republic of Korea	F 55.7	2,329	1.8	80.1	0.7	0.3	2.2	2.2	1.9	1.4
	M 54.8		0.1	10.1	0.7	1.3	0.5	–		
Burma	F –	2,011	1.9	74.9	4.7	0.3	1.7	3.6	3.3	12.7
	M –		1.4	0.3	8.0	1.4	1.8	–		
Thailand	F 64.4	2,226	3.8	72.5	5.3	0.7	0.9	5.9	4.6	6.9
	M 58.7		0.8	3.0	1.6	2.2	3.3	–		
Cambodia	F –	2,231	2.7	73.6	8.2	0.2	1.8	2.2	3.1	10.1
	M –		0.4	0.7	1.9	4.2	4.1	–		
Means with standard deviation in parentheses		2,230	3.3	68.3	5.1	0.5	2.0	5.3	4.3	10.6
		(133)	(2.0)	(8.5)	(3.9)	(0.5)	(0.8)	(4.1)	(2.1)	(5.6)
			1.0	5.1	5.5	2.1	1.8			
			(0.7)	(3.9)	(2.9)	(1.2)	(1.4)			

are shown by China (11.0% of total calories) and by the Republic of Korea (10.1% of total calories).

Eggs (tables I, III, V, VII and VIII) contribute negligable amounts of calories to the diet. Expressed as a percentage contribution to the total calories in the diets named the values arranged in descending order are as follows: meat, milk, 1.4 ± 0.4; maize, 1.0 ± 0.1; high-calorie wheat, 0.9 ± 0.8; rice, 0.5 ± 0.5, and low-calorie wheat, 0.4 ± 0.2.

Fish also tends to be a minor contributor to the total calories but the proportions in different countries show it to be more variable than any other minor food component. The percentage contributions to the total calories in the diets named are as follows: rice, 2.1 ± 1.2; meat, milk, 1.7 ± 1.3, high-calorie wheat, 0.5 ± 0.5; low-calorie wheat, 0.6 ± 0.4, and maize, 0.2 ± 0.1. The three highest values were Cambodia 4.2%; Iceland, 4.0%, and Japan, 3.5%.

Arranged in descending order the contributions of vegetables to the total calories of the diet groups (tables I, III, V, VII and VIII) are as follows: high-calorie wheat, 2.1 ± 1.0; rice, 2.0 ± 0.8; low-calorie wheat, 1.7 ± 0.5; meat, milk, 1.3 ± 1.8, and maize, 0.7 ± 0.3. The range extends from 3.7 (Japan) to 0.2% (Iceland) based on the total calories.

Fruit (tables I, III, V, VII and VIII) is shown to contribute in most cases more calories to the diet than vegetables. In the diets listed the percentage contribution to the total calories is ranked as follows: high-calorie wheat, 3.2 ± 1.7; meat, milk, 3.0 ± 1.0; low-calorie wheat, 3.0 ± 1.2; maize, 1.9 ± 0.3, and rice, 1.8 ± 1.4. High values expressed as a percentage of total calories are shown for Switzerland (5.2), Greece, (5.0) and Italy (5.0).

Pulses along with nuts and seeds provide a variable contribution to the total calories (tables I, III, V, VII and VIII) to the diets named as follows: maize, 6.5 ± 3.4; rice 5.3 ± 4.1; high-calorie wheat, 3.3 ± 1.2; low-calorie wheat, 2.5 ± 0.5, and meat, milk, 1.8 ± 1.0. As already mentioned the pulses component because of the inclusion of nuts provides 14.8% of the total calories in Sri Lanka.

Butter, which is included already under the oils and fats component, is of interest in that it provides 4.9 ± 1.0% of the total calories in the meat, milk countries but is largely excluded from the diets of other countries. The small amount in the Japanese diet in 1964–1966 of 1.4% of the total calories (table VIII) is shown to decrease to 0.4% in 1977–1979 (table IX). In New Zealand in 1964–1966 the level was 10.8% of the total calories.

Table IX. Food supply patterns of various countries. Intakes of food items expressed as a percentage of total calories. Derived from FAO [1984] Food Balance Sheets 1977–1979 Averages. Countries with rice diets and many with relatively low female life expectancy at birth. World Statistics in brief. United Nations [1985]. Data for 1983. Data for Taiwan and Cambodia not available for 1979–1981. For footnotes see table I

	Life expectancy at birth (years)	kcal per day	Meat Milk[1]	Cereals Starchy roots[2]	Sugars Oils and fats	Eggs Fish	Vege-tables Fruit	Pulses[3] Butter[4]	Total meat, milk	Total sugar, oils and fats
Japan	F 79 M 74	2,852	6.7 3.5	45.9 2.6	9.6 12.2	2.4 7.2	2.7 2.1	5.1 0.4	10.2	21.8
Sri Lanka	F 69 M 66	2,251	0.4 2.2	57.4 4.2	7.8 3.7	0.2 1.4	0.7 6.9	15.1 –	2.6	11.5
China	F 69 M 66	2,426	7.6 0.5	66.5 12.2	1.7 3.6	0.7 0.4	1.7 1.2	3.9 –	8.1	5.3
Republic of Korea	F 73 M 66	3,056	3.8 0.5	71.6 2.2	4.2 4.0	0.9 2.3	5.1 1.0	4.4 –	4.3	8.2
Burma	F 57 M 53	2,420	1.7 0.6	81.2 0.4	2.1 5.8	0.2 1.0	1.3 1.7	4.0 –	2.3	7.9
Thailand	F 65 M 61	2,330	3.8 0.4	67.0 2.7	12.6 2.5	0.3 1.6	1.6 4.2	3.3 –	4.2	13.1
Means with standard deviation in parentheses		2,556 (321)	4.0 (2.7) 1.3 (1.3)	64.8 (12.0) 4.1 (4.2)	6.3 (4.4) 5.3 (3.3)	0.8 (0.8) 2.3 (2.4)	2.2 (1.6) 2.9 (2.3)	6.0 (4.5)	5.3 (3.2)	11.6 (5.8)

Table X. Extreme values for percentage contribution to total calories of food components shown in tables I, III, V, VII and VIII

	Maximum		Minimum	
Meat	Canada	19.7	Sri Lanka	0.6
Cereals	Republic of Korea	80.1	Iceland	19.7
Sugar	Iceland	20.0	Republic of Korea	0.7
Eggs	UK	1.9	Taiwan	0.1
Vegetables	Japan	3.7	Iceland	0.2
Pulses, nuts and seeds	Sri Lanka	14.8	Denmark	1.0
Total sugar, oils and fats	Netherlands	41.5	Republic of Korea	1.4
Milk products	Norway	17.0	Republic of Korea	0.1
Starchy roots	China	11.0	Burma	0.3
Oils and fats	Netherlands	25.1	Republic of Korea	0.7
Fish	Cambodia	4.2	Yugoslavia	0.1
Fruit	Switzerland	5.2	China	0.3
Total meat, milk products	Canada	31.7	Republic of Korea	1.9
Butter	Iceland	6.3	Many countries	<0.1

Comparing the FAO [1971] and [1984] Food Balance Sheets there was no evidence that the mean values of the groups studied had changed significantly between 1964–1966 and 1979–1981. However, within the same country there appeared to be significant changes ($p < 0.05$) in some food items. In Iceland, for example, between the periods mentioned oils and fats dropped from 20.0% of the total calories to 10.5%. Correspondingly, in Greece and Italy meat consumption which was 5.2 and 6.1% of the total calories in 1964–1966 rose to 11.3 and 12.1%, respectively.

The diets described in tables I, III, V, VII and VIII give insights into the variations in food patterns. For convenience the maximum and minimum values are collected together in table X. The differences between maxima and minima in 11 out of 14 items fall approximately within the range of 15- to 40-fold. Cereals show a 4-fold range whereas milk products have a 170-fold range. It is perhaps significant that countries with the highest life expectancies, Iceland and Japan, should exhibit respectively the lowest and the highest intakes of vegetables. Iceland has the highest intake of sugar being more than twice that of Japan. Iceland ranks second to Canada in terms of meat, milk intake amounting to 31.3% of the total calories. In contrast the meat, milk intake is low in Japan at 4.7% of the total calories. The common feature of Iceland and Japan is that their consumption of fish at 4.0 and 3.5% of the total calories is in excess of that of other developed countries. The outstanding increase in fish consumption in these countries to 6.4 and 7.2% of the total calories, respectively in 1979–1981, is in keeping with their increasing life expectancy. These marked increases in fish consumption, however, fall short of reaching statistical significance at the ($p < 0.05$) level.

In Iceland as described by Cleave and Campbell [1966] the diet in 1850 was 80–85% protein and fat. With the replacement of fats and protein by refined carbohydrates (white flour and sugar) their level in the diet had fallen to a total of 45% in 1940 and the sugar consumption had risen to nearly 45 kg/head/year. The sugar consumption is currently 50 kg/head/year. The point made by Cleave and Campbell [1966] is that whereas neither diabetes nor obesity occurred to any great extent in Iceland formerly it is now prevalent. The US Senate Select Committee on Nutrition and Human Needs [1977] has recommended a reduction in the amount of sugar in the diet and reliance on highly refined foods. This defect in Iceland which is less marked in Japan may well place Japan ahead of Iceland in longevity in the future.

Other Dietary Patterns

The extremes in the consumption of food items shown in table X are greatly extended by the inclusion of diets not mentioned in the FAO [1971, 1984] Food Balance Sheets. For example, the diet of Eskimos in their native state comprises essentially the flesh of fish and marine mammals, the other food items shown in table X being absent. The diet of Pukapukans is based largely on coconut which provide 36% of the total calories. Such a contribution to the pulses, nuts and seeds item is several times that of any other country listed in the Food Balance Sheets. The remaining items expressed as a percentage of the total calories include: cereals, 25; taro, 20; meat and fish, 13, and sugar, 2 [Prior et al., 1966]. The intakes of male and female adults were estimated at 1,862 and 1,804 kcal/day. The fat, protein and carbohydrate intakes comprised respectively, 35, 13 and 52% of the total calories. Interest in the Pukapukan diet rests on the fact that despite the high intake of saturated fat in the form of coconut oil the mean cholesterol levels for males 20–29 years were low at 160 mg/100 ml serum rising to 185 mg/100 ml at 50–59 years but falling to 162 mg/100 ml at 70 years and over. The pattern for females showed 175 mg/100 ml at 20–29 years rising to 201 mg/100 ml at 50–59 years but falling to 171 mg/100 ml at 70 years and over. The Polynesians from Pukapuka were found to compare favourably with those from Rarotonga and especially with those from New Zealand (Maoris) where the diets had become increasingly Westernised and blood pressure along with cholesterol levels increased with age [Prior et al., 1966].

The atherogenic effects of saturated fatty acids may depend on their chain length. In the Western diets palmitic acid is the main saturated fatty acid but in the Pukapukan diet lauric (12:0) and myristic (14:0) make up respectively 43 and 20% of the total fatty acids. Shorland et al. [1969] found that consistent with the results for rats and other mammals the Pukapukans on the coconut oil diet contained in their depot and blood lipids a lowered ratio of lauric/myristic acid compared with coconut oil, possibly owing to chain extension of lauric acid following ingestion. In contrast, chickens fed coconut oil contained in their depot fats similar levels and proportions of lauric and myristic acid to those present in coconut oil [Shorland and Czochanska, 1970].

As will be discussed in section V, the intake of fat by the Eskimo in the native state is high but its composition is different from that of the West being marine based. The fatty oils which make up the fats of fish and marine mammals are derived via the plankton from linlenic acid or ω3-octadecatrienoic acid giving rise to substantial amounts of ω3-eicosapentaenoic acid. CHD is seldom found in Eskimos whose diet is substantially marine based. ω3-Eicosapentaenoic acid is a precursor [Vane, 1979] for a type of prostacyclin (PGI_2) in the vessel wall which has a direct anti-aggregatory activity on platelets. It is therefore suggested that the replacement of the normal precursor (arachidonic acid obtained from linoleic acid in vegetables and arachidonic acid in farm animals) of the clotting agent thromboxane with a more PUFA ω3-eicosapentaenoic acid would swing the thrombotic/antithrombotic equation beneficially [Vane, 1982]. This view is supported by the experimental work of Hay et al. [1982].

In sharp contrast to the flesh-eating Eskimos, the Pari tribe in the Highlands of New Guinea studied by Hipsley and Kirk [1965] have been found to live on a largely vegetarian diet. Expressed on a percentage of total calories basis the diet comprised: sweet potato, 77; taro, 6; banana, 4; other vegetables, 4; beans and corn, 3; leafy greens, 2; pig meat/pig fat, 2, and peanuts, 1. The intake of food was assessed at less than 2,000 kcal/person/day. The women were lactating effectively on 1,600 kcal/day. In physical strength, the men, though somewhat smaller than the average Caucasian, approached the standards required for the Australian Air Force, suggesting that the diet was satisfactory. In addition to the Pari tribe, Hipsley

Table XI. Protein and energy intakes of persons living on a fruit diet. Based on Jaffa [1901]

	Age, years	Weight, kg	Daily intake	
			protein, g	energy, kcal
Woman	33	40.8	23	1,300
Woman	30	47.2	25	1,040
Girl	13	34.2	26	1,235
Boy	9	19.5	27	1,255
Girl	6	13.8	24	1,190

and Kirk [1965] examined the diet of the Kaporaka tribe on the New Guinea Coast. The diet expressed as a percentage of total calories was as follows: yam, 51; coconut, 15; imported food, 12; cassava/sweet potato, 11; banana, 6; fish/shell fish, 3, and fruit and other vegetables, 2. The health of the population was judged to be as good if not better than that of the Pari tribe.

That a starchy root diet is adequate is suggested by the work of Hindhede [1913]. His group on a diet consisting almost entirely of potatoes over a period of 300 days remained in excellent health as judged by examination by the Medical School in Copenhagen. In such a vegetarian diet one could expect vitamin B_{12} deficiency but no evidence of anaemia was indicated. In his publication designed to show that the current standards for protein requirements were much in excess, Hindhede [1913] refers briefly to the work of Jaffa [1901] on fruitarians in California. The group examined was made up of two adult women and three children as shown in table XI.

The adults had lived on fruit for the past 7 years as had the children except during babyhood. The family ate two meals a day. The first was at 10 a.m. consisting of nuts and fruit and the second at 5 p.m. comprised fruit with honey and olive oil. As indicated in table XI, the persons involved were below average weight and were all of diminutive growth. The energy intake was also remarkably low. Nevertheless, it was claimed by the women that they were in better health and capable of more work than ever before. The children were adjudged to be healthy and active and unusually free from colds and other ailments. The evidence suggests further comparisons are needed to determine how far high calorie diets of today are conducive to a high standard of health and performance compared with a diet of lower energy intake adequately endowed with vitamins and minerals.

Further variations in diet customs are given by Pyke [1971]. These include eating insects, fresh or cooked, or eating maggots, with examples from Africa, Japan, China and Australia. He also touches on the effects of religion on dietary practices. Examples include the Hindu opposition towards eating flesh from cattle and that of the Muslim towards eating pig meat not to mention the Mosaic prohibition against the consumption of animals which do not chew their cud.

Orr and Gilks [1931] studied the diets of the Kikuyu and the Masai in Africa. The Kikuyu were a settled agricultural people living mainly on a vegetarian diet composed of cereals, tubers, legumes, plantain and green vegetables. Their neighbours, the Masai, were a pastoral community. They ate maize, bananas, beans and cereals. They consumed also milk and the blood of cattle which they drew without harm to the animal from time to time. Eventually the meat from the animals was eaten.

The Kikuyu in their predominantly carbohydrate diet were observed by Orr and Gilks [1931] to be lethargic, lacking in stamina and subject to disease. The Masai were on average 5 inches taller, 23 pounds heavier, and had 50% greater muscular strength. Bone defects, dental decay, anaemia, ulcers and bronchitis were more common among Kikuyu than the Masai.

However, despite the above evidence indicating the virtues of animal protein the diets of the centenarians in the Andes (Southern Ecuadorians), the Caucasus (Abkhasians) and the Hunza people living in the Hunza region North of Pakistan were largely based on cereals, such as wheat, maize and buckwheat [Shorland, 1978]. The evidence indicates that the centenarians grow their own crops which they processed for their food without recourse to modern food technology. The use of whole grain flour together with fruit, vegetables and limited supplies of milk and cheese fits into the pattern of the best diets encountered by McCarrison [1944], as outlined in his Cantor Lectures to the Royal Society of Arts in London in 1936. Though the evidence as to the precise age of the centenarians may not have been established beyond all doubt, their health patterns appear to be superior to those of Western countries. As recorded by the Harvard gerontologist Leaf [1977], who led medical teams into the areas mentioned above, the life-styles of the centenarians resulted in superb body tone and cardiovascular condition with low blood pressure and low levels of serum cholesterol. Coronary attacks, broken bones and senility were very rare in these lands.

McCarrison [1944] considered that nowhere in the world is the profound effect of food on physical efficiency more strikingly exemplified than in India. Because of racial, religious, and geographical considerations the diets in different regions differ sharply in their characteristics. The races of northern India are essentially wheat-eaters, the wheat being eaten whole after being freshly ground into coarse flour and made into cakes called chapattis. This McCarrison [1944] considered preserves all the nutrients with which Nature has endowed it. The second most important ingredient of the diet in northern India was milk and the products of milk, the third was dhal (pulse) and the fourth vegetables and fruit. Some ate meat sparingly, if at all; others, such as the Pathans, used it in considerable quantity. In conformity with the composition of their diets the races of northern India were found to be the finest races of India so far as their physique was concerned.

A decline in nutritive value of the diets was observed on passing to the east, south and west of India, being especially apparent in certain parts of the Madras Presidency. This was attributed to the change in the staple diet from whole wheat to rice which is a poor cereal at best. When, as was the case, the rice was parboiled, milled or polished, often all three, much of the proteins, minerals and vitamins was removed. The Bengali or Madrassi uses relatively little milk or milk products, fresh vegetables or fruit and is by religion a non-meat eater. One does not therefore have to look far to understand the poor physique that, in general, characterises him.

To assess the relative value of Indian diets seven groups of young rats selected for uniformity of age, sex distribution and body weight were fed under similar conditions in roomy cages and under ideal hygiene conditions for a period of 140 days. This period was approximately equivalent to 12 years for humans. Each group was fed a diet that was prepared and cooked to correspond to that of the national diet being tested. As judged from the weights in each group the diets arranged themselves in the descending order of nutritive value as follows: Sikh, Pathan, Maharatta, Goorkha, Kanarese, Bengali and Madrassi. Needless to say, McCarrison's [1944] order of nutritive value is based on weight gains, the validity of which is discussed in section III.

The results indicated the adequacy of the diets of northern India, particularly that of the Sikhs which McCarrison [1944] decided to use as the diet for the stock rats comprising about 1,000 in number. Over a period of 5 years there was no case of illness, no death from natural causes, no maternal or infant mortality. During the same period several thousand deficiently fed rats developed a wide variety of ailments. He found that if the milk component of the diet was cut out and, especially, if in addition the consumption of fresh vegetables was limited, respiratory diseases, gastro-intestinal diseases, and maladies consequent on degenerative changes in mucous membranes and other structures of the body became frequent.

In addition to evaluating the diets of India, McCarrison [1944] also compared the Sikh diet with that of the diet commonly used by the poorer classes in England and Europe. The latter diet consisted of white bread, margarine, over-sweetened tea with a little milk, boiled cabbage and boiled potato, tinned meat and tinned jam of the cheaper sorts. The first thing noticed was that the well-fed group lived happily together and flourished, whereas the other group did not increase in weight. Growth was stunted and they lived unhappily together. By the 60th day they began to kill and eat the weaker ones, thus necessitating segregation. At 187 days, corresponding to 16 years in man, they were killed. On the poor class British diet gastro-intestinal diseases as well as diseases of the lung were much more common than in the well-fed group. The animals, in fact, fared little or no better than those fed on a diet in common use in Madras. The maladies they suffered were much the same. On the other hand, the group on the Sikh diet were virtually free from disease. The average initial body weights of the groups were 125 g and the final weights for the Sikh and the poor European diets being 185 and 118 g, respectively.

It was found that peptic ulcers were 58 times more common in the south of India than in the north where it is rare. The relationship to diet was again suggested by the peptic ulcer incidence in rats fed Sikh, Madrassi and Travancore diets of nil, 11 and 29%, respectively. It was further considered that gastric and duodenal ulcers which were also common in Britain would not occur with a perfectly constituted diet.

In general, it has been customary to set the vitamin and mineral deficiency diseases as separate entities. McCarrison [1944], using epidemiological evidence and animal experimentation, greatly broadened the connections between diet and disease patterns of the human. Unfortunately, today, momentum has been lost. No obvious attempts are being made to test national diets as to their suitability for health promotion.

In the present section it is shown that the diets for the majority of humans in historical times have been largely cereal-based with the wealthy having access to a more varied diet, including meat, fish, vegetables and fruit. The meat of prehistoric times would have contained aside from proteins mainly structural lipids providing PUFA, including eicosapentaenoic acid with presumably anti-atherosclerotic properties compared with the meat of today in which the protein has been partly replaced by depot and intramuscular fat. In addition, it appears that the structural lipids are now devoid of eicosapentaenoic acid.

With the discovery of the Americas the diet of the poor has been enriched to some extent by the inclusion of the potato supplemented in some cases by the inclusion of maize and as always the rich have benefited to a even greater extent. For the great majority in the developed world the diet of today is immensely varied in comparison with the past. Using as a basis the FAO [1971, 1984] Food Balance Sheets, it has been possible to divide the diets in common use into meat, milk, high-calorie wheat, low-calorie wheat, maize and rice groups. The meat, milk group has significantly higher proportions of meat and milk products and of sugar, oils and fats, but significantly lower proportions of cereals than the other groups. Further differentiation occurs through the nature of the cereal, i.e. whether wheat, maize or rice.

Using longevity at birth as a basis for evaluation of the nutritive value it is shown that the meat, milk groups now attain up to 80 years for the female and 74 years for the male as shown by Iceland. The data for Norway, Netherlands, Sweden, and Switzerland approach within 1 year the longevity achieved by the Icelandic people. Other dietary groups generally fall far short by several years the standard set by Iceland. However, Japan, with female life expectancy of 79 years and male expectancy at 74 years now ranks next to Iceland, and because of the rate of improvement in life expectancy could be expected to overtake the Icelandic achievement. This suggests that high level cereal diets supplemented by modest intakes of animal proteins may in fact be superior to the meat, milk diets of the West as indeed is indicated by the high cereal intake diets of centenarian countries. The high fish intakes in Japan and Iceland at 7.2 and 6.4% of the total calories may be a significant factor in promoting longevity.

In many countries the use of longevity at birth is impaired by the factor of high infant mortality. Thus, when the low-calorie wheat countries, such as Algeria, Tunisia and Chile, are compared with the meat, milk countries in terms of life expectancy after the age of 20 years, it is found that particularly in later years their life expectancies may rise to nearly double that of the meat, milk groups.

The fact that Iceland and many other countries with high life expectancies depend on sugar and fat as their main dietary component runs counter to the national dietary goals such as those set by the US Senate Select Committee on Nutrition and Human Needs [1977]. The sugar component now reaches 55 kg/head/year in Iceland compared with negligible amounts a century ago. Associated with this increase diabetes, which was formerly rare, has now become prevalent [Cleave and Campbell, 1966]. The question could well be asked as to whether or not the observance of the dietary goals would further improve the health of these countries and whether it is not more important to maintain a high level of fish consumption. Iceland, in showing the lowest intakes of vegetables, fruit and pulses (tables I–IX), again runs counter to national dietary goals.

The great range and diversity of diets covered in this section suggest that good standards of health are achievable on meat, milk diets but that the levels of animal fat should be lowered and the proportions of fish should be raised to counter the problem of CHD. The Japanese experience of supplementing the rice diet which provides a relatively poor quality protein with relatively minor amounts of meat and dairy products along with relatively high levels of fish suggests that such diets are at least equivalent to the meat, milk diets. However, neither the meat, milk nor the rice diet as described above gave evidence of high life expectancies in later years found in low-calorie wheat or corn diets. The testing of such diets under the relatively high standard conditions of the West involving low infant mortality and adequate hygiene has not been carried out. Likewise, vegetarian diets comprising root crops, coconut or fruit, although seemingly possible as healthy alternatives, have not been adequately tested. As pointed out by Kummerow [1985] using USA as the model the amount of vegetables, fruit and milk that would be required for everyone to become a vegetarian is not available for 218 million Americans 365 days/year. Diets, as recently shown by Japanese experience, alter markedly such properties as height, not to mention physiological characteristics which as described in section IV include the onset of maturity, lactation capability and menstruation. Until the human race knows precisely what is desirable it is not feasible to prescribe what is needed in terms of dietary modification.

In most countries the role of government health regulations relating to food seems to be limited to the question of contamination by toxic substances, such as heavy metals, bacteria or pesticides. Whatever foods are placed on the markets provided they have been in use over the years regardless of the level of processing are deemed safe. Dietary goals recommend limitations on levels of salt and sugar but no control is imposed by health regulations.

As indicated by McCarrison [1944] at the time of his investigations, the diseases comprising those of the digestive system and of the respiratory system amounted in England and Wales to about one third of all recorded diseases with heart disease amounting to less than 2% of the total. If sufferers from purely tropical diseases were removed from the calculation, he assessed that diseases of the two systems mentioned would also account for one third of all sickness in Madras. McCarrison [1944] established that the poor diet was associated with the occurrence of the diseases of the digestive and respiratory systems. It could be similarly argued that with today's knowledge of the relationships between diet and CHD, it would be possible to reduce the level of CHD which appears to be related to affluence rather than to poverty. The costly investigations into CHD, such as those of Dayton et al. [1969], have reduced serum cholesterol levels by replacing in the Western diet the saturated animal fat with polyunsaturated oil rich in linoleic acid. Success has been achieved in lowering serum cholesterol levels but it now seems likely that linoleic acid which is the ultimate precursor of thromboxane would unfavourably alter the thromboxane/PGI_2 ratio that is the clotting/anticlotting ratio. The process overall appeared to do little towards the prevention of the disease and nothing towards saving lives.

Today, dietary goals and dietary allowances are the subject of committee meetings rather than of experimentation. It would seem that with the meticulous collection of dietary data by FAO in the form of Food Balance Sheets on a worldwide basis that an up-to-date McCarrison should be evaluating the national diets by means of rat feeding experiments. It is recognised that rat results are not necessarily applicable to the human but they can provide guidelines in the design of an experiment to be applied to the human as opportunity arises. Unless information is thus collected it cannot be claimed that our knowledge of human nutrition is soundly based.

III. Recommended Daily Dietary Allowances

Shorland [1983a] scrutinised the RDA on the basis of three main criteria: (1) the extent of changes in RDA of the US National Research Council's Food and Nutrition Board between successive six yearly revisions; (2) lack of agreement between the US and other national RDA, and (3) lack of relationship between conformity with RDA and health patterns. Data for discussion of relevant criteria are collected together in table XII. Further

Table XII. Per capita intake of nutrients in New Zealand, Algeria, Tunisia and Nicaragua compared with the US RDA values for 18- to 22-year-old males [Shorland, 1978]

US RDA values	1968	1974	1980	New Zealand	Algeria	Tunisia	Nicaragua
Kcal	2,800	3,000	2,900	3,454	1,892	2,205	2,253
Protein, g	60	54	56	110	56	63	61
Fat, g		117[1]		154	29	55	49
Calcium, mg	800	800	800	1,110	148	242	396
Phosphorus, mg	800	800	800	2,044	316	557	900
Magnesium, mg	400	350	350	389	113	156	275
Iron, mg	10	10	10	26	14	16	20
Zinc, mg		15	15	16	3	4	9
Iodine, μg	140		150				
Vitamin A, IU	5,000	5,000	1,000[2]	8,235	627	3,000	700
Vitamin D, IU	400	400	10[3]	64	5	6	15
Vitamin E, IU	30	15	10	12	11	12	14
Thiamine, mg	1.4	1.5	1.5	2.0	1.7	2.2	3.1
Riboflavin, mg	1.6	1.8	1.7	2.5	0.8	1.3	2.8
Niacin, g	18	20	19	33	21	26	32
Vitamin C, mg	60	45	60	163	56	97	113
Vitamin B_6, mg	2.0	2.0	2.2	3.0	1.8	1.3	3.1
Vitamin B_{12}, μg	5.0	3.0	3.0	8.7	0.7	1.0	1.9
Folacin, μg	400	400	400	200	151	181	217

1 Suggested.
2 Expressed as retinol equivalents = 1 μg retinol or 6 μg β-carotene.
3 10 μg cholecalciferol = 400 IU vitamin D.

support for the present author's contentions is provided by the postponement of the 1986 US RDA edition because of an impass between the Committee of the US National Research Council Food and Nutrition Board and the appointed scientific reviewers. The Committee has realised that its primary focus on the avoidance of nutritional deficiencies may be neither sufficient nor appropriate. There has been during the past 5 years a deepening understanding of the interplay between nutritional factors and health, especially the importance of these factors in the ageing process and the susceptibility to chronic diseases. Neither the present Committee nor the Committee responsible for the previous edition was asked to consider these issues. Nonetheless, reviews of the report strikingly suggest that the scientific developments in the past 5 years relating nutrition to health should be considered [Press, 1985].

RDA are taken seriously by dieticians and nutritionists in the belief that their use will lead to the formulation of an ideal diet. Unfortunately, exactly what the RDA are recommended for is not given. Is it for longevity, athletics, body building or to ensure freedom from disease? In much of the testing for the optimum level of nutrients weanling rats are used, the optimum level being deemed to coincide with the maximum growth rate. Such a criterion is applicable to meat production where the objectives, such as the production from the hatched egg of a number 6 chicken in the shortest possible time, are straight forward. The nutrient levels required for this purpose are known and applied. For the human the objectives are not clearly defined, hence the required diets cannot be specified [Shorland, 1983b]. There seems little doubt that the objective in New Zealand, as perhaps elsewhere, was to fatten the baby as if the dinner plate was in line with poultry nutrition. This is no longer advocated. It would appear that there are no agreed guidelines for human nutrition. Nevertheless, I believe that few would disagree that the objective of human nutrition is to achieve a long and useful life free from ill health. As reviewed by Shorland [1978, 1979], the maximum growth rate diet would not achieve this objective. In all the many species tested, including insects, life expectancy is increased by as much as nearly 50% by dietary restriction compared with full feeding. In humans dietary restriction is automatically achieved without experiencing hunger because of stomach size if the diet is based on bulky foods such as fruit, vegetables and potatoes which contain less than 1 kcal/g. In contrast, refined high-calorie foods made up of white flour, sugar and fat separately or in combination, the products of food technology, allow overeating. Health is difficult to define but as an index to the problem one can measure the causes of death data. As indicated earlier now that the infections diseases and deficiency diseases are to considerable extent under control life expectancy may also be used as an index of health.

Table XII compares three successive revisions of the US Food and Nutrition Board with the mean per capita intakes of nutrients in New Zealand and with those of three other countries characterised by high life expectancy after correction for infant mortality. The intakes of nutrients have been calculated from the FAO [1971] Food Balance Sheets in association with the food composition tables of McCance and Widdowson [1960] as previously described by Shorland [1978].

Changes in RDA with Successive Revisions

It is significant that changes in RDA in successive six yearly revisions by the Food and Nutrition Board of the US Academy of Sciences are determined by consensus opinions of committees rather than by experiment. The RDA for vitamin E which has no proven value for humans, though it has an antisterility function in rats, has moved down from 30 mg in 1968 to 10 mg in 1980. Its protective value in maintaining tissue integrity is indicated by early work [Dam, 1944] which showed that rats fed a fatally low protein diet survived only 75.0 days on a diet free from vitamin E compared with 93.6 days when supplemented with vitamin E.

That there could be other functions besides antisterility and anti-oxidant activity for vitamin E is indicated by Shorland et al. [1981] at Michigan State University. It was found that veal calves fed milk in which the butterfat was replaced by coconut oil contained in their depot fats highly significantly greater levels of stearic acid (18:0) but correspondingly lower levels of lauric (12:0), myristic (14:0), and palmitic (16:0) acids when supplemented with vitamin E. It is postulated that vitamin E may be involved in the chain extension of lauric, myristic and palmitic acids to form stearic acid. Therefore it could well be that the setting of a reliable RDA for vitamin E is not possible without a more complete understanding of its functions. In New Zealand, as elsewhere in the West, much (about 50%) of the vitamin E comes from wheat even though this cereal provides approximately only 25% of the total calories.

The RDA for vitamin C is shown to move down from 60 mg in 1968 to 45 mg in 1974 and then up to 60 mg in 1980. The fact that vitamin C has other functions beside the prevention of scurvy, such as its effect on cytochrome P-450 level and iron absorption, suggests that the RDA for this vitamin should also take into account its multi-functional nature.

Vitamin B_{12} over the period studied has moved down from an RDA of 5 to 3 μg. The fact that vegetarian diets in which vitamin B_{12} is absent support humans suggests that this vitamin is provided by microbial fermentation in the gut.

The RDA levels for vitamin A have remained essentially unchanged between successive revisions. However, whereas formerly the RDA for vitamin A was expressed as international units in 1980, the RDA is shown as retinol equivalents = 1 μg retinol or 6 μg β-carotene. As with the other vitamins discussed, it appears that vitamin A has many functions, some of which because of their long-term nature would not be taken into account in determining the RDA level. Furthermore, whereas vitamin A is known to be toxic at high levels, β-carotene is generally believed to be innocuous.

As reviewed by Goodman [1984], retinoids exert powerful effects on cell growth and cell division, suggesting that they prevent or inhibit the transformation of normal cells to cancer cells. Further, Lichti and Yuspa [1985] claim that the retinoids as shown by animal studies are most effective as anticarcinogens in the 'post-initiation portion of carcinogenesis'.

Epidemiological studies by Wald et al. [1980] indicate that low serum vitamin A levels are associated with the risk of developing cancer. However, Willett et al. [1984] in a relatively shorter-term study (5 years compared with 16 years) found no such association.

Shekelle et al. [1981] reported an inverse relationship between dietary carotenoids and development of lung cancer over a period of 19 years. β-Carotene exerts an effect as a 'quencher' of oxidative radicals that may be of biological relevance. Clearly, the levels of vitamin A appropriate to the prevention of cancer should be more accurately determined so that this factor can be incorporated into future RDA.

Variations in RDA between Nations

The constancy of some RDA over periods of six yearly revisions could give the impression that certainty has been reached. However, as indicated by Hughes [1971], the variations in RDA set by Canada, Japan, UK, USA and FRG for the young adult male cover a wide range. The constant value of 800 mg calcium set by USA may be compared with 500 mg set by Canada and UK. Even wider variation is shown for vitamin C. For Canada and UK the RDA is 30 mg compared with 75 mg for FRG. Similar lack of national agreement is shown for thiamine, riboflavin and niacin. Extreme differences cover a range for thiamine of 0.9 mg (Canada) to 1.7 mg (FRG) and for niacin 9 mg (Canada) to 18 mg (UK, USA and FRG).

The RDA for folacin in USA has remained constant at 400 μg but calculations based on FAO [1971] Food Balance Sheets and Food Composition Tables of McCance and Widdowson [1960] indicate that national diets as in New Zealand would provide no more than 200 μg, which is the RDA set in the UK. To raise the intake of folacin to 400 μg would require the dietary addition of about 200 g of lamb's liver. By seeking special dietary items, however, there is the risk of moving into the hypervitaminosis areas.

In the 1913 Mawson Antarctic expedition after the loss of the food supply down a crevasse, it became necessary to eat the Greenland huskies for food, the most edible portion being the liver. The ingestion of this organ gave rise to acutte vitamin A toxicity causing the death of a member of the team [Beckel, 1977].

The specific functions of some vitamins, such as folic acid, which is involved in the growth and reproduction of cells requiring the synthesis of thymine, the methylated pyrimidine for RNA, call for increased levels during pregnancy. Thus, the US RDA for folacin and iron are raised to twice the normal levels in this situation by supplementation. Justification for such increased levels is based on clinical evidence such as was found by Thompson and Pack [1980] concerning gingivitis in pregnancy.

Lack of Relationship between Conformity with RDA and Health Patterns

It is perhaps the discrepancies between the RDA and health patterns which indicate most markedly that RDA are not the total answer to human nutrition, which seems to have been assumed by many nutritionists and indeed seemed to be the basis of the Himsworth argument for abandoning nutrition research [Shorland, 1980]. As shown in table XII the mean levels of nutrients in the New Zealand diet are in excess of the RDA; except folacin, the levels of which are at least comparable with those of most Western diets. It could be expected, therefore, that compared with Nicaragua, Tunisia and Algeria where the levels of certain nutrients, such as calcium, zinc, magnesium and vitamin B_{12} and vitamin A are well below the RDA, the health in New Zealand would be superior. However, in these countries after the age of 20 years life expectancy is several years in excess of that found in New Zealand [Shorland, 1978] where the main causes of death (as elsewhere on the West) are CHD, cancer and cerebrovascular disease.

Of special concern is the high-protein RDA now set at 56 g which as discussed in the next section dealing with the protein saga has little relevance to the experimental evidence. The high levels of fat set in the RDA in 1974 amount to 35% total calories which is an excess of the 30% fat calories recommended by the US Senate Select Committee on Nutrition and Human Needs [1977]. The RDA seem to take no account of the fact that Eskimos in their natural environment, eating a high-calorie high-fat diet are relatively free from the Western type diseases as are populations in the developing countries, notably rural Africa where the diets are rich in dietary fibre [Burkitt and Trowell, 1975]. In fact, the question of dietary fibre is not addressed in the Setting of RDA though it is taken notice of in the recommendations of the US Senate Select Committee on Nutrition and Human Needs [1977] in terms of advocating the use of less refined foods, such as whole meal grain products together with vegetables and fruit. In short, the RDA do not encompass the recommendations of the above-mentioned Committee nor do they take fully into account, let alone explain, the anomalies introduced by the high-fat Eskimo diet and the foods which are low in fat but rich in dietary fibre as a means of preventing or lowering the incidence of the Western type diseases. The lack of attention to the requirements for essential fatty acids and their long chain polyunsaturated metabolites provides a further example of the defects in the current RDA system.

IV. The Protein Requirement Saga

Table XIII provides an outline of the salient points of the protein saga. With few exceptions the trend has been to promote the concept that relatively high levels of protein in the diet are desirable. This trend appears to have originated during the last century when Voit in Germany claimed without providing satisfactory experimental evidence that during muscular exertion protein is used up. To compensate for the loss of protein Voit considered that the working man required a daily allowance of 340 g beef [Hindhede, 1913]. Despite Hindhede's criticism, Voit's concepts gained widespread acceptance and his influence remains to some extent even to the present day.

Max Rubner, who with Voit and Atwater had been largely responsible for the era of energy metabolism, became advisor to the German army in World War I. Following the concepts of Voit he insisted that the army could not fight without the 340 g daily ration of beef. This meant that agricultural land normally used for grain and potatoes was diverted to meat production. Because it took four times as much land to feed a population on meat compared with grain and potatoes the food supply became inadequate and the war was drawn to a close earlier through widespread starvation than would otherwise have occurred [Mickelsen, 1964].

Preoccupation with protein became an important feature of the United Nations policy for feeding the third world as epitomised in the publication 'International Action to avert the Impending Protein Crisis' [United Nations, 1968]. McLaren [1974], who had worked on the problem, described the protein crisis under the heading of the 'Great Protein Fias-

the W.O. Atwater Lecture, Chittenden at Yale in 1904 challenged the ideas of Voit and his colleagues who had set the requirement of protein for heavy work as ranging from 145 to 165 g/day. Chittenden convinced a number of faculty members, including Mendel as well as a group of Yale athletes and a detachment from the US Army to participate in a low-protein diet over a period of 8 months. This near vegetarian diet provided 35–50 g protein per day. All participants were certified to be in good physical condition at the end of the study. One of the athletes was named the all-round Intercollegiate Champion of America during the dietary period.

Chittenden thought he had demonstrated that a protein intake of less than 50 g/day was not only nutritionally adequate but that there were economic, social and psychological benefits from this near-vegetarian regime. As pointed out by Hegsted [1985], Chittenden's work is never mentioned these days in reviews of protein requirements, but the hundreds of nitrogen balance trials that have been completed since then have not disproved his thesis.

It could also be claimed that the work of Hindhede [1913] on protein requirements using a diet based solely on potatoes, as mentioned in section II, has likewise been ignored. The nitrogen balance records indicate the protein adequacy even though the intake was about 21 g protein per day. Hindhede's results were confirmed by Kon and Klein [1928]. The largely vegetarian diet of the Pari tribe of the Eastern Highlands of New Guinea [Hipsley and Kirk, 1965] mentioned previously also provided two levels of protein intake. This was associated with good health, the women lactating more effectively on about 22 g protein per day than many of their Caucasian counterparts living on high protein levels. These observations are consistent with those of Breirem et al. [1961], who reported that animals fed rations that do not produce maximum growth rate are superior in lactational performance to animals fed more liberal rations.

Coinciding with the dietary changes in the West involving partial replacement of wheat with animal protein there have been physiological changes. Such changes have already been noted in section II in connection with the recent small increases in meat and dairy product intakes in Japan. Over the past 70 years, 5- to 10-year-old children in England were found by Tanner [1962] to be 5–10 cm taller with an adult stature increase of 5 cm. Whereas full height was formerly not reached before 26 years it is now attained at 18 years [Morant, 1950]. The concept of the value of attaining full growth potential has been approved by such leading nutritionists as Leveille [1977].

The supernutrition of today based on animal protein has not only made us bigger but it has also hastened maturity so that the young are ready earlier for top-grade athletics, adult work and mature study. Other notable changes have been the onset of menstruation which has been reduced in time at the rate of 4 months per decade for the past 100 years [Tanner, 1962]. The relationship to supernutrition is again indicated by Bruch [1941] who concluded from a study of obese girls that puberty is hastened by overfeeding. However, as reviewed by Davidson and Passmore [1966] dietary restriction in all species tested including insects is associated with increased life expectancy. It cannot therefore be assumed, as recently implied by Kummerow [1985], that optimising the growth rate which is the basis of meat production necessarily provides the best model for human nutrition. The fast-grown domestic beef and sheep not only contain undesirably high levels of fat but also are lacking in eicosapentaenoic acid providing anti-atherogenic potential, whereas the less fatty wild ruminants contain in their lipids some 4% of this acid [Crawford et al., 1969].

In agreement with the effective lactational performance of the women of the Pari tribe on a sparse protein diet mentioned above, Breirem et al. [1961] reported that animals fed rations that do not produce maximum growth are superior in lactational performance to animals fed more liberal rations. Further, Ross [1959] found that rats fed high-calorie, high-protein diets, characteristic of the Western nutrition, showed early degeneration and lowered life expectancy. As reviewed previously [Shorland, 1979] the high plane of nutrition provided by the meat, milk diets of today may be an important factor in promoting the Western type diseases and premature ageing. In contrast, the centenarian populations remain vigorous through life.

From the many observations relating to protein nutrition, it may be concluded that the definitive experiment to determine the absolute requirements for the achievement of a long and useful life free from ill health has not been carried out. Hindhede's [1913] observations using the potato as the sole source of protein in a diet containing adequate caloric intake indicates that as little as 21 g protein per day is enough to secure a nitrogen balance over an extended period of 300 days. However, as reviewed by Markakis [1975], the potato protein in well endowed with essential amino acids. The need for higher protein levels therefore in the case of cereals, such as rice or wheat, which have lower levels of essential amino acids, such as lysine, is understandable. Thus, the recommendation of 45 g of protein per day by the Joint FAO-WHO Expert Group [1965] is not necessarily in conflict with Hindhede's [1913] observations if applied to a cereal diet.

As to the recommendations for the upper limits for protein for the human the situation is less clear, particularly in the case of the Western diets, where the caloric intake of nutrients provides an excess of energy requirements. The rapid growth associated with the Western high-protein diets may carry with it disadvantages, including lowered lactational ability, early senescence and perhaps an enhanced propensity to chronic diseases not to mention reduced life expectancy. The extent to which these disadvantages occur will require more definitive experimentation to decide. There remains unanswered the question as to whether a population living largely on fish, which is often low in fat and therefore mainly protein, is subject to the disadvantages just mentioned. If such disadvantages are not evident, can this be ascribed to such factors as the protective effect of the marine type of fat including that of eicosapentaenoic acid?

In the final assessment of the upper safe limits for protein intake, it may be necessary to define these in terms of the nature of the protein involved as well as in terms of other dietary components. The fact that plant and animal proteins have different properties in relation to their effects on serum cholesterol levels [Carroll, 1974] further indicates that in defining protein levels one needs to have regard not only to the level of protein but also to the nature of the protein involved. The future recommendations will therefore need to be more specifically defined than has been the case in the past.

Research into protein requirements for the human is hampered by the lack of recognition of the experimental evidence as it comes to hand. Oliver et al. [1977], for example, found that in the Montreal Olympics some teams continued to use diets that contained several times the protein (including especially animal protein) content of the typical national diets with a view to improved performance. In text books recent advances in protein nutrition are seldom mentioned. We find, for example, Moran et al. [1980] in dealing with environmental science and Orten and Neuhaus [1975] in describing human biochemistry continue to record the inadequacy of wheat and other plant proteins and to make the distinction between the first-class animal proteins and the second-class plant proteins. The fact that the results apply to the rat and not to the human is lost sight of.

The United Nation's policy of promoting the need for protein in the developing countries not only misinforms the public but is also the driving force behind scientists like myself taking up projects that have little to do with the solution of the world hunger problems. The International Biological Programme supported the publication 'Food Protein Sources' edited by N.W. Pirie, FRS [1975]. In it are collected some 26 papers including my own on the conversion of wool into edible protein. The theme is essentially to make more protein available for the Third World. Two questions may be asked: (1) Why seek more protein when the problem is a shortage of calories? (2) Why make protein concentrates from leaves and other plant sources, thereby removing dietary fibre which may be the most important component lacking in the context of developed world nutrition?

V. Coronary Heart Disease and Nutrition

Nature of Coronary Heart Disease

In CHD the basic abnormality is atherosclerosis. This affects the coronary arteries in particular but also involves the large and medium arteries in general. In this condition the arteries contain lipid material in the subintimal area with fibrosis and hyperplasia of the intima or inner layer and disorganisation of the internal lamina. There is a successive development from fatty streaks which are typically found in Western populations as early as the second and third decades of life, followed by atherosclerotic plaques through to ulcers. When there is an acute occlusion of the arteries through thrombus formation, the blood supply is cut off and the part of the heart muscle (myocardium) thus affected dies. Such an event is popularly known as a heart turn. Similar atherosclerotic abnormalities in other parts of the body, as in the head, give rise to a stroke, or to the dilation of an artery or aneurism or again to gangrene as in the foot.

As an indication of the current state of knowledge, we find that there remain those who doubt that CHD is caused by atherosclerosis per se but concede that it provides an infrastructure for CHD, myocardial infarction and sudden death. The critical process is considered to be the thrombotic occlusion of a coronary artery [Mitchell, 1985] and that in sudden death, often in association with plaque disruption, it is also the critical underlying event [Davies and Thomas, 1984]. As will be described later, thrombus formation is mediated by the nature of the dietary fat.

As outlined by Florey [1963], whereas infectious diseases have a common cause many chronic diseases including CHD have no such unifying thread. It is not surprising, therefore, that progress in the understanding of

CHD is difficult. Nevertheless, from a variety of sources there are important indications as to how the disease may be made less prevalent. The importance of CHD in the Western industrialised countries is indicated by the fact that it remains the main cause of death. That atherosclerosis should be found in the fragments of the aorta of Egyptian mummies dating from between 1500 BC and AD 525 is perhaps not surprising as the wealthy of Egypt would, as mentioned earlier, have had access to an affluent diet. These and other historical aspects have been touched on in a previous report [Royal Society of New Zealand, 1971] with which the present author was associated.

Saturated Fat-Cholesterol Theory

It is not possible here to give a detailed account of CHD. The present aim is to discuss some of the current theories relating nutrition to the onset of the disease with a view to assessing their adequacy. The widely accepted theory of the relationship of diet to CHD follows the sequence:

High saturated fat levels in the diet → hypercholesterolaemia → atherosclerosis → heart attacks.

The epidemiological evidence for a relationship between high serum cholesterol levels and the incidence of CHD has been compelling. However, the attempts to establish the theory by lowering serum cholesterol levels in controlled experiments on humans by means of dietary modification or by drugs, such as clofibrate, have been encouraging but not entirely convincing. The Lipid Research Clinics Program [LCR-CPPT, 1984] has now established that a decrement in serum cholesterol induced by cholestyramine treatment in middle-aged men at risk correlates significantly with a reduction in CHD incidence. The diet theory of CHD causation has thus been strengthened. However, the problem that the death rate in the experimental group through other causes did not differ significantly from the control group remains. It is useful to indicate how the diet theory finds its place in the assessment of other competing hypotheses concerning the cause of CHD. In this connection the review of the Office of Home Economics [1982] states: 'Cigarette smoking is considered by many authorities to be potentially the major risk factor for CHD. The pooled results of several US studies [PPRG, 1978] suggest that one out of every three 40-year-old men who smoke 20 cigarettes or more per day will suffer a major heart attack before they reach the age of 65 years. Unanimity of opinion is less marked with regard to the role of dietary factors in CHD than is the case with cigarette smoking. Debate has ranged, for example over the significance of alcohol, salt, sugar and cereal fibre. The principal debate in the context of diet and CHD has centered, however, on the contention that diets rich in saturated fats are a cause of elevated levels of serum cholesterol and that the latter constitute a major risk factor for CHD. Support for the hypothesis may be drawn from epidemiological investigation. Intercountry comparisons have revealed positive associations between CHD mortality rates and both serum cholesterol and certain dietary factors, particularly the proportion of energy derived from saturated fats. Positive associations have also been demonstrated between the latter and serum cholesterol concentrations. Intranational studies have similarly established that for individuals the risk of subsequent CHD increases directly with plasma cholesterol levels: the risk for men in the top quintile of cholesterol distribution is 2.4 times that in the lowest two quintiles [PPRG, 1978]. But surveys within communities have generally failed to relate disparities in plasma cholesterol concentrations between individuals to difference in dietary intakes [Morris et al., 1963; Kannel and Gordon, 1970].'

The explanation of serum cholesterol elevation by high saturated fat levels lies in the pathways of utilisation of acetylcoenzyme A (acetyl-CoA) which arises from the metabolism of fats, carbohydrates and proteins. As shown in figure 3, acetyl-CoA thus formed may (1) enter the citric acid cycle for degradation to CO_2 and H_2O, (2) combine with CO_2, under the influence of acetyl-CoA carboxylase to form malonyl-CoA. Malonyl-CoA under the influence of fatty acid synthetase condenses with acetyl-CoA which, with the loss of CO_2, forms acetoacetyl-CoA. With the successive head-to-tail addition of six further malonyl-CoA units followed by loss of CO_2, there is formed palmityl-CoA, or (3) acetoacetyl-CoA may unite with acetyl-CoA to form mevalonic acid. Mevalonic acid is transformed with loss of CO_2 to isopentenyl pyrophosphate and dimethylallyl pyrophosphate to provide (C_5) isoprenoid units which, through successive condensations, elongate to squalene (C_{30}). This hydrocarbon cyclises to form the steroid ring structure leading to the biosynthesis of cholesterol.

The rate-limiting factor in fatty acid synthesis (the major pathway for acetyl-CoA) is the level of the enzyme acetyl-CoA carboxylase. A decrease of acetyl-CoA carboxylase levels by 50% may inhibit fatty acid synthesis by as much as 99% owing to concurrent dissociation of the enzyme which is reactivated by citrate. Bortz and Lynen [1963] found that long chain fatty acids, such as palmitic acid, inhibit acetyl-CoA carboxylase activity and are competitive in regard to citrate. Under these circumstances more

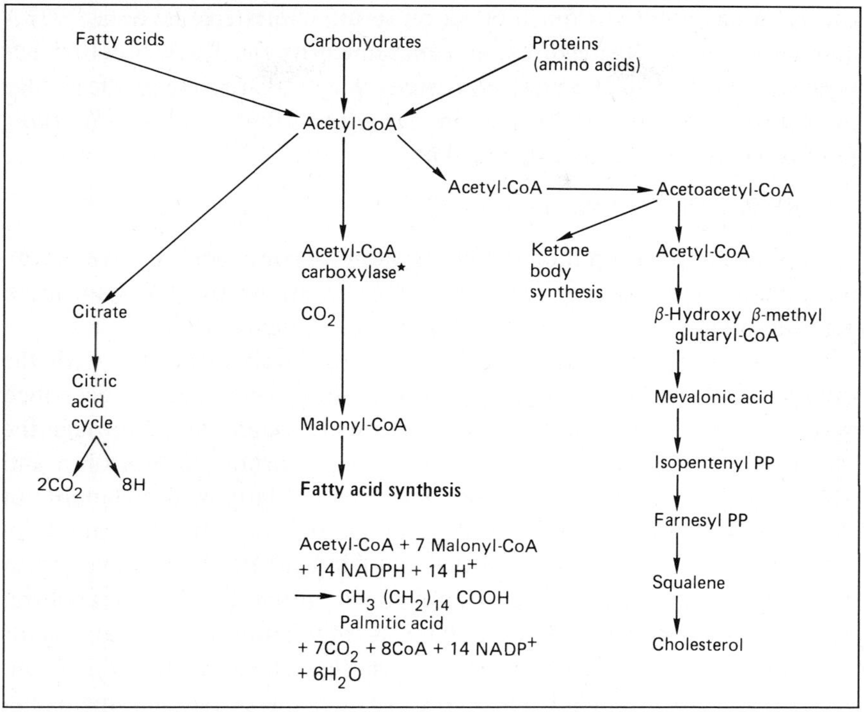

Fig. 3. Major pathways in the formation and utilisation of acetyl-CoA. * Denotes rate-limiting step.

acetyl-CoA will be directed towards cholesterol synthesis via the mevalonic acid pathway as shown in figure 3. Thus, saturated fatty acids, such as palmitic acid, elevate serum cholesterol levels by promoting cholesterol synthesis. In contrast PUFA, such as linoleic acid, lower serum cholesterol levels. As shown by Gerson et al. [1957] this is achieved by altering the distribution of cholesterol whereby more cholesterol is taken up in the tissues reducing the levels in the blood.

As a guide to the effects of saturated fatty acids and PUFA on serum cholesterol levels, Keys et al. [1957] developed the following predictive equation:

$$\Delta\text{Cholesterol} = 2.74\ \Delta S - 1.31\ \Delta P.$$

Where ΔS and ΔP are the changes in the percentage calories derived respectively from saturated fatty acids and PUFA. Saturated fatty acids are shown to have twice as much effect on serum cholesterol levels as PUFA and act in the opposite direction. Subsequently, the Keys equation has been refined to include dietary cholesterol where ΔC represents the change in dietary cholesterol expressed in decigrams [Report of the Working Group on Arteriosclerosis, 1981]. Thus:

$$\Delta \text{Cholesterol} = 2.16\ \Delta S - 1.65P + 6.77\ \Delta C.$$

Contrary to popular opinion dietary cholesterol contributes on average no more than 10% to serum cholesterol concentrations and the association between dietary cholesterol and CHD is weak [Oliver, 1976].

Whereas the increased serum cholesterol levels associated with the intake of dietary saturated fatty acids are readily explainable, as described above, the mechanism of lowering of serum cholesterol levels through the intake of PUFA is still somewhat obscure. According to Horrobin and Manku [1983] γ-linolenic acid, the first essential fatty acid metabolite of linoleic acid, has cholesterol-lowering actions about 170 times greater than the parent molecule, suggesting that linoleic acid must be converted to γ-linolenic acid to exert its desirable effects on cholesterol metabolism. Ageing, sex, diabetes mellitus, alcohol, catecholamines, *trans* fatty acids and saturated fats can all modulate the γ6-desaturase enzyme which converts linoleic to γ-linolenic acid. This provides a possible unifying explanation for the actions of these known risk factors in cardiovascular disease. Consistent with the unifying explanation, arachidonic acid, an essential fatty acid metabolite, has a much greater serum cholesterol lowering effect than linoleic acid [Kingsbury et al., 1961].

Dietary Control of Coronary Heart Disease

Attempts to control CHD experimentally by lowering serum cholesterol in apparently healthy humans at risk, notably males aged 50 years and over, in which the required conditions of randomisation and of double-blind techniques have been met, are few in number. Three such trials preceding the US Lipid Research Clinics Coronary Primary Prevention Trial [LRC-CPPT, 1984] have been reported thus: (1) The Los Angeles Veterans' Home involving 846 males [Dayton et al., 1969] in which serum cholesterol levels were reduced in the trial group by replacement of the saturated fats (40% of the total calories) in the control group by polyunsaturated oils. The trial lasted 7 years. (2) Helsinki Mental Hospital Study [Miettinen et al., 1972] involved 922 patients. As above the saturated fats of the control group were replaced in the trial group by polyunsaturated oils to lower serum cholesterol levels. The experiment continued for 12 years and included a cross-over design. (3) WHO trial. Serum cholesterol was lowered by clofibrate over a 5-year period [Committee of Principal Investigators, 1980]. This was the largest experiment yet conducted on CHD with more than 15,000 men at risk.

The principal findings from these trials include (1) a reduction in serum cholesterol levels of 9–15%; (2) a significant reduction in non-fatal myocardial infarctions in two of the trials but a non-significant result though a similar trend in the Los Angeles experiment; (3) in all trials there was no significant reduction in fatal myocardial infarction; (4) the increased number of non-CHD deaths in the trial groups resulted in a non-significant difference in death rates. Oliver [1981] concluded that the lipid hypothesis had been partly proved and that the case for lowering high serum cholesterol levels in otherwise healthy young men was strong. The non-CHD mortality increase in the trial groups was a cause for concern.

The recently completed LRC-CCPT [1984] experiment extended the evidence in favour of lowering serum cholesterol levels to control CHD. In the experiment 3,806 asymptomatic middle-aged men with primary hypercholesterolaemia were divided into a control group and an experimental group using the double-blind technique with cholestyramine resin which absorbs cholesterol to reduce serum cholesterol levels. The cholestyramine group experienced average plasma total cholesterol (TC) and low-density lipoprotein (LDC-C) reductions of 13.4 and 20.3%, respectively, which were 8.5 and 12.5% greater reductions than those obtained in the placebo group over the 7-year period. The cholestyramine group experienced a significant reduction of 24% definite CHD deaths and of 19% non-fatal myocardial infarctions. The risk of death was only slightly but not significantly reduced in the cholestyramine group. The non-CHD deaths in the placebo group totalled 27 compared with 36 in the cholestyramine group, the differences being mainly attributed to accidents, homicide and suicide amounting to 11 in the cholestyramine group compared with 4 in the placebo group.

In commenting on the violent and accidental deaths the authors consider that as no plausible connection could be established between cholestyramine treatment and violent or accidental deaths it is difficult to conclude that this could be anything but a chance occurrence. However, as other trials involving the control of CHD by reduction of serum cholesterol levels by means of polyunsaturated oils or by drugs gave a similar result, doubt may be expressed on the validity of the LRC-CPPT [1984] conclusion. This does not necessarily endorse the conclusion by Oliver [1985] that all intervention trials based on drugs or diet would show an increase in non-cardiovascular deaths. It is conceivable, for example, that diets which restrict fat intake, as in the Pritikin [1979] diet described below, may be conducive to longevity as well as to the prevention of CHD.

Comparing the LRC-CCPT with other clinical trials, the results of 8 of the 11 studies closely fit the regression line which indicates a reduction in CHD of 15.3% for diet and of 20.9% for drug treatment, respectively, per 10% decrement in TC level.

The LRC-CCPT results show that cholesterol lowering has saved 12 deaths in a population of 1,900 leaving 32 CHD fatalities for which the treatment was of no avail. When one adds another 9 non-coronary deaths to the group treated with cholestyramine, the difference between the control and the experimental groups falls to 3. The question arises as to the effectiveness of the experiment in practical terms and of the theory upon which it is based.

As found by Pritikin [1979] in his objective to eliminate atherosclerosis and other degenerative diseases by means of diet and exercise, it is possible to reduce serum cholesterol levels more substantially than in the LRC-CPPT experiment. Further, the dietary means include a reduction in fat levels rather than by the use of high levels of polyunsaturated oils which appear to increase the risk of cancer [Committee on Diet, Nutrition and Cancer, 1982]. The conflict between cancer causation and CHD control through polyunsaturated oils is also referred to by Morrison [1983] (table XIV).

The Pritikin [1979] diet contains 5–10% fat, 10–15% protein and 80% carbohydrate compared with the average US diet made up of 40–45% fat, 15–20% protein and 40–45% carbohydrate expressed on the basis of total calories. It was found during a 26-day course involving 900 patients that the serum cholesterol levels fell from 235 to 175 mg/100 ml or 25% compared with a mean of 8% for the cholestyramine resin treatment. That the Pritikin diet is effective is suggested by the fact that Pritikin himself was afflicted by a heart attack some 30 years ago when he subjected himself to his diet and exercise programme. He died last year. The postmortem report published by Hubbard et al. [1985] states: 'In a man of 69 years old, the near absence of atherosclerosis and the complete absence of its effects are remarkable. In 1958, Mr. Pritikin had a malignant lymphoma. He died from this problem in February 1985 after several complications of therapy. Whereas in December 1955 his serum cholesterol was high at 280 mg/100

Table XIV. Pritikin [1979] list of foods to use and to avoid (abbreviated)

Category	Foods to use	Foods to avoid
Fats, oils, sugars		avoid
Poultry, fish, meat	lean fish, meat (limit to 100 g/day)	fatty meat
Dairy foods	non-fat milk (limit to 230 g/day)	
Eggs	7 per week maximum	
Beans, peas, nuts, seeds	limit 680 g/week chestnuts	soybeans all other nuts
Vegetables	limit those high in oxalic acid: spinach, rhubarb	
Fruits	5 servings/day	cooked, canned or frozen with added sugar
Grains	all whole or lightly milled grains (unlimited quantity)	extracted wheat germ
Salt	limit salt intake to 3–4 g by eliminating table salt	
Beverages	mineral water, carbonated water, milk	alcoholic beverages, coffee, tea, cococola

ml the later readings presumably following the effects of his diet. By 1958 it had fallen below 200 and by November 1984 it had fallen to the very low value of 94.'

The saturated fat-cholesterol theory of the causation of atherosclerosis has been shown to have some relevance to CHD but the evidence includes certain unsatisfactory features, such as the increased non-coronary death rate which requires more adequate explanation. The theory also tends to obscure the effect of other dietary components, such as notably the effect of the nature of the protein on serum cholesterol levels. In the rabbit for example, Hamilton and Carroll [1976] found that semisynthetic diets containing animal proteins, such as casein, gave higher plasma cholesterol levels than did those from plants. Epidemiological data on human populations show that mortality from CHD is correlated as strongly with animal protein intake as with dietary fat [Connor and Connor, 1972; Yudkin,

1957]. It should be pointed out, however, that the correlation between CHD incidence and protein level is counterindicated by the fact that the protein level in the traditional diet of the Eskimo who was relatively unaffected by CHD was several times greater than in the meat, milk countries with a high CHD incidence.

The Significance of Thrombosis in Coronary Heart Disease and Its Prevention

In reviewing the literature on CHD the present author has been impressed by the significance of the thrombus or clot in the coronary arteries as the prime cause of a heart attack. Atherosclerosis occurs generally in mammals and birds but, under natural conditions, with the exception of primates, the formation of a thrombus is extremely rare [Finlayson et al., 1962]. In recent years there has been considerable progress in the understanding of the factors which control thrombus formation. These factors involve the prostaglandins which are produced in nanogram quantities from the long chain PUFA present in the phospholipids of cell membranes. Some of these substances contract and others relax smooth muscle, making possible induction of labour at term or first-trimester abortion. Some affect blood pressure. Of interest to the present topic, however, is the fact that prostaglandins can also promote or retard platelet aggregation or blood clotting. The practical issue in the present context is that the composition of the long chain PUFA determines whether or not the prostaglandins formed favour or retard the clotting process. There is now considerable epidemiological evidence to show that populations having access to marine sources of food are protected against CHD because of their intake of certain PUFA, such as eicosapentaenoic acid, mentioned earlier in connection with the Eskimo diet. Before considering in detail the relationships between the long chain PUFA and prostaglandin synthesis, a brief survey of epidemiological evidence will now be given.

Epidemiological Evidence

As summarised in the Lancet [1983], the Eskimos on their traditional marine type diet were free of chronic degenerative diseases, such as CHD, cancer, diabetes, diverticulitis, ulcerative colitis and rheumatoid arthritis. The more recent records (1950–1974) of a hospital in Upernavik, Greenland, involving a population of whalers and sealers show changes. Kroman and Green [1980] compared these records with those of Denmark and found higher levels of apoplexy and epilepsy and similar levels of cancer but of different types. The near absence of acute myocardial infarction (CHD) and of diabetes mellitus, however, in view of the increasing European way of life with access to Danish food was considered remarkable. The importance of the marine type diet is further indicated by the low death rates from CHD in Japan [Keys, 1980]. This is attributed by Kromhout et al. [1985] to the high per capita intake of fish estimated at about 100 g/day, which is much higher than in the West. The lowest death rates are found on the island of Okinawa where fish consumption is about twice as high as on the mainland [Kagawa et al., 1982]. Similarly, Kromhout et al. [1985], quoting unpublished data, indicated that mortality from CHD was significantly lower in the fishing village than in the farming area in Japan.

Recent studies by Bang et al. [1980] provide a further comparison between the traditional Eskimo diet and that of today's Westernised Eskimo living in the settlement of Idlorssuit in northwestern Greenland. The Eskimo diet of 1855, which was essentially carnivorous, was estimated at 377 g protein, 59 g carbohydrate, and 162 g fat per person per day, corresponding to 47.1, 7.4 and 45.5%, respectively, of the total calories. In the 1976 survey made up from 50 Greenlander fishermen and/or hunters and their wives, the diets contained 23% protein, 39% carbohydrate and 38% fat based on the total calories. To the intake of marine food (whale and seal meat) at about 400 g/person/day there was now added 700 kcal sugar, 447 kcal cereals (mainly white flour) and 37 kcal potatoes. Despite the drop in protein intake to half that of the traditional eskimo, it was still double that of the average Dane consuming the meat, milk products diet. The outstanding difference concerned the high level of PUFA in the dietary fat of the Eskimo compared with that of the Dane (19.2 versus 12.7%) with high levels of eicosapentaenoic acid (4.6 versus 0.5%). Despite the partial Westernisation of the Greenland diet, CHD comprised only 3.5% of the total deaths even though the life span was more than 60 years. Eskimos were seldom found to be obese, hypertension was uncommon and diabetes mellitus unknown, whereas most Eskimos were heavy cigarette smokers. This contrasts with Iceland where as earlier mentioned there was a high incidence of diabetes associated with a high sugar intake. Smoking is regarded as a major CHD risk factor but as recorded by Keys [1980]: 'Japan had the highest proportion of heavy smokers ... However, the ten-year mortality could not be shown to be related to the smoking habits of these Japanese.' One could hypothesise from these data that if high levels of eicosapentaenoic acid are maintained through the marine type diet the commonly accepted risk factors of CHD are inhibited.

The Role of Long Chain Polyunsaturated Fatty Acids in Thrombosis

As shown in figure 4, the precursors of the long chain PUFA involved in prostaglandin synthesis are the dietary linoleic and α-linoleic acids. The basic pattern of PUFA is made up of double bonds separated by single methylenic groups (—CH=CH·CH$_2$·CH=CH—). The structures of PUFA are therefore defined by the position of the first double bond and conveniently described using linoleic acid as an example as follows: $C_{18:2\omega6}$. The number after the colon designates the number of double bonds, and the number following ω denotes the position of the first double bond from the methyl end of the fatty acid. Similarly, α-linolenic acid may be written $C_{18:3\omega3}$. As the chain extension occurs at the carboxyl end, the ω6 and ω3 positions remain intact during hepatic elongation and desaturation and the ω6 and ω3 series are not interconvertible.

In terrestrial animals the depot fats contain as a rule no appreciable amounts of C_{20} and C_{22} PUFA, the PUFA being represented typically by linoleic acid and sometimes with α-linolenic acid. These acids undergo desaturation and elongation in the liver as shown in figure 4 to give C_{20} and C_{22} PUFA. These long chain unsaturated fatty acids are largely confined to the phospholipids of the cell membranes where they appear to contribute to the local regulation of membrane microviscosity and more importantly they provide a source through the mediation of cyclo-oxygenases of prostaglandins. It is in this context that PUFA play a regulatory role in thrombosis.

In contrast, the fish and mammals that provide the traditional diet of the Eskimo depend for their depot fats ultimately on the phytoplankton which synthesise the marine type of fat containing as much as 40% C_{20} + C_{22} PUFA derived almost entirely from α-linolenic acid. Such acids therefore belong to the ω3 series. The depot fats consumed by Eskimos are thus of a uniform nature reflecting the pattern of the ingested fat.

The inclusion of the marine type of fat in the diet not only modifies the nature of the membrane lipids but also has a profound effect on the relative proportions of the prostaglandins produced from the long chain PUFA. In the absence of fish or other marine-based food, the main long chain PUFA will be arachidonic ($C_{20:4\omega6}$). The acid thus formed is stored in the membrane phospholipids to be released by phospholipase for conversion by cyclo-oxygenase into prostaglandin P_gG_2. From P_gG_2 the platelets synthesise as a metabolite thromboxane (TxA_2). TxA_2 is potently proaggregatory through its inhibitory effect on the membrane located enzyme, adenylate cyclase [Gorman, 1979]. It is proposed that the reduced supply of $C_{20:4\omega 6}$ and the inhibitory effect of $C_{20:5\omega 3}$ are factors responsible for inhibiting aggregation [Needleman et al., 1980].

Effect of Fish Oils on Platelet Aggregation, Membrane Lipid Composition, Blood Pressure and Eicosanoid Production

Siess et al. [1980] found that low-dose collagen-induced platelet aggregation was significantly reduced after one week of consumption of a high fish intake diet by volunteers. This was confirmed by Thorngren and Gustafson [1981] in a similar study over a period of 11 weeks. In addition the bleeding time was prolonged.

In other studies, platelet aggregation was lower in Japanese fishermen than in Japanese farmers [Hirai et al., 1980] and lower in Eskimos than in Danes and with increased bleeding times [Dyerberg and Bang, 1979]. Later studies by Sanders [1985] show that moderate intakes of fish oil not only alter membrane fatty acid composition but the bleeding time is also increased.

The blood pressure lowering effect in normotensive volunteers by a diet supplemented with fish oil has been described [Lorenz, 1983]. It has been shown by Singer et al. [1985] that a mackerel or a herring diet in which two cans of fish fillet were consumed daily over 2 weeks within a prescribed regimen produced markedly lower systolic and diastolic blood pressures in normotensives. In hypertensives and hyperlipaemic subjects only systolic blood pressure was significantly decreased. After the herring diet, which served as a control, changes in blood pressure were of a minor degree.

Fish oil supplements change not only the membrane fatty acid composition but also the composition of blood lipids. Bang and Dyerberg [1980] found that Eskimos living on traditional seafoods with 5 g eicosapentaenoic and 6 g docosahexaenoic acid in their daily diet have high levels of high-density lipoproteins, moderately low levels of low-density lipoproteins and very low levels of very low-density lipoproteins and low triglyceride levels in their blood compared with Eskimos living on a Western diet. The results are consistent with a low incidence of CHD in Eskimos.

The favourable dietary effects of fish oil are shown by Black et al. [1979] and by Culp et al. [1980] to extend to reducing cerebral infarction in cats and dogs, respectively.

Dietary fat source alters the fluidity of platelet membranes and hence the activity of all membrane-located enzymes and receptors involved in the aggregatory process. Hyslop and York [1980] found marked differences in the PUFA composition of membranes between lean and obese mice. The obese mice had significantly higher levels of $C_{22:6\omega3}$ with increased membrane fluidity and decreased activity of adenylate cyclase. Membrane fluidity may also affect TxA_2 levels. Cholesterol-enriched platelets produced twice as much TxA_2 as did control platelets. The data of Shattil and Cooper [1976] suggest that this is due to a decrease in membrane fluidity associated with an increased platelet cholesterol:phospholipid ratio. Clearly, hypercholesterolaemia has direct implications in both atherosclerosis and thrombosis.

Platelet aggregation and adhesion are mediated by prostaglandin metabolites (fig. 4). PGG_2, for example, forms TxA_2 which encourages platelet formation through its inhibitory effect on adenylate cyclase [Gorman, 1979]. PGI_2 is produced by arterial endothelial cells from arachidonic acid and inhibits platelet aggregation by its stimulatory effect on adenylate cyclase. The prevailing hypothesis is that the two prostaglandins have opposing influences on platelet aggregation [Moncada and Vane, 1979]. Healthy arterial tissue generates PGI_2 nearly twice as rapidly as arterial tissue with atherosclerosis ranging from fatty streaks to complicated lesions [Sinzinger et al., 1979]. On the other hand, drugs such as aspirin, indomethacin, and other anti-inflammatory drugs are potent inhibitors of cyclo-oxygenase involved in the conversion of arachidonic acid to cyclic endoperoxides are also anti-thrombotic agents [Mustard et al., 1980].

Eicosapentaenoic (20:5ω3) acid present in marine fats has been shown to be the precursor of TxA_3 and of PGI_3. TxA_3 has no platelet aggregatory effects in contrast to TxA_2. Dyerberg et al. [1978] therefore suggested that high levels of eicosapentaenoic acid and low levels or arachidonic acid may lead to an antithrombitic state in which active PGI_3 and inactive TxA_3 are formed. This explains the low rate of death from CHD amongst Eskimos. Evidence is also accumulating that people who ingest 4 g or more of eicosapentaenoic acid per day form TxA_3 and PGI_3.

The alternative hypothesis put forward by Hornstra et al. [1983] and Goodnight et al. [1981] that the low thrombogenicity of fish oils is mainly due to insufficient TxA_2 to maintain platelet aggregation discounts the importance of TxA_3 and PGI_3 in the process. Fischer and Weber [1983] reconciled the two hypotheses just mentioned by formulating that reduced platelet aggregatibility and increased bleeding times might be due to the formation of PGI_3 and TxA_3 in association with reduced synthesis of TxA_2.

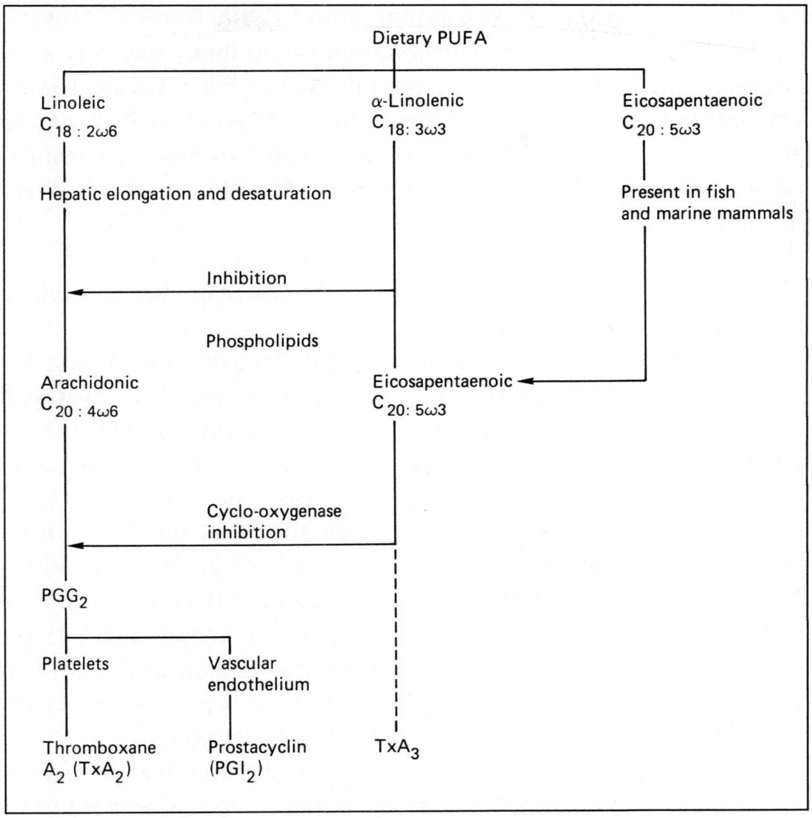

Fig. 4. Outline of the effects of ω3-PUFA on ω6-PUFA in relation to TxA_2 and prostacyclin levels.

On a more practical note Kromhout et al. [1985] made a longitudinal study over a period of 20 years beginning in 1960 in Zutphen, the Netherlands, based on 850 middle-aged men without CHD. During the period 78 died of CHD. Mortality from CHD was 50% lower ($p < 0.05$) amongst those who consumed at least 30 g fish per day than amongst those who did not eat fish. The risk for death from CHD decreased with increasing fish consumption. It was concluded that as little as one or two dishes of fish per week may be of preventative value against CHD. In the study the group with the highest fish intake consumed an average of 67 g fish per day equivalent to 0.4 g/day of eicosapentaenoic acid. The fact that the inverse relationship between fish consumption and death from CHD was seen over the whole range of fish consumption would imply that tiny amounts of eicosapentaenoic acid might have a protective effect against CHD. The fact that lean fish intake containing about 1.5% fat of which about 5% was eicosapentaenoic acid was also inversely related to mortality from CHD indicates that the relationship cannot be explained on the basis of eicosapentaenoic acid alone.

The Physiological Significance of the Structure of Polyunsaturated Fatty Acids

It was widely believed that linoleic acid alone provided totally for the observed effects of essential fatty acid requirements. The investigations into the effects of PUFA described above highlight differences between specific members of ω6- and ω3-polyunsaturated fatty acids, namely arachidonic and eicosapentaenoic on thrombosis. The fact that linoleic acid lowers serum cholesterol levels has been the basis for experiments on humans to lower the incidence of CHD. The results have shown indifferent effects in the control of CHD without significant differences in death rates between the control and experimental groups [Dayton et al., 1969]. In hindsight the result is perhaps not surprising as linoleic acid used to lower serum cholesterol is the precursor of arachidonic acid concerned with the formation of TxA_2 responsible for thrombus formation.

Studies on different types of ω3-fatty acids show that whereas 6.5 g α-linolenic acid taken daily by healthy volunteers for 2 weeks led to a very small increase in eicosapentaenoic acid, 2.5 g of preformed eicosapentaenoic acid produced a large increase in the proportion of eicosapentaenoic acid and a decrease in arachidonic acid in platelet lipids [Sanders and Younger, 1981].

The predominant effects of eicosapentaenoic and docosahexaenoic acid on eicosanoid production are probably as inhibitors of linoleic and arachidonic acid metabolism: they readily displace arachidonic acid from membrane lipids, inhibit the conversion of linoleic acid to arachidonic acid [Brenner and Peluffo, 1967] and are competitive inhibitors for cyclooxygenase [Lands et al., 1973; Corey et al., 1983].

Evidence for a specific requirement of α-linolenic acid for capuchin monkeys was obtained by feeding, as the sole source of fat, corn oil in a diet that was otherwise nutritionally complete. Corn oil is rich in linoleic acid but contains no α-linolenic acid. The monkeys lost hair, developed skin lesions and a fatty liver which was defined at biopsy, histologically and by biochemical analysis [Fiennes et al., 1973]. The condition was reversed by feeding linseed oil containing α-linolenic acid. Other instances of a specific need for a particular essential fatty acid are seen in nutritional encephalomalacia in chicks with diets low in tocopherol and containing linoleic acid. It was formerly believed to be due to lipid peroxidation [Machlin, 1963]. It is now known that the disease is dramatically arrested by replacement of linoleic acid with α-linolenic acid [Budowski et al., 1980]. A further instance of a requirement for PUFA of specific structures is the retinal rods of the rat. In this instance docosahexaenoic acid ($C_{22:6\omega 3}$) accounts for more than 60% of the phosphoglyceride fatty acids in the outer segments of the retinal rods where there is a requirement for rapid depolarisation and polarisation in response to individual photons of light; deficits of ($C_{22:6\omega 3}$) in the photoreceptors' decreased electrical transmission [Anderson et al., 1976].

Throughout the animal kingdom there is selection at various points of the fatty acids which find their way into the various lipid fractions including the triglycerides and the various categories of phospholipids as well as into the different parts of the body [Shorland, 1962], not to mention selective transport through the placenta of specific fatty acids that are transferred to the foetus. As reviewed by Crawford [1985], animals such as the dolphin and the zebra, with predominantly ω3-acids in the diet nevertheless have a high ratio of ω6/ω3 in the liver phospholipids. There is a trend for different species of mammals to have an approximately constant ratio of ω6/ω3-fatty acids in the structural lipids and liver of between 3:1 and 6:1 in their phosphoglycerides but nearer to 1:1 in the brain. A ratio of about 4.8:1 was found from random human milk samples taken from eight different countries. The brain stands out by exhibiting little variation in fatty acid composition between different species. Maternal essential fatty acid deficiency during gestation and lactation has been shown to reduce the levels of essential fatty acids in the brain of the offspring with permanent deficits in learning ability despite nutritional rehabilitation. The process of measuring the requirements of these acids by their effects, if any, on the growth rates of weanling rats is inappropriate. There will be a need to look for a particular physiological response such as was used to study the requirements of docosahexaenoic acid in the brain tissues of the rat based in this case on intelligence measurements as mentioned earlier in this section. It is further obvious that provision of the basic essential fatty acids, namely linoleic and α-linolenic acids, does not necessarily assure an adequate supply of the desired PUFA metabolite. This applies to the human requirement for eicosapentaenoic acids which, as in the case of the vitamins, must come preformed in the diet.

Nutrition can become a matter of conflict. For example, the use of a polyunsaturated oil diet to reduce serum cholesterol levels may conflict with the promotion of cancer. An Academy of Science Committee on Diet, Nutrition and Cancer [1982] considers that there is a relationship between diet and cancer justifying a recommendation for a reduction in fat consumption. As summarised by Hegsted [1983]: 'Briefly stated, the evidence is that there are many studies showing that animals fed a high-fat diet are more susceptible to both spontaneous cancer and cancers induced by a variety of carcinogens. These experimental data are consistent with epidemiologic data showing that a number of cancers – especially breast cancer and cancer of the lower bowel which are the two most prevalent cancers – are high in populations which consume large amounts of fat and the prevalence appears to be almost proportional to fat consumption. Whereas CHD correlates best with saturated fat and cholesterol consumption, the cancer data are much better correlated with total fat consumption.' However, as reviewed by Jansen [1982], none of the data discussed proved that dietary habits were responsible for the larger part of the current cancer incidence in developed countries. Nevertheless, Jansen [1982] considered there was good evidence to indicate the possibility of importantly reducing cancer incidence by possibly simple modifications of the diet; such measures might be as simple as yet to be specified anti-oxidants to yet unidentified fats. Ames [1983], in a review on oxygen radicals and degenerative diseases, considers that the human diet contains a great variety of natural mutagens and carcinogens which may act through the generation of oxygen radicals. Such radicals may also play a role as endogenous initiators of degenerative processes, such as DNA damage and mutation, that may be related to cancer, heart disease and ageing. One may therefore speculate that the earlier comment of Florey [1963] to the effect that the chronic diseases had as then no unifying thread to connect them may now find a unifying thread in the degenerative processes relating to the action of oxygen radicals.

The present author considers that if the Eskimo living on the traditional diet with high levels of fat is not susceptible to cancer, the Academy of Science Committee recommendation mentioned above is in conflict with the epidemiological evidence. It may well be that it is not so much the level of fat involved but that it relates to the fatty acid components present. Again the observations of Burkitt and Trowell [1975] on the inverse relationship between dietary fibre levels and the Western type diseases, including CHD and cancer, do not explain the absence of these diseases in the Eskimo living on a traditional diet. In terms of conventional knowledge one could use the Pritikin low-fat diet or the high-fat diet of the Eskimo as a means of prevention of these diseases. Our knowledge of human nutrition is moving in the direction of the prevention of chronic diseases but until the underlying mechanisms of the disease processes are adequately explained it is clear that our knowledge of human nutrition is not soundly based.

VI. Other Nutritional Considerations

There are areas of concern in which the extent of nutritional involvement has not been clearly defined owing to lack of experimental proof. Such areas nevertheless by reason of animal experimentation and/or epidemiology appear to involve nutritional considerations. Included in these areas are nutritional distortion, longevity and behaviour. The first two topics only will be dealt with here as the American Dietetic Association [1985] consider that there is still a great need for scientifically sound research on the relationship of diet and nutrition to behaviour.

Nutritional Distortion

Nutritional distortion is here used to indicate the addition to the diet of a component which has been selectively removed from plant or animal tissues, such as fats and oils or sugar, or alternatively the component removed from the tissue, e.g. bran and the residue (white flour) is then incorporated into the diet. The extent of nutritional distortion in diets of the West is indicated in table I, which shows that oils and fats and sugar amount respectively to the addition of 19.0 ± 2.9 and 15.9 ± 2.0% of the total calories. In contrast, the levels of these components in the rice-eating countries fall respectively to 5.5 ± 2.9 and 5.1 ± 3.9% of the total calories with intermediate values shown for the other diets. In the Republic of Korea oils and fats and sugar provide respectively only 0.7% of the total calories. It is not possible to calculate the nutritional distortion caused by the removal of bran from cereals but an extraction rate of up to 70% for wheat is not uncommon, indicating that up to 30% of the product is removed. In the production of polished rice, which is commonly used in the East, there would also be a substantial change in composition from that of the whole rice. In the diets of the West cereals comprise (table I) 23.1 ± 2.5% but in the rice diets the levels rise (table VIII) to 68.3 ± 8.5%, offering considerable scope for nutritional distortion. Salt provides a further example of nutritional distortion which, according to Eckholm and Record [1977], continues in the industrialised countries at a level of at least 10 times the bodily needs.

In setting the US dietary goals the Senate Select Committee on Nutrition and Human Needs [1977] has recommended a reduction in fat consumption from 40 to 30% of the total calories. In the industrialised nations it is clear that the removal from the diet of oils and fats now added would achieve a reduction to about 20% of the total calories. The level of sugar intake would also fall as recommended if the processed foods of high caloric content including cakes, pastries and biscuits were removed from the diet.

The availability of sugar promotes its use in commercially produced food. Isaacson [1979] found that nearly all of 60 such foodstuffs contained added sugar. Examples with the percentage of added sugar in parentheses included canned fruit (6–8), yoghurt (10.5), biscuits (11.2), cakes and pies (32.2), sweetened condensed milk (45.3) and chocolate (69.0). Even higher levels are provided by jam at 69% [McCance and Widdowson, 1960].

Many of the conventional foods of the West are made up from white flour in combination with fat and sugar to make pastries, cakes, biscuits and puddings. Sometimes, as in chocolates, the components are largely fat and sugar or as in sweets largely sugar. The above-mentioned foods, along with fatty meat, provide important sources of calories (often with 3–5 kcal/g). Starling [1918] quoted by Longenecker [1944] recognised that the size of the stomach normally controlled the upper limit of intake. However, this mechanism failed if the food was made up of concentrated calories. It seems evident that much of the obesity of the West is owing to the availability of high-calorie content foods. The effect of cooking fat is seen using as an example potatoes. Whereas boiled potatoes contain but 0.8 kcal/g, potato crisps may contain as much as 5.6 kcal/g. The use of oils and fats for cooking compared with casseroling or steaming is obviously adding to the level of fat intake.

According to Burkitt and Trowell [1975], the relative absence of dietary fibre in the Western diets is associated with the occurrence of the Western-type diseases including CHD, cancer, cerebrovascular disease, diabetes, diverticulitis, cholecystitis, hiatus hernia and appendicitis. These diseases are prevalent in the West but rare in rural Africa and in the underdeveloped world generally where the intake of dietary fibre is much higher. Although the theory is not experimentally proven it is reflected in the US dietary goals previously mentioned which advocate increased use of whole grain products. Tissue disruption which is involved in the production of white flour from grain causes changes in the properties of the components. Whole ground rice, in which dietary fibre and starch are still in close physical relationship, was about 4 times as effective in lowering blood levels and glucose as an equal amount of the fibre of rice bran when this was mixed again with the refined flour from which it was removed [Vijayagopalan and Kurup, 1970]. The addition of moderate amounts of fibre-rich wheat bran as distinct from whole wheat cereal appears not to alter the serum cholesterol levels in man [Burkitt and Trowell, 1975].

Tissue disruption in the production of oils and fats may change the nutritional quality of the product. The inclusion of (polyunsaturated) corn oil as a milk fat replacer in the diet of veal calves was associated with poor growth rates and mortality necessitating replacement of some of the animals in the early stages of the experiment. On the other hand, veal calves fed (saturated) coconut oil as a milk replacer grew normally [Shorland et al., 1981] as did calves fed polyunsaturated milk from cows receiving protected polyunsaturated oils [Wrenn et al., 1973]. The unsatisfactory growth of calves fed rations containing highly unsaturated oils was ascribed by Adams et al. [1959] to the development of rancidity. The indications are that polyunsaturated oils taken out of context of the tissues in which they reside may have adverse nutritional effects. However, rancid polyunsaturated oils fed to cows appeared to have no adverse effects on the animal or on the quality of the carcase [Hartman et al., 1968]. Likewise harmful effects of ingestion of polyunsaturated oils out of context of the tissues in which they reside has not been demonstrated in humans. Nevertheless, any process which is associated with the generation of free radicals is not without potential risk.

Insights into the effects of disturbance of tissue structures are given by Pearson et al. [1977] in a review on warmed-over flavour. Warmed-over flavour is a term which was first used by Timms and Watts [1958] to describe the rapid development of oxidised flavour in refrigerated cooked meat. At 4 °C the rancid or stale flavours usually become apparent within 48 h. This process is catalysed by ferrous iron and by ascorbate in the tissues. This is in contrast to the slow onset of rancidity in refrigerated raw intact meat and fatty tissues not normally apparent until stored for weeks or even months. Warmed-over flavour also occurs in poultry and fish and has been shown to apply to ground or minced uncooked tissues. Phospholipids make up about 0.8% of fresh meat and contain, especially in the phosphatidyl ethanolamine and phosphatidyl choline fractions, high concentrations of C_{20} and C_{22} highly unsaturated fatty acids. These phospholipids form an integral part of the cellular membrane lipoprotein structure. The stability of such structures is indicated by the preservation of intact mammoths in the frozen Arctic as well as by the minimal indications of autoxidation in intact beef stored for 18 months at −18 °C [Shorland, unpublished]. Such changes are conveniently measured by the thiobarbituric acid (TBA) value of Tarladgis et al. [1960] which reacts with malonaldehyde released from the methylenic double bonds to give a red colour during autoxidation. In table XV is shown the effect of mincing beef on the development of autoxidation over a period of 14 days at −18 °C. Invariably, when intact beef is thus stored, as shown by many experiments, the TBA value remains unchanged. The phospholipids used in table XV were freshly extracted from the beef tissues and added in the same proportions as were present in the intact beef. In the minced sample it was clear that considerable auto-oxidation had taken place which would not have occurred in the intact tissues under the conditions used.

Interest in warmed-over flavour stems from the fact that in the fast food business it becomes necessary to prepare cooked food in readiness for rapid reheating as may be required on airlines. At that stage the acceptability of the product may be of prime concern rather than the effects on nutritive value.

Similar considerations apply to national and international organisations involved in food production. It is not hard, however, to visualise that in future there will be an increasing awareness of the need to provide for nutritional needs, such as for example the provision of the appropriate levels of essential fatty acids and their polyunsaturated fatty acid metabolites. Evidence of increased nutritional concern was displayed at the International Dairy Federation 69th Annual Sessions held in Auckland in October 1985. There were included projects to investigate the effects of *trans* and branched chain fatty acids on human nutrition. Rat experiments had already shown that *trans* acids affect essential fatty acid requirements as well as those of energy, not to mention serum cholesterol levels. In another project it was asserted that a fat-free diet would not only lead to an essential fatty acid deficiency but it would be unpleasant to eat. It was proposed to identify a useful proposal for work in the area. One could suggest that the necessity for fat as a basis for acceptibility may not be entirely true. It

Table XV. Effect of adding lipids from 1. dorsi muscle of beef to intact and minced tissues of the same muscle on the development of rancidity (TBA values) during frozen storage for 14 days at – 18 °C[1]

	TBA value
Before storage	
Intact beef	0.27
Minced beef	0.28
After storage	
Minced beef with added phospholipids	14.8
Intact beef with added phospholipids	8.4
Effect of mincing (grinding)	6.4
Ground beef with neutral fat	7.7
Intact beef with neutral fat	1.3
Effect of mincing (grinding)	6.4

[1] Unpublished results.

would not apply, for example, to fruit. The dairy industry provides an example of nutritional distortion to give products which meet a public demand rather than a nutritional requirement. One finds that the fat is extracted from milk to make butter to add to the fat calories. In contrast, there is provision for low-fat milk for those who wish to lower their fat intake. In New Zealand nearly twice as much milk fat is consumed as butter as in the form of milk [Shorland, 1978]. The dairy industry has been channelled to provide the population with enhanced levels of fat in direct opposition to the US Dietary Goals mentioned previously.

Longevity and Nutrition

It is clear that if premature mortality from chronic diseases of the West, including CHD, stroke and cancer, were eliminated the average age at death would be greatly increased. If one took, for example, the hypothetical case that half the population died on average through an atherosclerotic event at the age of 60 years and the remaining half had an average life expectancy of 80 years. The elimination of atherosclerotic events could raise the mean life expectancy from 70 to 80 years. The possibility of moving in the direction of such an achievement is suggested by the results of the Pritikin diet and more particularly by the traditional Eskimo diet applied under the conditions of the Westernised industrial society. Life span is distinguished from life expectancy as the maximum attainable age of a member of a species which would not necessarily be changed by the elimination of a chronic disease. As documented the life span of the human is estimated at about 115 years [Fries, 1980].

As reviewed by Munro [1981] who cites Hayflick [1977], in the ageing process there appears to be an inexorable programme embedded in the genome. This is evidenced by the finding that human fibroblasts in tissue culture can undergo only a finite number of cell divisions which are fewer and fewer as the age of the donor increases. Munro [1981] further postulates that with the ageing, cells may have less capacity to transport nutrients. Lung fibroblasts cultured until cell division had almost ceased showed a decline in zinc uptake of 40%. The uptake of zinc by isolated fat cells from testicular pads of 24-month-old rats compared with 12-month-old rats was 40% less [Sugarman and Munro, 1980a, b]. The uptake of vitamin C in the white cells of the blood of the elderly was less than in those of the young [Andrews et al., 1969].

Perhaps the most marked changes with age are associated with essential fatty acid metabolism. Body and Shorland [1974] noted low levels of C_{18} PUFA in association with high levels of C_{20} PUFA in foetal lamb phospholipids compared with the adult sheep; this is consistent with Brenner's [1971] observation that the ability of the rat to desaturate to form C_{20} + C_{22} PUFA falls off with age. Testicular degeneration has been reported in rats maintained on diets deficient in essential fatty acids [Aaes-Jørgensen and Høelmer, 1969]. Hall and Burdett [1975], in a more detailed study of Tuck/Wistar rats, found that the rate of conversion of $C_{18:2\omega6}$ to $C_{18:3\omega6}$ decreased consecutively when measured at 1.5, 7.5 and 17.5 months of age as did the conversion into C_{20} and C_{22} PUFA. The essentiality of the PUFA for testicular development mentioned above focuses attention on their role in nutrition. Testicular lipids are characterised by their high contents of polyunsaturated C_{20} and C_{22} acids. These acids in terrestrial mammals as a rule are confined to the phospholipids, which in turn, apart from blood lipoproteins, are found largely in cell membranes, where they appear to have an essential role. Other specific requirements for the essential fatty acids and their long chain of polyunsaturated C_{20} and C_{22} metabolites have been described in section V. The phospholipid membranes depend not only on the presence of essential fatty acid precursors in the form of linoleic and α-linolenic acids in the absence of which the longer chain polyunsaturated acids, such as arachidonic (C20:4ω6) and docosahexaenoic (C22:6ω3) will not be synthesised, but also on the presence of dietary protein. In the absence of such protein, as shown by Gerson [1974], chain elongation of linoleic and linolenic acids is restrained in such membranes as the outer mitochondrial and the endoplasmic reticulum of rat liver cells. It can be argued that if these PUFA are essential, they need to be protected against oxidation, to which the polyunsaturated acids C_{20} and C_{22} are particularly susceptible. Further, oxidation leads to the production of free radicals, with destruction of mitochondrial and other cell membranes. It was earlier shown by Dam [1944] that rats fed a fatally low-protein diet survived 75 days in the absence of vitamin E compared with 94 days when supplemented with this vitamin. At the time he was unable to explain the result. However, in the light of present discussion it may be hypothesised that in the absence of adequate protein the mitochondrial and other cell membranes are disrupted with exposure and possible release of PUFA, which are then amenable to auto-oxidation against which vitamin E offered some protection.

Combs et al. [1975] have discussed the mechanisms of action of selenium and vitamin E in the protection of biological membranes. They refer to evidence showing the existence of peroxides in vivo in adipose tissue and the probability of controlled lipid peroxidation as a continous process in all tissues. In particular, erythrocyte plasma membranes were cited as being quite liable to lipid peroxidation, owing to their high PUFA content and to their direct exposure to molecular oxygen. Peroxidation therefore readily leads to haemolysis of these cells.

As reviewed by Ames [1983], the human diet contains a great variety of natural mutagens and carcinogens, many of which may act through the generation of oxygen radicals. He highlights, in addition, the role of the oxidised lipids which may form a considerable part of the ingested food. The lipid oxidation chain reaction (rancidity) yields a variety of mutagens and carcinogens, such as fatty acid hydroperoxides, cholesterol hydroperoxide, endoperoxides, cholesterol and fatty acid epoxides, enals and other aldehydes and alkoxy and hydroperoxy radicals.

Peroxisomes oxidise an appreciable percentage of the dietary fat. The removal of each two carbon unit generates one molecule of hydrogen peroxide (a mutagen promoter and carcinogen). Some hydrogen peroxide escapes the catalase in the peroxisome. The significance of the above-mentioned lipid oxidation products is that they relate to the generation of free radicals, including oxygen radicals. For example, hydroperoxides generate oxygen radicals in the presence of iron-containing hydroperoxides in the cell. Oxygen radicals, in turn, can damage DNA and start the rancidity chain reactions which lead to the production of the mutogens and carcinogens listed above.

The enzymatic systems involved in scavenging free radicals in higher organisms include superoxide dismutase, catalase, and glutathione peroxidase which detoxify the superoxide radical, hydrogen peroxide, and lipid hydroperoxides. In addition to these enzymes, free-radical scavengers are present, such as vitamins E and C, cysteine and glutathione [Leibovitz and Siegel, 1980].

Studies on the activity of superoxide dismutase have not shown any consistent change with ageing. However, a survey of different animal species showed that the longest living species – the human – had the highest blood and tissue levels [Tolmasoff et al., 1980]. There is no evidence that diet supplementation would prolong life since oral ingestion did not augment the levels in blood or tissue [Zidenberg-Cherr et al., 1983].

To reduce the generation of free radicals one may vary the levels of PUFA. Decreased life expectancy was found with increased dietary unsaturated fat levels in certain mouse or rat strains [Harman, 1971; French et al., 1953]. The anti-oxidant properties of vitamins A, C and E have led to increased consumption of these vitamins by a highly selected group of people over 65 without evidence of dose-related response between mortality and levels of vitamin supplementation. In fact, increased mortality was observed in people who consumed very high levels of vitamin E – more than 1,000 IU per day [Estrom and Pauling, 1982].

As reviewed by Ames [1983], the significance of oxygen radicals not only concerns the mechanism of mutagenic and carcinogenic action but it relates also to the ageing process and the occurrence of chronic diseases including cancer and CHD.

The protection of DNA against oxidative processes would undoubtedly assist in the prevention of chronic diseases and enhance life expectancy. If, however, the ageing process is made up of an inexorable programme embedded in the genome limiting the number of cell divisions, it seems that the protection of DNA against oxidation processes may do little towards increasing life span. Nevertheless, Walford [1983] considers the life span of 115 years currently assigned to the human will be considerably exceeded. Walford's diets for humans, though possessing low-calorie contents, are nevertheless designed to provide adequate levels of essential nutrients. A prominent feature in his diets is the inclusion of free radical scavengers, for which he gives evidence as to their effectiveness in promoting longevity. This applies even to synthetic anti-oxidants, such as BHT. An interesting aspect is the observation that the annual fish in its natural habitat, Brazil, lives for about a year at a temperature of 68 °F. If kept at 59 °F the fish lives twice as long. If, in addition, the diet is restricted the life expectancy is increased threefold. Similar considerations apply to fruit flies and lizards. Life extension is thus consistent with the slowing down of the metabolic processes.

The present author suggests that the phenomenon of warmed-over flavour in cooked meat possesses features in common with the ageing process, especially in regard to the need for maintenance of lipoprotein structures of the cell membranes. If the structure is disrupted the highly unsaturated fatty acids are unprotected and the oxygen radicals can initiate the lipid oxidation chain reaction. In the living cell this promotes the oxidative processes leading to DNA damage. In the intact meat the membranes are disrupted and the enzymes are released, resulting in autolysis of the tissues.

Much of the information on the effect of nutrition on longevity comes from the studies of McKay et al. [1939]. Severe food restriction on rats from weaning to 300 days increased the mean life span of rats to 949 days compared with 656 days for the ad-libitum-fed group. As reviewed by Schneider and Reed [1985], numerous studies have verified the life-prolonging effect of food restriction in various strains of rats and mice. It has been shown that with dietary restriction certain chronic diseases, including cancer, occur less frequently or later, immunologic response is improved, occurrence of auto-antibodies is diminished, as is collagen cross-linking. Further, calorie-restricted rats do not have the same age-related changes in serum [Masoro et al., 1983] and hepatic lipid [Yu, 1984] concentrations and serum insulin levels [Reaven and Reaven, 1981] as sedentary control rats.

Before calorie restriction can be recommended for the human it seems necessary to ascertain more precisely the relationship of weight to health. However, Nutrition Reviews [1985] notes that overweight people tend to die sooner than average-weight persons. This is especially true for those who are overweight at younger ages. The weights associated with greatest longevity tend to be below the average weights of the populations as long as such weights are not associated with concurrent illness or a history of significant medical impairment.

VII. Concluding Remarks

This review indicates that much of our present-day knowledge of human nutrition has not come directly from controlled experiments on humans. Such experiments, in many cases, would require extreme conditions that conflict with ethical considerations, not to mention the problems of genetic variation and of human behaviour. Contemporary knowledge of human nutrition has perforce slowly evolved imperfectly on the fragile basis of assuming, often at the risk of generating faulty hypotheses, that the human response is similar to that of the animal. For example, the inadequacy of wheat protein as found for rats was applied wrongly as if valid for the human. Human nutritional knowledge has been greatly supplemented by epidemiology which is usefully suggestive rather than final in outcome. The understanding of the biochemical mechanisms behind nutritional phenomena is likely to play an ever-increasing role in the promotion of our knowledge of human nutrition. The diets of the Western industrialised world have evolved largely from grain, especially wheat, over the past several thousand years. Although the wealthy have had ready access to meat, fish, fruit and vegetables, much of the world even today is largely dependent on cereals. Most of the change towards the varied diet of today's industrialised world, including the population as a whole, has taken place mainly during the present century. To within the past 100 years in Europe and Britain wheat generally remained the dominant source of calories. Dupin et al. [1984], for example, assessed the bread consumption in France in 1880 at 600 g/person/day. This would be equivalent to about 1,500 kcal/person/day or considerably more than half the total caloric intake.

In this review the contemporary diets have been broadly categorised into meat, milk; high-calorie wheat (consumption ca. 3,000 kcal/person/day); low-calorie wheat (ca. 1,900–2,500 kcal/person/day); maize and rice groups. Other diets, such as those of the traditional Eskimo, consisting almost entirely of the flesh of marine mammals and fish through to the almost entirely vegetarian diet of the Pari tribe in New Guinea based largely on root crops, have also been considered. The industrialised nations of the West generally belong to the meat, milk group having the means to purchase the relatively expensive meat, milk products to form some 27.5% of the total calories. A substantial amount (34.9%) of the remaining calories comes from sugar, oils and fats with only 23.1% from cereals. In the remaining groups cereals generally make up more than 50%

of the total calories, with meat and milk products comprising less than half that of the meat, milk group based on the period under review (1964–1966). However, during the subsequent 15 years in the high-calorie wheat group, wheat consumption fell from 54.7 to 42.5% and the meat, milk products rose from 12.7 to 18.0% of the total calories, the rise in meat consumption in Greece and Italy being significant at the $p < 0.05$ level. This change is consistent with the evolution of the high-calorie wheat diet towards the meat, milk diet. In the meat, milk group apart from the significant drop in oils and fats intake in Iceland from 20.5 to 10.5% of the total calories, no other significant changes over the 15-year period were observed. In the rice group no significant changes were noted in the diet over the 15-year period studied. However, the continued downturn in rice consumption in Japan was shown by its decline from 54.7 to 42.5% of the total calories.

During the 15-year period studied, life expectancy in the meat, milk group increased by 2–3 years, the maximum values being achieved by Iceland with female life expectancy at 80 years and male at 74 years. Norway, the Netherlands, Sweden and Switzerland closely followed to within one year the Icelandic achievement. In the other groups only Japan achieved comparable longevity, being ranked second to Iceland at the end of the 15-year period studied, with life expectancies of 79 and 74 years for the female and male, respectively. The relatively poor performance by the other diet groups appears to be related to the absence of adequate medical care, giving rise to high infant mortality. This is suggested by the life expectancy in Algeria, Tunisia (low-calorie wheat) and Nicaragua (maize) which, at 80 and 85 years, is nearly double that of the meat, milk group.

Over the 15-year period, life expectancy in Japan has increased by approximately 5 years, indicating that this country will readily overtake the meat, milk countries in this regard in the near future. Longevity in Japan and Iceland is associated with the highest fish intakes found in the developed countries. Furthermore, over the 15-year period reviewed, these intakes have increased in Iceland and Japan from 4.0 to 6.4% and from 3.5 to 7.2% of the total calories, respectively. The relative unimportance of vegetables in the context of longevity is suggested by the fact that of the countries studied, Japan had the highest consumption at 3.7% compared with 0.2% (lowest) recorded for Iceland.

The fact that on diets covering a wide range from the flesh-based food of the traditional Eskimo through to the almost completely vegetarian, root-based, diet of the Pari tribe, the human survives and often thrives makes it difficult to prescribe what is ideal. The collection of Food Balance Sheets by FAO serves to provide useful information on the composition of national diets throughout the world, but there remains the need to test the nutritive value of such diets and to rank them. Such an evaluation based on rat feeding experiments would provide some information which could be further tested as the opportunity arises by experiments carried out on humans. Only then can it be considered that our knowledge of national diets is soundly based. Our diets as in the past are still largely based on what is available and acceptable without regard to nutritional quality.

The publication of the 1986 10th edition of the US Recommended Dietary Allowances has been delayed on the grounds that the appointed reviewers consider that the primary focus on the avoidance of nutritional deficiencies is neither sufficient nor appropriate. Consideration must also be given to the effect of nutritional factors on the ageing process and on the susceptibility to chronic diseases. In the present review the following additional defects become apparent: (I) What the RDA are recommended for is not stated. Are they recommended for a long and active life free from ill health? (2) The vitamins, in particular, have functions other than to prevent deficiency diseases. They may be involved in cancer prevention or in the protection against free radicals, for example. The levels needed for these purposes may be higher than prescribed by the RDA. (3) The RDA do not include the levels or the proportions of the essential fatty acids. Further, the RDA should include the levels of the metabolic chain extension products of these acids, such as eicosapentaenoic acid, which the human cannot readily synthesise from dietary essential fatty acids. Eicosapentaenoic acid appears to be anti-thrombotic as well as protecting against diabetes and CHD induced by smoking.

The assessment of the protein requirements of the human has undergone many changes. As described by Hegsted [1985], Voit considered during the past century that the adult male engaged in hard work required 145 g protein/day. In contrast, Hinhede [1913] found that adult males engaged in agricultural work were maintained in nitrogen balance on a potato diet for 300 days at the level of 20 g protein/day. The current value of the US RDA is set at 56 g.

Evidence as to the effects of high protein intake by the human appears to be lacking. However, the fact that rats fed high-calorie, high-protein diets compared with those fed normal rations exhibited early degeneration and lowered life expectancy [Ross, 1959] may have relevance to the human. In contrast, the traditional Eskimo diet would have contained about 377 g protein/day without incurring degenerative diseases from which the Eskimo was notably free. Evidently, our knowledge of the effects of protein levels on human health has not been clarified. In stipulating protein requirements there appears to be a need to specify the protein source – whether plant or animal and whether terrestrial or derived from planktonic sources.

The literature on the attempts to control the incidence of CHD by lowering serum cholesterol by means of polyunsaturated oils, rich in linoleic acid, or by means of drugs, have tended to be disappointing. Though the correlation between the incidence of coronary events and the extent of reduction of serum cholesterol levels has been established by the LRC-CPPT [1984], there remains the difficulty in securing an overall improvement in the level of mortality. Invariably, the non-CHD deaths are higher in the experimental group than in the control group. There is evidence to suggest that dietary restriction in association with a low fat intake with special reference to saturated animal fats would be more effective in the control of CHD as in the Pritikin [1979] diet.

Probably the most important contribution to the solution of the CHD problem comes from the knowledge of the effects of prostaglandins on the clotting process. It is postulated that the thrombotic process is controlled by the ratio of thromboxane/PGI_2 or the clotting factor/anticlotting factor. The ratio is favourably influenced by the presence of ω_3-eicosapentaenoic acid which interferes with the course of synthesis of TxA_2 from arachidonic (ω_6-eicosatetraenoic) acid derived in turn from linoleic acid. The absence of CHD in Eskimos on their traditional diet based on marine animals and fish is now explainable on the basis of eicosapentaenoic acid content which is generally low or absent in the diets of the West unless supplemented with fish. The longitudinal experiment by Kromhout et al. [1985] involving 850 middle-aged asymptomatic men over a period of 20 years has established that the mortality from CHD amongst those who ate as little as 30 g/day was 50% lower ($p < 0.05$) than amongst those who did not eat fish. Epidemiological evidence from Japan and elsewhere continues to support the view that fish play a role in the control of CHD.

In this review the term nutritional distortion has been introduced to signify the addition to the diet of a component, such as fat or sugar, which has been extracted from a food source or alternatively a component such as bran is removed from a food source such as wheat prior to its use as a dietary item. The extent of nutritional distortion in the West is indicated in the diets of the meat, milk group where 34.9% of the total calories comes from sugar, oils and fats. It is not readily possible to calculate the distortion arising from the extraction of bran from wheat but an extraction rate for wheat of 70% is common and the prevalence of white rice suggests that much of the rice has been similarly treated. If nutritional distortion had not occurred the recommendations of the US Senate Select Committee on Nutrition and Human Needs [1977] requiring a reduction of fat consumption from 40 to 30% of the total calories would be readily met as would the requirements for increased whole grain and reduced intake of sugar.

Nutritional distortion involves tissue disruption which may alter the properties of food components. The inclusion of (extracted) polyunsaturated corn oil as a milk replacer in the diet of veal calves was associated with poor growth rates and mortality [Shorland et al., 1981], whereas calves fed polyunsaturated milk from cows receiving protected polyunsaturated oils [Wrenn et al., 1973] grew normally. The adverse nutrition effects on calves receiving polyunsaturated oils have been ascribed by Adams et al. [1959] to rancidity. Intact meat tissues store with minimal changes under refrigeration. In contrast, even under refrigerated conditions cooked or minced meats undergo rapid development of oxidised or warmed-over flavour [Pearson et al., 1977].

Longevity as reviewed by Munro [1981], who cites Hayflick [1977], appears to be limited by the inexorable programme embedded in the genome so that cells may undergo only a finite number of divisions. Throughout life there is controlled lipid peroxidation which affects the lipoprotein cell membranes. These contain the phospholipids with long chain PUFA that are amenable to oxidative attack as well as a source for prostaglandin synthesis. The enzymatic systems involved in scavenging the free radicals concerned with the oxidation process include the enzymes superoxide dismutase, catalase, and glutathione peroxidase which detoxify the superoxide radicals, hydrogen peroxide and lipid peroxide. In addition, vitamins E and C, cysteine, and gluthione are also free radical scavengers.

The protection of DNA against oxidative processes would assist in the prevention of chronic diseases, such as cancer, and enhance life expectancy. There is already some evidence to show that the addition of vitamin E and synthetic anti-oxidants will prolong the life of animals to a small degree. However, the most successful results have so far been achieved through dietary restriction in which the life span of the rat was extended from a mean of 656 to 949 days. The application of dietary restriction to the human is already the concern of certain groups, such as the weight watchers. It cannot be ascertained in advance that the human could prolong life as successfully as indicated by the rat feeding experiments. Nevertheless, there is enough evidence to show that the contemporary overeating occasioned by the meat, milk diet could be immediately countered by omitting the addition of oils, fats and sugar and increasing the whole grain components in terms of the US Select Senate Committee on Nutrition and Human Needs [1977], emphasising the need to increase the intake of fish to protect against CHD. Our understanding of human nutrition as shown by the examples of its influence on the ageing processes and on chronic diseases is merely suggestive. It has not reached the stage of being soundly based.

References

Aaes-Jørgensen, E.; Høelmer, G.: Essential fatty acid deficient rats: growth and testes development. Lipids *4:* 501–506 (1969).

Adams, R.S.; Gander, J.E.; Gullickson, T.W.; Sautter, J.H.: Some effects of feeding various filled milks to dairy calves. 3. Blood plasma tocopherol and vitamin A levels, diet storage effects, and evidence of toxicity. J. Dairy Sci. *42:* 1569–1579 (1959).

American Dietetic Association: Position paper on: diet and criminal behaviour. J. Am. diet. Ass. *85:* 361–362 (1985).

Ames, B.N.: Dietary carcinogens and anticarcinogens oxygen radicals and degenerative diseases. Science *221:* 1256–1263 (1983).

Anderson, R.E.; Landis, D.J.; Dudley, P.A.: Essential fatty acid deficiency and renewal of rod outer segments in the albino rat. Investve Ophth. *15:* 232–236 (1976).

Andrews, J.; Letcher, M.; Brook, M.: Vitamin C supplementation in the elderly: a 17-month trial in an old persons' home. Br. med. J. *ii:* 416–418 (1969).

Bang, H.O.; Dyerberg, J.: Lipid metabolism and ischaemic heart disease in Greenland Eskimos. Advances in nutrition research, vol. 3, pp. 1–22 (Plenum Press, New York 1980).

Bang, H.O.; Dyerberg, J.; Sinclair, H.M.: The composition of Eskimo food in Northwestern Greenland Coast Eskimos. Am. J. clin. Nutr. *33:* 2657–2661 (1980).

Barnicoat, C.R.; Shorland, F.B.: New Zealand lamb and mutton. N. Z. J. Sci. Tech. sect. A *33:* 16–23 (1952).

Beckel, L.: This accursed land (McMillan, Melbourne 1977).

Black, K.L.; Culp. B.; Madison, D.; Randall, O.S.; Lands, W.E.M.: The protective effect of dietary fish oil on cerebral infarction. Prostaglandins Med. *5:* 257–258 (1979).

Body, D.R.; Shorland, F.B.: The fatty acid composition of the main phospholipid fractions of the rumen and abomasum tissues of foetal and adult sheep. J. Sci. Fd Agric. *25:* 197–204 (1974).

Bolourchi, S.C.; Friedemann, M.; Mickelsen, O.: Wheat flour as a source of protein for adult human subjects. Am. J. Nutr. *21:* 827–835 (1968).

Bortz, W.M.; Lynen, F.: The inhibition of acetyl-CoA carboxylase in long chain acyl-CoA derivatives. Biochem. Z. *337:* 505–509 (1963).

Brenner, R.R.: The desaturation step in the animal biosynthesis of polyunsaturated fatty acids. Lipids *6:* 567–575 (1971).

Brenner, R.R.; Peluffo, R.O.: Inhibitory effect of docosa-4,7,10,13,16,19-hexaenoic acid upon the oxidative desaturation of linoleic into gamma-linolenic acid and of alpha-linolenic into octadeca-6,9,12,15-tetraenoic acid. Biochim. biophys. Acta *137:* 184–186 (1967).

Brierem, K.; Ekern, A.; Homb, T.: Relation of nutrition of the young animal to subsequent fertility and lactation. Fed. Proc. *20:* suppl. 7, part III, pp. 275–283 (1961).

Budowski, P.; Hawkey, C.M.; Crawford, M.A.: *L*-Acide α-linolenique sur l'encephalomalacie chez le poulet. Annls Nutr. Aliment. *34:* 389–400 (1980).

Burkitt, D.P.; Trowell, H.C.: Refined carbohydrates, foods and disease (Academic Press, London 1975).

Call, L.: An estimate of caloric availability and consumption in the United States, 1909–1963. Am. J. clin. Nutr. *16:* 374–379 (1965).

Cleave, T.L.; Cambell, G.D.: Diabetes, coronary thrombosis and the saccharine disease (Wright, Bristol 1966).

Clements, S.; Rogers, J.F.: Nutrition handbook for pharmacists (Canberra Publishing, Canberra 1983).

Combs, G.F., Jr.; Noguchi, T.; Scott, M.L.: Mechanism of action of selenium and vitamin E in protection of biological membranes. Fed. Proc. *34:* 2090–2095 (1975).

Committee on Diet, Nutrition and Cancer. National Research Council (Natn. Academy of Sciences, Washington 1982).

Committee of Principal Investigators: FAO Clofibrate Trial. Lancet *ii:* 379–385 (1980).

Connor, W.E.; Connor, S.L.: The key role of nutritional factors in the prevention of coronary heart disease. Prev. Med. *1:* 49–83 (1972).

Corey, S.J.; Shih, C.; Cashman, J.R.: Docosahexaenoic acid is a strong inhibitor of prostaglandin but not leucotriene biosynthesis. Proc. natn. Acad. Sci. USA *80:* 3581–3584 (1983).

Crawford, M.A.: The balance between α-linolenic and linoleic acid; in Podley, Podmore, The role of fats in human nutrition, pp. 62–63 (Horwood, Chichester 1985).

Crawford, M.A.; Casperd, N.M.; Sinclair, A.J.: The long chain metabolites of linoleic and linolenic acids in liver and brains of herbivores and carnivores. Compar. Biochem. Physiol. *54B:* 395–401 (1976).

Crawford, M.A.; Gale, M.M.; Woodford, M.H.: Linoleic and linolenic elongation products in muscle tissue of *Syncerus caffer* and other ruminant species. Biochem. J. *115:* 25–27 (1969).

Culp, B.R.; Titus, B.G.; Lands, W.E.M.: Inhibition of prostaglandin biosynthesis by eicosapentaenoic acid. Prostaglandins Med. *3:* 269–278 (1978).

Dam, H.: Vitamin E and the length of life of rats fed a diet with a fatally low protein content. Proc. Soc. exp. Biol. Med. *55:* 55–56 (1944).

Davidson, F.; Gilmour, E.: The Carterton dietary survey, part I. J. N.Z. Diet. Ass. *23:* 5–12 (1969).

Davidson, L.S.P.; Passmore, R.: Nutrition and dietetics; 3rd ed. (Livingstone, Edinburgh 1966).

Davies, M.J.; Thomas, A.: Thrombosis and acute coronary artery lesions in sudden death. New Engl. J. Med. *310:* 1137–1140 (1984).

Dayton, S.; Pearce, M.L.; Hashimoto, S.; Dixon, W.J.; Tomiyasu, U.: A controlled clinical

trial of a diet high in unsaturated fat in preventing complications of atherosclerosis. Circulation *40:* suppl. 11, pp. 1–62 (1969).
Dupin, H.; Hercberg, S.; Lagrange, V.: Evolution of the French diet: nutritional aspects. Wld Rev. Nutr. Diet., vol. 44, pp. 57–84 (Karger, Basel 1984).
Dyerberg, J.; Bang, H.O.: Haemostatic function and platelet polyunsaturated fatty acids in Eskimos. Lancet *ii:* 433–435 (1979).
Dyerberg, J.; Bang, H.O.; Stoffersen, E.; Moncada, S.; Vane, J.R.: Eicosapentaenoic acid and prevention of thrombosis and atherosclerosis? Lancet *ii:* 117–119 (1978).
Eaton, S.B.; Konner, M.: Palaolithic nutrition: a consideration of its nature and current implications. New Engl. J. Med. *312:* 283–289 (1985).
Eckholm, E.; Record, F.: The affluent diet. A worldwide health hazard. Futurist *11:* 32–42 (1977).
Estrom, J.E.; Pauling, L.: Mortality among health-conscious elderly Californians. Science *221:* 1256–1268 (1982).
FAO: Food balance sheets (FAO, Roma 1971).
FAO: Food balance sheets (FAO, Roma 1984).
Fiennes, R.M.; Sinclair, T.W.; Crawford, M.A.: Essential fatty acid studies in primates linolenic acid requirement of capuchins. J. med. Primatol. *2:* 155–169 (1973).
Finlayson, R.; Symons, D.; Fiennes, R.M.: Atherosclerosis: a comparative study. Br. med. J. *i:* 501–510 (1962).
Fisher, S.; Weber, P.C.: Thromboxane A_3 (TXA_3) as formed in human platelets after dietary eicosapentaenoic acid. Biochem. biophys. Res. Commun. *116:* 1091–1099 (1983).
Florey, M.: Atherosclerosis. Endeavour *22:* 107–111 (1963).
French, C.E.; Ingram, R.D.; Uram, J.A.; Barron, J.P.; Swift, R.W.: The influence of dietary fat and carbohydrate on growth and longevity in rats. J. Nutr. *51:* 329–339 (1953).
Friend, B.: Nutrients in the United States food supply. A review of trends, 1907–1913 to 1965. Am. J. clin. Nutr. *20:* 907–914 (1967).
Fries, F.J.: Ageing, natural death, and the compression of morbidity. New Engl. J. Med. *303:* 130–135 (1980).
Gerson, T.: A comparison of the effects of dietary protein and lipid deprivation on lipid composition of liver membranes in rats. J. Nutr. *104:* 701–709 (1974).
Gerson, T.; Shorland, F.B.; Livingston, M.; Bell, M.E.: The effect of dietary fatty acid constituents on the body cholesterol of rats. Archs Biochem. Biophys. *68:* 313–318 (1957).
Goodman, D.S.: Vitamin A and retinoids in health and disease. New Engl. J. Med. *310:* 1023–1031 (1984).
Goodnight, S.J., Jr.; Harris, W.S.; Connor, W.E.: The effects of dietary ω3 fatty acids on platelet composition and function in man: a prospective, controlled study. Blood *58:* 880–885 (1981).
Gopalan, C.; Narasinga, R.: Dietary allowances for Indians. Special report Ser., No. 60 (Indian Council of Medical Research, Hyderabad 1968).
Gorman, R.R.: Modulation of platelet function by prostacyclin and thromboxane A_2. Fed. Proc. *38:* 83–88 (1979).
Hall, D.A.; Burdett, P.E.: Age changes in the metabolism of essential fatty acids. Biochem. Soc. Trans. *3:* 42–47 (1975).

Hamilton, R.M.G.; Carroll, K.K.: Plasma cholesterol in rabbits fed low-fat, low-cholesterol diets: effects of dietary proteins, carbohydrates and fibre from different sources. Atherosclerosis *24:* 47–62 (1976).

Harman, D.: Free radical theory of ageing: effect of amount and degree of unsaturation of dietary fat on mortality rate. J. Geront. *26:* 451–457 (1971).

Hartman, L.; Shorland, F.B.; Czochanska, Z.; Woodhams, P.; Kirton, A.H.: The effects of drenching cows with oxidised oils on the composition of the fat and the quality of the meat. N.Z. J. Sci. *11:* 122–130 (1968).

Hay, C.R.; Durber, A.P.; Saygnor, R.: Effect of fish oil on platelet kinetics in patients with ischaemic heart disease. Lancet *i:* 1269–1272 (1982).

Hayflick, L.: In Finch, Hayflick, Handbook of the biology of aging, pp. 159–186 (Van Nostrand, New York 1977).

Hegsted, D.M.: The potential of wheat for meeting man's nutrient needs; in Role of Wheat in World's Food Supply. Report on Conf., Albany 1962 (US Department of Agriculture, Western Regional Laboratories, 1962).

Hegsted, D.M.: Dietary guidelines. Proc. Int. Conf. Oils, Fats and Waxes, Auckland 1983, pp. 221–226 (Duromark, Auckland 1983).

Hegsted, D.M.: Nutrition: the changing scene. W.O. Atwater Memorial Lecture. Nutr. Rev. *43:* 357–367 (1985).

Hindhede, M.: Protein and nutrition: an investigation (Seymour, London 1913).

Hipsley, E.H.; Kirk, E.: Studies on dietary intake and expenditure by New Guineans (South Pacific Commission, Noumea 1965).

Hirai, A.; Hamazaki, T.; Terano, T.; Nishikawa, T.; Tamura, Y.; Kumagai, A.; Sajiki, J.: Eicosapentaenoic acid and platelet function in Japanese. Lancet *ii:* 1132–1133 (1980).

Hollingsworth, D.: Changing patterns of consumption in Britain. Nutr. Rev. *32:* 353–359 (1974).

Hornstra, G.; Haddeman, E.; Kloeze, J.; Verschuren, P.M.: Dietary fat-induced changes in the formation of prostanoids of the 2 and 3 series in relation to arterial thrombosis (rat) and atherosclerosis (rabbit). Adv. Prostaglandin Thromboxane Leucotriene Res. *12:* 193–202 (1983).

Horrobin, D.F.; Manku, M.S.: How do polyunsaturated fatty acids lower plasma cholesterol levels? Lipids *18:* 558–562 (1983).

Hubbard, J.D.; Inkeles, S.; Barnard, R.J.: Nathan Pritikin's heart. New Engl. J. Med. *313:* 52 (1985).

Hughes, R.E.: Human dietary patterns and technological change; in Head, Lowenstein, Oxford biology readers, pp. 3–16 (Oxford University Press, London 1971).

Hyslop, P.A.; York, D.A.: Membrane fluidity and adenylate cyclase activity in genetically obese mice. Biochem. biophys. Res. Commun. *92:* 819–823 (1980).

Innami, S.; Mickelsen, O.: Nutritional status – Japan. Nutr. Rev. *27:* 275–278 (1969).

Isaacson, C.: The sweetness that's turned sour. Here's Health *23:* 29–32 (1979).

Jaffa quoted by Hindhede (1913): Bull. No. 107 (US Department of Agriculture, Washington, DC, 1901).

Jansen, J.D.: Nutrition and cancer. Wld Rev. Nutr. Diet., vol. 39, pp. 1–22 (Karger, Basel 1982).

Joint FAO-WHO Expert Group: Protein requirements. WHO Tech. Rep. Ser., No. 301 (WHO, Genève 1965).

Kagawa, Y.; Nishizawa, M.; Suzuki, M.; et al.: Eicosapolyenoic acids of serum lipids of Japanese islanders with low incidence of coronary heart diseases. J. Nutr. Sci. Vitaminol. Tokyo *28:* 441–453 (1982).

Kannel, W.B.; Gordon, T.: The Framingham Study: an epidemiological investigation of cardiovascular disease, sect. 24. The Framingham diet study. Diet and its regulation of serum cholesterol (National Institute of Health, US Department of Health, Education and Welfare, Washington 1970).

Keyfitz, N.; Flieger, W.: Population facts and methods of demography (Freeman, San Francisco 1971).

Keys, A.: Seven countries: a multivariate analysis of death and coronary heart disease (Harvard University Press, Cambridge 1980).

Keys, A.; Anderson, J.T.; Grande, F.: Prediction of serum cholesterol response of men to changes in fats in the diet. Lancet *i:* 959–966 (1957).

Kingsbury, K.J.; Morgan, D.M.; Aylott, C.; Emmerson, R.: Effects of ethyl arachidonate, cod-liver oil, and corn oil on the plasmacholesterol level. A comparison of normal volunteers. Lancet *i:* 739–744 (1961).

Kon, S.K.; Klein, A.: The value of the whole potato in human nutrition. Biochem. J. *22:* 258–267 (1928).

Kromann, N.; Green, A.: Epidemiological studies in the Upernavik District, Greenland. Acta med. scand. *208:* 401–406 (1980).

Kromhout, D.; Rosschieter, E.B.; Coulander, Cor de Lezenne: The inverse relation between fish consumption and 20-year mortality from coronary heart disease. New Engl. J. Med. *312:* 1205–1209 (1985).

Kummerow, F.A.: Optimum nutrition through better planning of world agriculture. Wld Rev. Nutr. Diet., vol. 45, pp. 1–41 (Karger, Basel 1985).

Lancet: Eskimo diets and diseases. Lancet *i:* 1139–1141 (1983).

Lands, W.E.M.; Le Tellier, P.R.; Rome, L.H.; Vanderhoek, J.Y.: Inhibition of prostaglandin biosynthesis. Adv. Biosci. *9:* 15–18 (1973).

Leaf, A.: A doctor examines modern Methuselahs. Futurist *11:* 24 (1977).

Leibovitz, B.E.; Siegel, B.V.: Aspects of free radical reactions in biological systems: ageing. J. Geront. *35:* 45–56 (1980).

Leveille, G.A.: Issues in human nutrition and their possible impact on foods of animal origin. J. Animal Sci. *41:* 723–731 (1975a).

Leveille, G.A.: Dietary fiber in human nutrition and disease. Proc. 28th Annu. Reciprocal Meat Conf. of the Am. Meat Science Ass., pp. 166–176 (1975b).

Leveille, G.A.: Establishing and implementing dietary goals. Food Nutr. News *49:* 1–4 (1977).

Lichti, U.; Yuspa, S.H.: Inhibition of epidermal terminal differentiation and tumour promotion by retinoids. Ciba Fdn Symp. *113:* 77–86 (1985).

Longenecker, H.E.: Fats in human nutrition. J. Am. diet. Ass. *20:* 83–85 (1944).

Lorenz, R.; Spengler, H.; Fischer, S.; Duhm, J.; Weber, P.: Platelet function, thromboxane formation and blood pressure control during supplementation of the Western diet with cod liver oil. Circulation *67:* 504–511 (1983).

LRC-CPPT: I. Reduction in incidence in coronary heart disease. II. The relationship of reduction in incidence of coronary heart disease to cholesterol lowering. J. Am. med. Ass. *251:* 351–374 (1984).

Machlin, L.J.: The biological consequences of feeding polyunsaturated fatty acids to antioxidant deficient animals. J. Am. Oil Chem. Soc. *40:* 368–371 (1963).
Markakis, P.: The nutritive quality of potato proteins; In Mendel Friedman, Protein nutritional quality of foods and feeds. 2. Quality factors – plant breeding, composition, processing and anti-nutrients (Dekker, New York 1975).
Masoro, E.J.; Compton, C.; Yu, B.P.; Bertrand, H.: Temporal and compositional dietary restrictions modulate age-related changes in serum lipids. J. Nutr. *118:* 880–892 (1983).
McCance, R.A.; Widdowson, E.M.: The composition of foods. Med. Res. Council Spec. Rep. Ser., No. 297; 3rd rev. ed. Spec. Rep. No. 235 (HMSO, London 1960).
McCarrison, R.: Nutrition and national health. Cantor Lectures to the Royal Society of Arts 1936 (Faber & Faber, London 1944).
McKay, C.M.; Maynard, L.A.; Sperling, G.; Barnes, L.L.: Restricted growth, lifespan, ultimate body size, and age changes in the albino rat after feeding diets restricted in calories. J. Nutr. *18:* 1–13 (1939).
McLaren, D.S.: The great protein fiasco. Lancet *ii:* 93–96 (1974).
Mendel, L.B.: Nutrition: the chemistry of life (Yale University Press, Newhaven 1923).
Mickelson, O.: Nutrition science and you. A vistas of science book (Scholastic Book Services. A division of Scholastic Magazines, New York 1964).
Miettinen, M.; Turpeinen, O.; Karvonen, M.J.; Elosuo, R.; Paalvilainen, E.: Effect of cholesterol-lowering diet on mortality from coronary heart disease and other causes. Lancet *ii:* 835–838 (1972).
Mitchell, J.R.A.: Diet and arterial disease – the myths and the realities. Proc. Nutr. Soc. *44:* 363–369 (1985).
Moncada, S.; Vane, J.R.: The role of prostacyclin in vascular tissue. Fed. Proc. *38:* 66–71 (1979).
Moran, J.M.; Moran, M.D.; Wiersma, J.H.: Introduction to environmental science (Freeman, San Francisco 1980).
Morant, G.M.: The heights of British people. Biology human Affairs *16:* 20–26 (1950).
Morris, J.N.; Marr, J.W.; Heady, J.A.; Mills, G.L.; Pilkington, T.R.E.: Diet and plasma cholesterol in 99 bank men. Br. med. J. *i:* 571–576 (1963).
Morrison, S.D.: Nutrition and longevity. Nutr. Rev. *41:* 133–142 (1983).
Munro, H.N.: Nutrition and ageing. Br. med. Bull. *37:* 83–88 (1981).
Mustard, J.F.; Kinlough-Rathbone, R.L.; Packham, M.A.: Prostaglandins and platelets. Annu. Rev. Med. *31:* 89–96 (1980).
National Research Council: Recommended dietary allowances; 9th ed. (Natn. Academy of Sciences, Washington 1980).
Needleman, P.; Whitaker, M.O.; Wyche, A.; Watters, K.; Sprecher, H.; Raz, A.: Manipulation of platelet aggregation by prostaglandins and their fatty acid precursors: pharmacological bases for a therapeutic approach. Prostaglandins *19:* 165–168 (1980).
Nutrition Reviews: Special report: body weight, health and longevity: conclusions and recommendations of the workshop. Nutr. Rev. *43:* 61–63 (1985).
Office of Health Economics: Coronary heart disease. The scope for prevention (Office of Health Economics, London 1982).
Oliver, J.H.; McKasen, D.; Percy, I.C.: Experience of the Canadian medical team at the 21st Olympiad. Can. med. Ass. J. *117:* 609–616 (1977).

Oliver, M.F.: Dietary cholesterol, plasma cholesterol and coronary heart disease. Br. Heart J. *38:* 214–218 (1976).
Oliver, M.F.: Diet and coronary heart disease. Br. med. Bull. *37:* 49–58 (1981).
Oliver, M.F.: Strategies for preventing coronary heart disease. Nutr. Rev. *43:* 257–262 (1985).
Orr, J.G.; Gilks, J.L.: Med. Res. Council. Spec. Rep. Ser., No. 155, 1931; quoted by Pyke (1971).
Orten, J.M.; Neuhaus, D.W.: Human biochemistry (Mosby, St Louis 1975).
Parowski, W.; Patchett, N.: Cereals and potatoes, a study of patterns of production in New Zealand from 1886 to 1960. J. N.Z. diet. Ass. *24:* 9–11 (1970).
Pearson, A.M.; Love, J.D.; Shorland, F.B.: 'Warmed-over' flavour in meat, poultry, and fish. Adv. Food Res. *23:* 2–74 (1977).
PPRG (Pooling Project Research Group): Relationship of blood pressure, serum cholesterol, smoking habits, relative weight and ECG abnormalities to incidence of major coronary events. Final Report of the Pooling Group. J. chron. Dis. *31:* 201–306 (1978).
Press, F.: Postponement of the 10th ed. of the RDAs. J. Am. diet. Ass. *85:* 1644–1645 (1985).
Prior, I.A.M.; Harvey, H.P.B.; Neave, M.N.; Davidson, F.: The health of two groups of Cook Island Maoris. N.Z. Dept. of Health Spec. Rep. Ser. *26:* 1–44 (1966).
Pritikin, N.: The Pritikin program for diet and exercise; 16th print. (Bantam Books, New York 1979).
Pyke, M.: Food and society (Murray, London 1968; reprinted 1971).
Reaven, G.M.; Reaven, E.P.: Prevention of age-related hypertriglyceridemia by calorie restriction and exercise training in the rat. Metabolism *30:* 982–986 (1981).
Report of the Working Group on Arteriosclerosis of the National Heart, Lung and Blood Institute: Arteriosclerosis, US Department of Health and Human Sciences, Public Health Service, National Institute of Health, NIH Publication No 81–2034, June 1981.
Ross, M.H.: Protein, calories and life expectancy. Fed. Proc. *18:* 1191–1207 (1959).
Royal Society of New Zealand: Coronary heart disease; in Shorland, McGillivray, Miles, Prior, Wigley, Report of a Committee (Royal Society of New Zealand, Wellington 1971).
Rynearson, E.H.: Americans love hogwash. Nutr. Rev. suppl., pp. 1–14 (1974).
Sanders, T.A.B.: Influence of fish oil supplements on man. Proc. Nutr. Soc. *44:* 391–397 (1985).
Sanders, T.A.B.; Younger, K.M.: The effects of supplements of ω3 polyunsaturated fatty acids on the fatty acid composition of the platelets and plasma choline phosphoglycerides. Br. J. Nutr. *45:* 613–616 (1981).
Schneider, E.L.; Reid, J.D.: Life extension. New Engl. J. Med. *312:* 1150–1168 (1985).
Shattil, S.J.; Cooper, R.A.: Membrane microviscosity and human platelet function. Biochemistry *15:* 4832–4837 (1976).
Shekelle, R.B.; Lepper, M.; Liu, S.; et al.: Dietary vitamin A and risk of cancer in the Western Electric Study. Lancet *ii:* 1185–1190 (1981).
Shorland, F.B.: Comparative aspects of fatty acid occurrence and distribution; in Florkin, Mason, Comparative biochemistry, vol. 111, pp. 1–102 (Academic Press, London 1962).

Shorland, F.B.: How good is the diet of today? A study of food in relation to life expectancy, with reflections on the ageing process. N.Z. J. Sci. *21:* 3–40 (1978).
Shorland, F.B.: Can nutritional knowledge affect the shape of agriculture and food technology in New Zealand? Proc. Nutr. Soc. N.Z. *4:* 173–192 (1979).
Shorland, F.B.: Do we really know anything about human nutrition? The fifth Murel Bell Memorial Lecture. Proc. Nutr. Soc. N.Z. *4:* 1–39 (1980).
Shorland, F.B.: Is our knowledge of human nutrition based on faulty premises? Nutr. Hlth *2:* 85–87 (1983a).
Shorland, F.B.: Do recommended daily dietary allowances stand up to scrutiny? Nutr. Hlth *2:* 105–109 (1983b).
Shorland, F.B.; Czochanska, Z.: The fatty acid composition of hens fed on coconut meal: differences in fat metabolism between birds and mammals. Aust. J. Sci. *32:* 336 (1970).
Shorland, F.B.; Czochanska, Z.; Prior, I.A.M.: Studies on the fatty acid composition of adipose tissue and blood lipids of Polynesians. Am. J. clin. Nutr. *22:* 594–605 (1969).
Shorland, F.B.; Igene, J.O.; Pearson, A.M.; Thomas, J.W.; McGuffey, R.K.; Aldridge, A.E.: Effects of dietary fats and vitamin E on the lipid composition and stability of veal during frozen storage. J. Agric. Fd Chem. *29:* 863–871 (1981).
Siess, W.; Scherer, B.; Bohlig, B.; Roth, P.; Kurzman, I.; Weber, P.C.: Platelet-membrane fatty acids, platelet aggregation, and thromboxane formation during a mackerel diet. Lancet *i:* 441–449 (1980).
Singer, P.; Jaeger, W.; Wirth, M., et al.: Lipid and blood pressure lowering effect of mackerel diet in man. Atherosclerosis *49:* 99–105 (1983).
Singer, P.; Wirth, M.; Gödicke, W.; Heine, H.: Blood pressure lowering effect of eicosapentaenoic acid-rich diet in normotensive, hypotensive and hyperlipemic subjects. Experimentia *41:* 462–464 (1985).
Starling, E.H.: Br. med. J. *ii:* 105 (1918); quoted by Longenecker (1944).
Sugarman, B.; Munro, H.N.: Altered accumulation of zinc by aging human fibroblasts in culture. Life Sci. *26:* 915–920 (1980a).
Sugarman, B.; Munro, H.N.: Altered [65-Zn] chloride accumulation by aged rats' adipocytes in vitro. J. Nutr. *110:* 2297–2307 (1980b).
Sukatme, P.V.: Size and nature of the protein gap. Nutr. Rev. *28:* 223–226 (1970).
Tannahill, R.: Food in history (Paldin Frogmore, St Albans 1975).
Tanner, J.M.: Growth and adolescence; 2nd ed. (Blackwell, Oxford 1962).
Tarladgis, B.G.; Watts, B.M.; Younathan, M.T.; Duggan, L.R.: A distillation method for the quantitative determination of malonaldehyde in rancid foods. J. Am. Oil Chem. Soc. *37:* 44–48 (1960).
Tepstra, A.H.M.; Hermus, R.J.J.; West, C.E.: The role of dietary protein in cholesterol metabolism. Wld Rev. Nutr. Diet., vol. 42, pp. 1–55 (Karger, Basel 1983).
Thompson, M.E.; Pack, A.R.C.: Effects of topical and systemic folate supplementation during pregnancy. Proc. Nutr. Soc. N.Z. *5:* 100–106 (1980).
Thorngren, M.; Gustafson, A.: Effects of 11-week increase in dietary eicosapentaenoic acid on bleeding time, lipid and platelet aggregation. Lancet *ii:* 1190–1193 (1981).
Timms, M.J.; Watts, B.M.: Protection of cooked meats with phosphates. Food Technol. *12:* 240–243 (1958).

Tolmasoff, J.M.; Ono, T.; Cutler, R.G.: Superoxide dismutase: correlation with life-span and specific metabolic rate in primate species. Proc. natn. Acad. Sci. USA *77:* 2777–2781 (1980).

United Nations: International action to avert the impending protein crisis (United Nations, New York 1968).

United Nations: Statistics in brief (United Nations, New York 1985).

US Senate Select Committee on Nutrition and Human Needs. Dietary Goals for the United States; 2nd ed. (Government Printing Office, Washington 1977).

Vaghefi, S.B.; Makdani, D.D.; Mickelsen, O.: Lysine supplementation of wheat proteins. A review. Am. J. clin. Nutr. *27:* 1231–1246 (1974).

Vane, J.R.: Fats and atheroma: an inquest. Br. med. J. *i:* 484–485 (1979).

Vane, J.R.: Private communication in reference (Office of Health economics, 1982).

Vijayagopalan, P.; Kurup, P.A.: Effect of dietary starches on the serum aorta and hepatic lipid levels in cholesterol fed rats. Atherosclerosis *11:* 257–264 (1970).

Wald, N.; Idle, M.; Boreham, J.; Bailey, A.: Low serum vitamin A and subsequent risk of cancer: preliminary results of a prospective study. Lancet *ii:* 813–815 (1980).

Walford, Roy L.: Maximum life span (Norton, New York 1983).

Willett, W.C.; Polk, B.F.; Underwood, B.A.; et al.: Relation of serum vitamins A and E and carotenoids to the risk of cancer. New Engl. J. Med. *310:* 430–434 (1984).

Wrenn, T.R.; Wyant, J.R.; Gordon, C.H.; et al.: Growth, plasma lipids and fatty acid composition of veal calves fed polyunsaturated fats. J. Anim. Sci. *37:* 1419–1427 (1973).

Yu, B.P.; Wong, G.; Lee, H.C.; Bertrand, H.; Masoro, E.J.: Age changes in hepatic metabolic characteristics and their modulation by dietary manipulation. Mech. Age. Dev. *24:* 67–81 (1984).

Yudkin, J.: Diet and coronary thrombosis – hypothesis and fact. Lancet *ii:* 155–162 (1957).

Zidenberg-Cherr, S.; Keen, C.L.; Lonnerdahl, B.; Hurley, L.: Dietary superoxide dismutase does not alter tissue levels. Am. J. clin. Nutr. *37:* 5–7 (1983).

Dr. F.B. Shorland, Department of Biochemistry, Victoria University of Wellington, Private Bag, Wellington (New Zealand)

Wld Rev. Nutr. Diet., vol. 57, pp. 214–274 (Karger, Basel 1988)

ω3-Fatty Acids in Health and Disease

P. Budowski[1]

Faculty of Agriculture, The Hebrew University of Jerusalem, Rehovot, Israel

Contents

[1] I thank S.A. Reed, P. Green and R. Karmali for providing information on recent publications on ω3-FA.

I. Introduction

We are witnessing an amazing surge of interest in ω3-fatty acids (ω3-FA) which, less than a decade ago, were of concern only to a few specialists. Today, ω3-FA provided by fish oils are attracting the attention of nutritionists, physiologists, biochemists and medical doctors. Some marketing operators have also been quick to seize up the situation.

The purpose of this review is to examine the developments that have taken place in the area of ω3-FA over the past decade. Older work will be referred to to the extent that it helps to put the more recent studies in proper perspective and provides the necessary background information. The emphasis is on human studies. Animal experiments will be discussed insofar as they serve as models and contribute to an understanding of the mechanisms involved.

II. What Are ω3-FA?

The ω3-family of polyunsaturated fatty acids (ω3-PUFA or ω3-FA) comprises α-linolenic acid and its metabolic conversion products found in animal tissues and blood. The other important PUFA family occurring in

Scheme 1. Chemical structures of linoleic and α-linolenic acids

Linoleic acid:

$CH_3(CH_2)_4CH{:}CHCH_2CH{:}CH(CH_2)_7COOH$

α-Linolenic acid:

$CH_3CH_2CH{:}CHCH_2CH{:}CHCH_2CH{:}CH(CH_2)_7COOH$

nature is made of ω6-FA whose parent FA is linoleic acid. The chemical structures of linoleic and α-linolenic acid are shown in scheme 1.

Omega, the last letter of the Greek alphabet, symbolizes the last carbon of the FA chain, the first being the carboxyl carbon, according to the official system [139]. The designation ω3-FA means that in these FA the first double-bond is situated between carbons 3 and 4, *counted from the methyl end of the FA chain.* The chemical structures of individual FA are described by the shorthand ω-notation, e.g. 18:2ω6 and 18:3ω3 for linoleic and α-linolenic acid, respectively. The notation shows the chain length, followed (after the colon) by the number of double-bonds and the position of the double-bond proximal to the methyl group. Instead of ω3, etc., the symbols n-3 etc., are often used, e.g. 18:3n-3. Two implicit assumptions are that the double-bonds are arranged according to the usual methylene-interrupted sequence and that they all have the *cis* configuration. The advantages of the ω-notation in the nutritional and metabolic context will become clear below.

The parent PUFA, linoleic and α-linolenic acids, are formed only in the vegetable kingdom and cannot be synthesized de novo by animals. They can, however, undergo alternating desaturation and chain elongation in animals, thus giving rise to the two PUFA families already mentioned. Scheme 2 shows the main conversion reactions.

Two more families of FA are known, based on oleic and palmitoleic acids (18:1ω9 and 16:1ω7, respectively) but conversions within these two families become significant only in animals receiving fat-free or PUFA-free diets. No interconversion between different FA families takes place in the animal kingdom.

The formation of double-bonds and the addition of two-carbon units in the above conversion reactions take place on the carboxyl side of the FA, so

Scheme 2. Main conversion pathways of linoleic and α-linolenic acids

ω6 or linoleic acid family:

18:2ω6 → 18:3ω6 → 20:3ω6 → 20:4ω6 → 22:4ω6 → 22:5ω6

ω3 or α-linolenic acid family:

18:3ω3 → 18:4ω3 → 20:4ω3 → 20:5ω3 → 22:5ω3 → 22:6ω3

that the saturated ω-moiety remains intact and constitutes a characteristic feature of each FA family, one that is immediately recognizable in the ω-notation, hence biogenic relationships are readily apparent. This important advantage is lost in the convention endorsed by IUPAC-IUB [139] in which the carbon atoms are counted from the carboxyl group. The latter system is used in a chemical context, or when the position of the double-bonds in relation to the carboxyl group is of biochemical significance. For instance, the first, third and fifth reactions in the two conversion sequences shown in the above scheme are referred to as Δ6, Δ5 and Δ4-desaturations, respectively, on account of the specificity of the corresponding desaturases.

Beside shorthand notations, trivial names are also used to designate the more common PUFA. The alpha is often omitted from α-linolenic acid, but in print and in speech, linolenic acid is easily confused with linoleic acid, and a distinction should also be made between α-linolenic acid and its isomer γ-linolenic acid or 18:3ω6. Other common names are *timnodonic acid* for 20:5ω3 and *clupanodonic acid* for 22:6ω3. These two FA are also referred to by their chemical names *icosapentaenoic acid* (IPA) and *docosahexaenoic acid* (DHA). IPA is often spelled eicosapentaenoic acid and abbreviated EPA. Such ambiguity complicates the indexing and retrieval of information. The Latinized spelling of the Greek root for C_{20} FA endorsed by IUPAC-IUB [139] is *icosa.*

III. ω3-FA in Historical Perspective

The nutritional significance of PUFA was first recognized by Burr and Burr [51, 52] in their work on deficiency symptoms induced in rats by fat-free but otherwise nutritionally adequate diets. Linoleic and arachidonic acids prevented the symptoms and were termed 'essential fatty acids' (EFA). α-Linolenic acid was also named as a possible EFA, but it soon became clear that this FA did not prevent all the symptoms caused by fat-free diets. For instance, according to the rat growth test under conditions of restricted water intake, α-linolenic acid had only 9% of the EFA activity of linoleic acid [279]. This, and the fact that Western diets usually contain far less α-linolenic acid than linoleic acid, caused nutritionists to focus their attention mainly on linoleic acid. The phrase 'anything α-linolenic acid does, linoleic acid can do better' probably sums up the opinion prevailing until the late 1970s, even though observations on the pronounced hypolipidemic effects of fish oils, epidemiological data, and the discovery that DHA is a major constituent of membrane lipids in brain and retina already pointed to possible biological functions and activities that were different from those of linoleic acid and derived FA.

The situation was to change drastically when Dyerberg et al. [78] suggested that IPA, found in foods of marine origin, might protect against thrombosis. By viewing the results of platelet aggregation measurements in the light of recently acquired knowledge on prostanoids formed from IPA and earlier observations on food habits, blood lipids, hemostasis and heart disease in Eskimos, the authors provided the trigger for a resurgence of interest in ω3-FA. It seems no exaggeration to say that this paper marks the beginning of the 'ω3 revolution'. Since then, a rapidly increasing number of publications on the effects of ω3-FA in health and disease has appeared, and the literature explosion still continues unabated. This is well illustrated by the small number – barely a dozen – of controlled trials with volunteers consuming fish, fish oils or concentrates of ω3-FA carried out before 1980 [103], while since then, well over 50 reports on the effects of ω3-FA on plasma lipids and platelet characteristics have been listed by Herold and Kinsella [118].

Sessions on ω3-FA have now become a regular feature at the annual meetings of the American Oil Chemists' Society, which also conducts short courses on ω3-FA [8, 9]. Since 1981, meetings on nutritional, metabolic and medical aspects of ω3-FA have been held in London [18], Hull [70], Reading [133], Oslo [203], Washington, DC [254] and St. Louis, Mo. [5]. A quarterly newsletter entitled 'n-3 News' has begun to make its appearance [185].

Recent reviews cover the following topics: the biological role of α-linolenic acid [171], α-linolenic acid deficiency [287], dietary requirements and functions of α-linolenic acid [285], the nutritional significance of ω3-

FA [40], the nutritional importance of IPA and DHA [234] and of fish oil supplements [235], and the prevention of atherosclerosis and cardiovascular disease by ω3-FA [73, 118].

In addition to the meeting proceedings published in book form [18, 254], recent books on seafoods are by Noelle [198], Nettleton [193] and Lands [163], the latter dealing extensively with the biochemical effects and nutritional importance of ω3-FA.

IV. Food Chains and Sources of ω3-FA

The distribution of α-linolenic acid and other ω3-FA in plants and animals has been extensively reviewed by Tinoco et al. [287] and Tinoco [285]. Only some salient points need to be discussed here.

Synthesis de novo of linoleic and α-linolenic acid takes place only in plants. While lower plants, such as ferns, liverwort, mosses and algae, also contain C_{20} and C_{22} conversion products, higher plants lack the capacity for further desaturation-elongation of C_{18} PUFA. Chloroplast lipids, especially phosphatidylgalactosides, are rich in α-linolenic acid, but fruits and seeds, including those used as raw materials for the production of edible oils, contain, as a rule, mainly linoleic acid, with little α-linolenic acid. Soybean oil, with about 8% α-linolenic acid and over 50% linoleic acid, is one of the few edible oils with significant amounts of α-linolenic acid. Rapeseed oil is another with some 9% 18:3ω3 and two or three times as much 18:2ω6. Linseed oil, not generally used as a food today but available in health food and specialty stores, is a good source of α-linolenic acid; it contains over 50% 18:3ω3 and 15–20% 18:2ω6.

Strict vegetarians and herbivorous animals therefore ingest C_{18}-PUFA, which are partly converted to long-chain PUFA, mainly 20:4ω6 and 22:6ω3. Omnivores and carnivores, on the other hand, receive preformed long-chain PUFA from their food and, in the case of felines, appear to have lost the capacity for producing them from C_{18}-PUFA [116, 225, 226]. High concentrations of long-chain ω3-PUFA are found in membrane lipids of brain, retinal photoreceptors, peripheral nerves, spermatozoa and testes of many species [285].

Unlike land species of plants and animals, in which the PUFA are generally dominated by ω6-FA, marine life forms exhibit a frank predominance of ω3-FA. This situation holds true all along the food chain, from phytoplankton and zooplankton through fish to marine mammals and applies also to birds and land mammals [1, 285] feeding on marine organisms. Fish caught in Northern latitudes (> 30 °N) have, on average, seven times as much ω3-FA as ω6-FA, whereas fish caught off the coast of Australia at 17 °S contain elevated levels of 20:4ω6 [207], in accordance with the higher 20:4ω6 levels along the food chain in these warmer waters [88, 98, 255].

The FA composition of different sea fish oils has been reviewed by Ackman [1]. ω3-FA make up 5–40% of the total FA of commercial fish oils. Menhaden oil, by far the major fish oil produced in the USA, typically contains 14% 20:5ω3 and 9% 22:6ω3. Other fish body oils also have an excess of 20:5ω3 over 22:6ω3, but the proportions are reversed in cod liver oil.

Marine oils, with an annual world production of 1.5 million metric tons [25], represent a huge potential source of ω3-FA. Ninety-seven percent of this amount are body oils from fatty fish such as menhaden, herring, sardine and many other species. Only a small percentage is produced from liver, mainly cod liver. Fish oils as such are not used as foods because of their poor shelf life and organoleptic properties which are due to the highly unsaturated PUFA. They are, however, widely used for margarine stock and some types of shortening, after partial hydrogenation which destroys ω3-FA. In the USA, fish oils and partially hydrogenated fish oils do not have the GRAS status (generally recognized as safe), and only recently was a petition to this effect filed for menhaden oil with the Food and Drug Administration [83].

The content and composition of lipids from 18 species of freshwater fish were reported by Kinsella et al. [151]. Representative samples of filets yielded an overall average of less than 2% lipid, not counting lake trout which had 7% lipid. The PUFA were dominated by ω3-FA, of which 22:6 was the major constituent, followed by 20:5. 20:4ω6 was also present. Unlike sea fish, freshwater species contained appreciable amounts of precursor PUFA 18:2ω6 and 18:3ω3. The ratio of ω6 to ω3-FA averaged 0.35, intermediate between the values for marine fish caught in cold and warm waters, respectively [255].

V. Metabolic Interactions

Interference with the metabolism of ω6-FA plays an important part in the way in which ω3-FA exert their effects on cell function. The interactions take place at different biochemical levels.

A. Δ6-Desaturation

An inhibitory effect of ω3-FA on the conversion of linoleic acid to arachidonic acid was first inferred by Machlin [175] from the hepatic FA composition of chicks receiving either ethyl linoleate (2 and 4% of the diet) or 10% linseed oil which provided approximately the same amount of linoleic acid as did 2% ethyl linoleate. The hepatic concentration of arachidonic acid was strongly depressed in chicks fed linseed oil, and the level of linoleic acid in these chicks was increased to twice the level found in the group fed 2% linoleate. Mohrhauer and Holman [180] reached a similar conclusion from liver and heart data in systematic rat experiments involving graded amounts of linoleic and α-linolenic acid. Conversely, the hepatic conversion of α-linolenic to its long-chain metabolites is partly suppressed by linoleic acid [222].

Brenner and Peluffo [33] showed, in vitro, that these mutual inhibitory actions take place at the Δ6-desaturase level, i.e. at the first enzymic step in the conversion sequences. Since the affinity of α-linolenic acid for the Δ6-desaturase is greater than that of linoleic acid, relatively small amounts of α-linolenic acid will effectively reduce the Δ6-desaturation of linoleic acid, whereas an excess of linoleic acid is required to inhibit the analogous desaturation of α-linolenic acid. The affinity of oleic acid, 18:1ω9, for the Δ6-desaturase is weak, so that this FA will not be desaturated as long as the diet supplies PUFA. Therefore, the appearance of 20:3ω9, which is the main conversion product of oleic acid in blood and tissues, is an early biochemical symptom brought about by a lack of dietary PUFA [90, 124].

B. Incorporation into Phospholipids

Membrane PUFA are almost exclusively located in the 2-position of phosphoglycerides, which imposes an upper limit on the amount of PUFA held in membrane phosphoglycerides. Hence, substrate competition for acyltransferases affects the PUFA composition of membrane phosphoglycerides. Since the incorporation of arachidonic acid and long-chain ω3-PUFA into these lipids proceeds at comparable rates, they extensively substitute for each other, according to the availability of dietary PUFA [136]. Brain lipids of young chicks provide a dramatic illustration of the strict regulation of total PUFA, in spite of dietary influences on the relative proportions of ω6 and ω3-FA [45]: after the chicks had received a diet containing either linoleic acid as safflower oil, or linseed oil rich in α-linolenic acid, the ω6/ω3 FA ratios of the cerebellar lipids were 2.6 and 0.4, respectively, but the total PUFA content was the same in both treatments, and a similar picture was seen in the cerebral lipids. Similar reciprocal replacements of ω6 and ω3-FA were reported for rat brain phospholipids [95, 159, 204], rat retina and retina and brain of the Rhesus monkey [195].

C. Icosanoid Formation

The term *icosanoids* refers to the metabolic oxygenation products formed from free arachidonic acid and other long-chain PUFA. They include the *prostanoids* (prostaglandins or PG, and thromboxanes or TX) produced via the cyclooxygenase pathway, and the hydroxy-FA and *leukotrienes* (LT) formed through the lipoxygenase pathway. Icosanoids act as cellular messengers and metabolic regulators and are produced by different cell types in response to physiologic and nonphysiologic stimuli. They are involved in such diverse physiopathologic processes as thrombosis and hemostasis, inflammation and immune responses, reproduction, renal function, and many others. Since icosanoids are ultimately derived from PUFA provided by the diet, it is clear that quantitative and qualitative changes in the dietary PUFA supply will have profound repercussions in the production of icosanoids by different tissues and cells.

The relationship between dietary PUFA and icosanoid formation has been reviewed [93, 110, 161, 172]. Scheme 3 illustrates the formation of icosanoids from arachidonic acid. The first step in the biosynthesis of icosanoids consists in the incorporation of molecular oxygen into the substrate FA to form peroxides which then undergo a series of enzymic and nonenzymic transformations to yield PG, TX, prostacyclins (PGI), hydroxy-FA and LT. For example, arachidonic acid 20:4ω6, the principal icosanoid precursor in cells, is converted by platelets mainly to TXA_2, a potent vasoconstrictor and platelet-aggregating agent, while the vessel epithelium specializes in the production of PGI_2, a PG with vasodilator and anti-aggregating properties. The PGI_2-TXA_2 balance is believed to play a role in thrombosis [120] and may be of significance in hypertension [202]. 20:3ω6 and 20:5ω3, which are normally present in membrane lipids in small amounts only, also serve as prostanoid precursors, giving rise to prostanoids of the 1- and 3-series, respectively (the subscripts in TXA_1, TXA_2, TXA_3 and other prostanoids refer to the number of double-bonds remaining in the side chains of the prostanoids).

IPA is a poor substrate for the cyclooxygenase [188], but is readily oxygenated when the concentration of peroxides in the incubation medium is elevated [65]. This peroxide effect has implications in situations in

Scheme 3. Main pathways of icosanoid production from arachidonic acid.

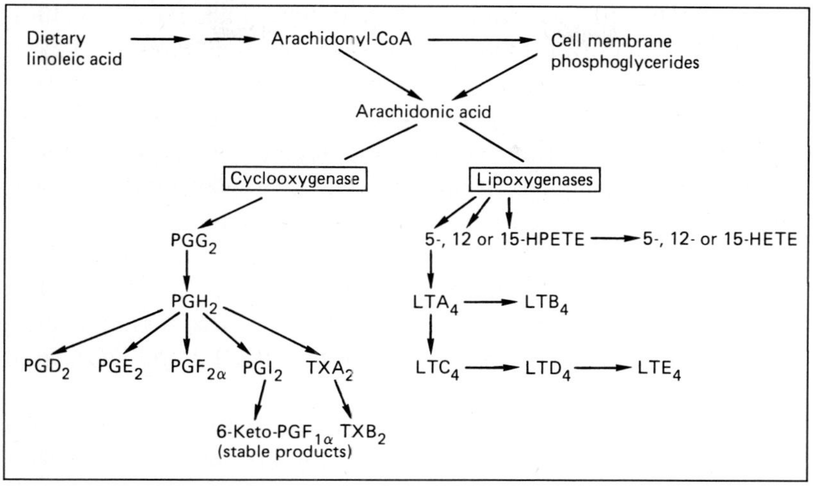

which the 'peroxide tone' is high, e.g. vitamin E deficiency. A claim according to which DHA is converted to a PG by trout gill [177] was later withdrawn [97]. While ω3-FA do not normally form prostanoids in amounts comparable to those produced by arachidonic acid, they strongly bind to the cyclooxygenase, thus inhibiting the cyclooxygenase-mediated oxygenation of arachidonic acid. IPA and DHA are particularly effective inhibitors [61, 164]. Results on prostanoid production in vivo and ex vivo in humans ingesting ω3-FA will be discussed in the section on platelet function.

Several lipoxygenases induce the oxygenation of arachidonic acid and other PUFA. The primary metabolite in the 5-lipoxygenase pathway is 5-hydroperoxyicosatetraenoic acid, the hydroperoxy derivative of arachidonic acid better known as 5-HPETE. This is reduced to the corresponding hydroxy compound 5-HETE, or dehydrated to the unstable epoxide LTA_4. LTB_4 is a hydrated derivative of LTA_4, whereas LTC_4, LTD_4 and LTE_4 are sulfopeptide conjugation products of LTA_4. Similar products are formed from IPA and their designations carry the subscript 5 (the subscript shows the number of double-bonds in the lipoxygenase substrate, a number that is preserved in the carbon skeleton of the LT produced; three of the double-bonds in the products are conjugated, hence the term 'leukotriene').

LT generated from arachidonic acid through the 5-lipoxygenase pathway are produced by leukocytes, lung and other cells and tissues. The biological effects of LT have been reviewed [214]. LTB_4 induces chemotaxis, chemokinesis and adhesion of leukocytes, and stimulates aggregation, degranulation and generation of superoxide. This LT is therefore an important mediator of inflammation. The sulfur-containing LTC_4, LTD_4 and LTE_4 exert spasmogenic effects on smooth muscle; they are especially potent bronchoconstricting agents, increase vascular permeability and stimulate mucus secretion. They are major constituents of the slow-reacting substance of anaphylaxis and are believed to contribute to the symptoms of asthma and other hypersensitivity reactions.

IPA, though a poor substrate for cyclooxygenase, is readily converted to LT of the 5-series by lipoxygenases in vitro [109, 140, 205, 297] and ex vivo [184]. More recently, it was shown that activated human neutrophils produce LTB_5 after dietary supplementation with IPA and DHA from fish oil [167, 216, 269, 275].

Dietary IPA was reported to reduce LTB_4 synthesis by human neutrophils [167, 216, 275], the action appearing to take place at the level of the LTA hydrolase which converts LTA_4 to LTB_4. Furthermore, the neutrophil-aggregating and chemotactic activities, and several other responses elicited by LTB_5, were lower by about one order of magnitude than those of LTB_4 [100, 169, 170, 216, 276]. LTC_5 equalled LTC_4 in smooth-muscle-contracting activity [168, 170].

Unlike IPA, DHA is not readily oxygenated by 5-lipoxygenase from rat basophilic leukemia-1 cells and only weakly interferes with LTB_4 synthesis [61]. In addition, the C_{22} analog of LTC_4 is virtually devoid of spasmogenic activity [61].

As a result of the various metabolic interactions outlined above, a dietary supply of ω3-FA will decrease the level of arachidonic acid-derived icosanoids, especially prostanoids, produced by different tissues. Such an effect has been observed in rat experiments, e.g. for cerebral cortex [94], clotting blood [132], heart and aorta [128], liver, thymus and spleen [178], and peritoneal macrophages [176]. Results on prostanoid production in vivo and ex vivo in humans ingesting ω3-FA will be discussed in the section on platelet function (section VIII).

VI. ω3-FA as EFA

One of the classical symptoms of EFA deficiency is increased water consumption due to trans-epidermal water loss [19]. It is a basic defect which may account for other features of EFA deficiency in young animals, such as growth retardation. The abnormality can be corrected or prevented by linoleic acid, but not by α-linolenic acid, apparently because the former, but not the latter, is incorporated into acylglucosylceramide and acylceramide which make up the epidermal water barrier [111]. Although arachidonic acid is also very effective in maintaining or reestablishing normal skin permeability, only linoleic acid is found in the epidermal sphingolipids, and there is evidence for retroconversion of arachidonic acid to linoleic acid [112]. It appears, therefore, that linoleic acid itself, rather than its C_{20} conversion product, plays an essential role here. When α-linolenic acid was applied topically [131], its activity in restoring normal water loss was 50% of that of linoleic acid, compared to only 6–10% in experiments in which the two PUFA were administered per os. It is possible that α-linolenic acid reaches the target organ only when allowed to bypass hepatic metabolism. Interestingly, the trans-epidermal water loss bears no direct relationship to membrane structure, since the epidermal sphingolipids responsible for the effect form an intercellular matrix [112].

While the essentiality of linoleic acid has been abundantly documented in numerous animal species [125] and normal growth and reproduction can be sustained by linoleic acid as the sole dietary PUFA over several generations, both in rats [159, 286] and guinea pigs [166], evidence for an absolute requirement for α-linolenic acid, not met by linoleic acid, has been scarce, at least until recently. For instance, Fiennes et al. [85] described skin symptoms and fatty liver in Capuchin monkeys fed on corn oil as the only source of dietary fat. In the diet of two of the animals, linseed oil was substituted for corn oil. This resulted in the normalization of liver histology. The skin pathology cleared up in one of the monkeys after some 2 months on the linseed oil regimen. This finding was not replicated in Rhesus monkeys under conditions of far more severe ω3-FA depletion [195]. Lamptey and Walker [159] reported that when rats were fed on a diet supplying only linoleic acid, the young of the second generation had impaired learning capacity in a simple black-and-white discrimination test, compared to rats also receiving α-linolenic acid in their diet. Growth and reproduction were normal in these animals, although there was substantial substitution of ω6-FA for ω3-FA in tissue phosphoglycerides, as also reported by Tinoco et al. [286]. Wheeler et al. [293] showed that α-linolenic but not linoleic acid restored normal electroretinographic responses in previously EFA-deficient rats. Therefore, impaired vision could account for the poor learning performance of the ω3-deficient rats in Lamptey and Walker's [159] experiment. A learning test that did not involve vision revealed that rats receiving 20%

soybean oil in a semisynthetic diet performed better than rats receiving lard or control animals on rat chow [62]. This result hints at some role of α-linolenic acid in brain function. Rat experiments in which sunflower oil was supplied to provide 1 g linoleic acid/100 g dry diet revealed impaired reproduction and lactation [89] and increased perinatal mortality [107], compared to animals receiving soybean oil which supplied linoleic acid with additional α-linolenic acid. However, no such effects were observed by Tinoco et al. [286] in their multigeneration rat experiments in which similar low amounts of linoleic and α-linolenic acid were provided as the pure methyl esters. A 6-year-old girl who had most of her small and large intestine removed and who was fed intravenously, developed neurological disturbances when an emulsion based on safflower oil was included in the infusion medium [126]. The symptoms disappeared after the emulsion was replaced by one having the FA composition of soybean oil. A membrane-bound enzyme of rat brain, 5′-nucleotidase, has a specific requirement for α-linolenic acid [22].

That ω3-FA may have specialized functions in the nervous system is suggested by the ubiquitous occurrence of DHA in high concentrations in brain gray matter [63] and retina of numerous mammalian species [6].

Neuringer et al. [195, 196] recently obtained strong evidence that Rhesus monkeys have an absolute requirement for ω3-FA for normal vision, a requirement that is met by α-linolenic acid but not by linoleic acid. The results have been discussed by Neuringer and Connor [194]. Pregnant females and their infants received a diet deficient in ω3-FA but containing linoleic acid as safflower oil. The control group received soybean oil. ω3-Deficient infants had subnormal visual acuity and prolonged recovery times of the dark-adapted electroretinogram after a saturating flash. Neuringer and Connor [194] suggest that there may be a slowing down of molecular events in the photoreceptors of ω3-deficient animals, as indicated by the defect in the rapid phase of dark-adaptation.

In fact, the association of ω3-FA with structures involving rapid molecular or ionic movement, or signal transmission, seems to be a general biological principle. Gudbjarnason et al. [106], in a discussion of the role of DHA in heart muscle function, thought that the spiral structure of DHA which is due to the ‘kinks’ at the *cis* double-bonds of the acyl chain, is subject to conformational changes upon polarization and depolarization, resulting in the opening and closing of cation-conducting trans-membrane channels. They observed that the heart rate of different mammals is related exponentially to the DHA content of cardiac muscle phospholipids. At one end of the spectrum, the fin whale, with 4.5% DHA, has a heart rate of 8 bpm, while at the other end, there is the mouse with the highest content of DHA, 40%, and a heart rate of 624 bpm. The above principle seems to apply to the vegetable kingdom where α-linolenic acid, the predominating FA of chloroplasts, is associated with photosynthesis: changes in photosynthetic competence of Chlorella, due to aging or to the illumination regimen, are paralleled by changes in the ratio of α-linolenic acid to chlorophyll [10].

The results indicating that ω3-FA play an essential role in the retinal function of infant Rhesus monkeys are relevant to human newborns. The ω3-FA status of preterm infants, as measured by the DHA content of erythrocytes, was reported to decline during the period of stomach-tube feeding [53]. With the start of breast-feeding, the DHA level increased again, but formula feeding sustained the decrease in DHA level. Breast milk provides DHA and other long-chain ω3-FA which are undetectable in formula milk products [60].

Another aspect of the retinal requirement for ω3-FA which may be relevant to human health concerns the relation between age and the DHA content of the retina. A recent rat study [232] has revealed a decrease in the retinal DHA level with age. Moreover, the results indicate that age does not affect the enzymic activities involved in the synthesis and turnover of the phospholipids and suggest that the age effect is due to a lower availability of DHA, since incorporation of labeled DHA in vitro into retinal phospholipids is more efficient for retinas of old rats than for those from young animals. The interesting possibility raised by the authors is that the dietary provision of preformed DHA might slow down the deterioration in retinal function that occurs in old age.

Minimum or optimum requirements for ω3-FA in human nutrition are not known. In view of the metabolic interactions already discussed (section V), any estimate will have to take into consideration the intake of linoleic acid.

In the case of a child on total parental nutrition [126], it was estimated that 0.54 cal% α-linolenic acid was required to maintain serum levels of ω3-FA metabolites. The apparent agreement of this figure with similar values arrived at in rat experiments [180, 221] is misleading, however, since the rat data were obtained in feeding experiments with purified α-linolenate ester, in the absence of linoleic acid. Laserre et al. [165] compared the effects of four different fats, supplied in a formula diet, on the serum lipids of healthy adult women. These authors thought that an intake of 0.5–1 cal% α-linolenic acid, together with 5–6 cal% linoleic acid, was necessary to maintain normal serum cholesterol and C_{20} ω6-FA levels. While the usefulness of the serum cholesterol value as a criterion for ω3-FA requirements is open to argument, the recommended dietary PUFA intake values represent a range of ω3/ω6 FA ratios which is close to the range of 1:4 to 1:10 considered prudent by Neuringer and Connor [194] and which also agrees with the ratio of 1:5, based on considerations of human milk and food selection by primitive man and wild animals [44].

The above attempts at estimating desirable ω3-FA intakes and ω3/ω6 FA ratios do not address the central question of the quantitative requirement for ω3-FA for normal development of brain and retina in the human fetus and infant. This difficult question is likely to be attacked in studies with nonhuman primates [194].

VII. The Hypolipidemic Action of ω3-FA

A. Early Work

Among the various biological properties of ω3-FA, the lipid-lowering action was the first to be recognized. The discovery that hypocholesterolemic effects could be achieved in humans by certain dietary vegetable oils [150] or vegetable diets [105] was followed by the recognition that fish oils were also effective, as first reported for sardine oil by Bronte-Steward et al. [35]. This effect of fish oils has since been abundantly confirmed. Peifer [212] and Stansby [265] have reviewed the early work on the subject. In his review, Peifer [212] discussed his own studies with rats in which he showed that the active fraction responsible for the hypocholesterolemic effect was the one containing C_{20} and C_{22}-PUFA of the ω3-family. He also pointed out that the cholesterol-lowering activities observed by various authors in mice, rats, chickens and humans were greater for fish oils than for linoleic acid-containing vegetable oils. Ahrens et al. [4] reported that menhaden oil, in addition to its cholesterol-lowering effect, also exhibited hypotriglyceridemic activity which exceeded that of corn oil, but this observation received little attention at the time.

B. Epidemiological Observations

Eskimos living in the arctic regions of Greenland, Alaska and Canada, whose traditional diet is composed primarily of fish and marine mammals, have long attracted the attention of physicians and nutritionists, because of the apparent absence of noninfective diseases prevalent in Western countries, especially ischemic heart disease, some forms of cancer, and diabetes [160]. For instance, a survey of the Upernavik district in Northwest Greenland, the site of one of the few remaining whaling and sealing populations, revealed that during 1950–1974 the incidence of acute myocardial infarction was 13 times less than expected from statistics in Denmark [157]. These authors also found a low incidence of chronic diseases such as psoriasis, bronchial asthma and diabetes mellitus, but a relatively high prevalence of apoplexy, epilepsy and cancer of the upper respiratory tract and salivary glands. Another survey of medical records for the period 1963–1978 was carried out by Dyerberg [72] in the UmanaK district which is also situated on the northwest coast of Greenland and whose population subsists mainly by hunting and fishing. An extremely low incidence of atherosclerotic heart disease and no reported cases of acute myocardial infarction were found.

Autopsies carried out on Alaskan natives revealed less severe atherosclerosis than found in Caucasians [247] and a low percentage of deaths due to cardiovascular diseases [12].

Sinclair [256], who earlier had closely observed the food habits of Canadian Eskimos and coastal Indians, noted their carnivorous habits and high cholesterol and fat intakes, and suggested a link between the absence of noninfective Western diseases and the elevated intake of fat of marine origin.

In the early 1970s, Bang et al. [15] and Bang and Dyerberg [14] published their data on plasma lipids and lipoproteins of Eskimos from the UmanaK district of Greenland. Cholesterol and triglyceride levels were much lower than in Danes, reflecting corresponding differences in low density lipoproteins (LDL) and very low density lipoproteins (VLDL) concentrations. High density lipoproteins (HDL) levels were higher in Eskimo males than in Danish men, and the age-dependent increase in plasma lipids generally observed in industrialized countries was not seen in Eskimos.

In a continuation of these studies, Dyerberg et al. [77] reported on FA analyses of plasma lipids in Greenland Eskimos. Very low concentrations of linoleic and arachidonic acid were found in Eskimos, compared to Danes, but IPA, present only in traces in plasma lipids of Danes, was a major PUFA in Eskimos. Native Greenlanders who had settled in Denmark and adopted Western food habits exhibited plasma FA profiles resembling those of Danes, an observation that strongly suggested an environmental influence.

A study of the Eskimos' diet by the double-portion technique [16, 17] showed that, while the total fat intake of Eskimos approximated that of Danes, the cholesterol intake was considerably higher (790 vs 420 mg/ 3,000 kcal), as was the dietary P/S ratio (0.864 vs 0.24). Of great interest was the pronounced difference in the ratio of ω3 to ω6-FA in Eskimo and Danish food (2.8 vs 0.3), due to the fact that the PUFA of the Eskimos' diet were dominated by 20:5ω3, 22:5ω3 and 22:6ω3, while the main PUFA in the Danish diet was linoleic acid, 18:2ω6.

Japanese, whose traditional diet is rich in fish, marine invertebrates and seaweed [149], have been the subject of numerous epidemiological studies [264]. The incidence of cardiovascular disease and mortality has long been known to be very low in Japan but rising in men of Japanese ancestry living in Hawaii or California [147]. The westernization of dietary habits is accompanied by increases in the level of serum lipids, especially triglycerides [147]. Japanese eating their traditional foods have elevated levels of ω3-FA, especially IPA, in their serum lipids [122, 271]. Within Japan, coastal people who eat more fish tend to have lower levels of plasma lipids and higher IPA concentration than farmers who consume less fish [122].

These observations on Eskimos and Japanese suggest a link between the intake of ω3-FA of marine origin and the level of serum lipids.

C. Recent Work

Results obtained in recent trials on the hypolipidemic effects of ω3-FA or fish oils have been discussed in reviews by Goodnight et al. [103], Herold and Kinsella [118] and Dyerberg [73]. The most important conclusion to emerge from these studies is undoubtedly that fatty fish, fish oils or concentrates of ω3-FA are powerful triglyceride-lowering agents, far more active than linoleic acid-rich vegetable oils.

This was demonstrated in an open trial with healthy volunteers in which a diet based on salmon and salmon oil was compared with a vegetable oil diet rich in linoleic acid and a control diet simulating a typical American diet [115]. The percentage of calories derived from fat, protein and carbohydrate, and the amount of cholesterol were the same for the three diets. The intakes of ω3-FA from the salmon diet and of linoleic acid from the vegetable oil diet were very high, 8 and 26% of the calories, respectively. After 4 weeks, plasma triglyceride concentrations dropped by 38% in the salmon oil group, compared to the control group, while the vegetable oil had no effect on the triglyceride level. Cholesterol concentrations decreased by only about 10% in both treatments. The changes in triglyceride and cholesterol concentrations reflected corresponding changes in the levels of VLDL and LDL. HDL cholesterol remained unchanged. Similar results were reported by Nestel et al. [192] for healthy volunteers receiving safflower oil, followed by fish oil, as 30% of the calories.

A different approach to the comparison between the hypolipidemic effects of fish oil and vegetable oils rich in linoleic acid is provided by encapsulated oils taken as supplements to the usual diets. Such an approach involves smaller amounts of oils than were used in the above trial by Harris et al. [115], but it has the advantage of permitting a double-blind crossover design. This design was used by Sanders and Hochland [236] and Mortensen et al. [182] in trials with healthy volunteers lasting 2 and 4 weeks, respectively. In both cases, ω3-FA were provided by MaxEPA capsules containing 18% IPA and 12% DHA, while the vegetable oil capsules contained a mixture of corn oil and olive oil with a linoleic acid content similar to the ω3-FA content of the fish oil. In both studies, the oils were supplied in amounts of 10 g/day. Total cholesterol remained unchanged in both treatments, but the fish oil supplement caused a drop in triglycerides by as much as 26% in the 4-week experiment, together with a fall in VLDL. The vegetable oil capsules did not affect the triglyceride level. HDL concentrations increased significantly after the MaxEPA treatment.

The remarkable triglyceride and VLDL-lowering activity of ω3-FA was reported by other investigators for normolipidemic subjects consuming fatty fish or seal [84, 174, 257, 259, 261, 263, 282], a diet rich in salmon and salmon oil [113, 134], cod liver oil [239, 245], ω3-FA concentrates [34, 71, 186, 274] and MaxEPA capsules [117, 237, 238, 242]. Only a few studies failed to find a statistically significant change in plasma triglycerides following ingestion of marine lipids, e.g. Lorenz et al. [173] in healthy volunteers consuming 40 ml cod liver oil during 25 days, or Bradlow et al. [31] in healthy subjects on a fish regimen during 8–21 days, but even in these cases the mean triglyceride level dropped by 20 and 33%, respectively.

The successful lowering of plasma triglycerides and VLDL by fish oils in healthy subjects prompted several trials with hyperlipidemic individuals. A double-blind crossover study was reported by Saynor [241]. Sixteen hypertriglyceridemic subjects were asked to take 20 g encapsulated Max-

EPA oil per day, or capsules providing 20 g/day of a corn oil-olive oil blend. Each oil was taken over a period of 2 months, with a washout period of one month between the two treatments. The fish oil supplement caused a 48% drop in serum triglycerides and a significant 8% reduction in cholesterol. The vegetable oil capsules resulted in a 13% decrease in triglyceride level, but the change in cholesterol was not significant. An open trial in which the same fish oil supplement was given to 92 patients with cardiovascular disease or hyperlipidemia over periods up to 2 years yielded essentially similar results [243]. In that study, it was found that the reduction in triglycerides was most rapid during the first month of fish oil supplementation, while the decrease in cholesterol was slower, reaching 5% at the end of 2 years.

Two short-term double-blind trials with hypertriglyceridemic patients taking 10 or 15 g of MaxEPA or matched capsules containing corn oil-olive oil yielded similar results, with less pronounced reductions in triglycerides and no change in cholesterol [237, 295].

Simons et al. [253] reported on a double-blind crossover study with MaxEPA (6 or 16 g/day) and matched placebo capsules containing olive oil. Each supplement was taken during 3 months. The subjects were patients with common lipid phenotypes and their diet was restricted in saturated FA and cholesterol. Compared to the placebo, the fish oil reduced the mean triglyceride value by 22% in the group with IIa phenotype, by 28% in the IIb patients and by 41% in type IV subjects. In one patient with phenotype V, triglycerides fell by 63%. The decrease in cholesterol was insignificant, except in the type V patient where it attained 26%. Single-blind observations showed that the triglyceride-lowering effect was maximal after one month on MaxEPA, and that the effect was completely lost one month after switching from MaxEPA to placebo. It was also noted that the higher the placebo plasma level of triglycerides, the greater the decrement in triglyceride concentration brought about by the fish oil.

Another trial involved 20 hypertriglyceridemic subjects with phenotypes IIb and V, which were put successively on a low-fat, low-cholesterol control diet, a salmon and fish oil diet, and a vegetable oil diet rich in linoleic acid [213]. The two experimental diets were balanced for cholesterol content. After 4 weeks of the fish oil diet, the mean plasma triglyceride levels decreased by 64% in the type IIb patients and by 79% in the type V subjects, whereas the cholesterol concentrations in these two groups fell by 27 and 45%, respectively. VLDL were dramatically reduced, and the fasting chylomicronemia present in some of the type V subjects disappeared. Replacement of the fish oil diet by the vegetable oil regimen led to a rapid rise in plasma lipids. When the concentrations of total triglycerides, VLDL-cholesterol and VLDL-triglycerides tripled in the type V patients and approached control values, the vegetable oil regimen had to be discontinued after 2 weeks. Lipid-lowering effects were also observed by Singer et al. [262] in patients with types IV and V hyperlipoproteinemia after a mackerel diet.

The experimental diets in these trials provided mixtures of ω3-FA, principally IPA and DHA. According to Sanders [235], purified ethyl esters of IPA and DHA both possess hypotriglyceridemic activity in rats. It appears therefore justified to relate the triglyceride-lowering activity of fish lipids to the total amount of long-chain FA.

In several trials, graded amount of fish oil or ω3-FA concentrates were tested in humans. Estimates of the minimum daily dose of total long-chain ω3-FA producing a significant reduction in serum triglyceride varied from 7 g in the case of a DHA concentrate taken by healthy volunteers during 4 weeks [34] to as little as 2 g in a 3-month experiment with hyperlipidemic patients taking MaxEPA capsules [253]. Sanders and Roshanai [238], in a 3-week dose-response study with healthy subjects, found that 10 g MaxEPA/day, or 3.4 g ω3-FA/day, were required to elicit a significant hypotriglyceridemic effect. Singer et al. [261, 263] obtained a similar value of 4 g ω3-FA/day from experiments with normolipidemic individuals receiving a mackerel diet during 2 weeks, but when these subjects consumed a herring diet providing only 2.8 g ω3-FA/day, the effects were not significant. However, this lower dosage of ω3-FA from a herring diet did cause a fall in serum lipids in hyperlipidemic subjects [262].

α-Linolenic acid is relatively ineffective under conditions under which ω3-FA from fish lipids produce significant effects. Thus, 20 ml linseed oil/day taken by healthy subjects during 2 weeks failed to alter the levels of total plasma cholesterol and triglycerides, while the same amount of MaxEPA oil caused a 43% drop in triglycerides [238]. The linseed oil FA contained 54% α-linolenic acid, whereas the value for ω3-FA in the fish oil was 37%. A large-scale Norwegian vegetable oil experiment, in which volunteers took 10 ml linseed oil or safflower oil/day, did not reveal any significant changes in plasma cholesterol after 6 months [187]. Much greater amounts of linoleic acid-rich vegetable oils are required to achieve hypocholesterolemic effects, and the same is true for α-linolenic acid from linseed oil [82].

D. Mechanism of Action

The mechanism involved in the hypolipidemic action of dietary ω3-FA has been investigated by observing changes in the metabolism of plasma lipoproteins.

A striking lowering of VLDL has been consistently found to accompany the fall in plasma triglyceride concentration. According to Nestel et al. [191, 192], this effect is due to a depressed hepatic production and secretion of VLDL, as shown by the considerable reduction in the fluxes of both VLDL apoprotein B and VLDL triglycerides, compared to the values found in individuals on a safflower oil regimen. A similar mechanism may operate in the attenuation, by fish oil, of the rise in plasma triglycerides and VLDL that follows a carbohydrate load in healthy subjects [114]. Inhibition of hepatic FA synthesis by dietary ω3-FA has been observed in rats [137, 296] and may play a role in the depression of VLDL synthesis.

LDL are remnants of VLDL catabolism and their concentration would be expected to decrease when VLDL synthesis is inhibited. This was found to be the case with high doses of fish oil providing over 20 g ω3-FA/day [114, 134, 213], though smaller doses used by others caused only slight, and sometimes insignificant, changes. Turnover studies on healthy volunteers established that fish oil reduced the synthesis of LDL apoprotein. High intakes of fish oil not only cause a decrease in LDL cholesterol, but also prevent the rise in LDL cholesterol that results from supplemental dietary cholesterol [190]. A special case is presented by hyperlipidemic subjects with type V phenotype which exhibit increased LDL-cholesterol levels after fish oil [213, 253], perhaps because of the very large concentration of VLDL whose cholesterol, after loss of triglycerides, accumulates in the LDL particles.

While the hypotriglyceridemic action of ω3-FA can be ascribed to the inhibition of the hepatic synthesis of VLDL, the cholesterol-lowering effect is still surrounded by controversy. The traditional view, according to which dietary PUFA cause an increase in fecal steroid excretion, has recently been challenged by Beynen and Katan [24]. Following a suggestion by Nestel et al. [192], Beynen and Katan [24] postulated that fish oil PUFA and vegetable PUFA enter the hepatic pathway of oxidation and ketogenesis, rather than esterification and VLDL production, thus raising fasting blood levels of ketone bodies. Since the PUFA carbons are exported as ketone bodies for utilization by the periphery, this process would leave no trail of cholesterol-carrying lipoproteins. The idea of ketogenicity increasing with the degree of unsaturation of dietary FA is open to argument [42] and contradicts older work with rats in vivo.

A diet rich in ω3-FA reduced plasma cholesterol in rats and increased the transfer of cholesterol into bile [13]. This means that LDL catabolism is increased in this animal model. Whether fish oils produce a similar effect in humans remains to be seen, since dietary linoleic acid-rich oils do not consistently result in increased fecal steroid excretion in man [39].

Some authors reported higher HDL-cholesterol levels after a fish oil regimen [117, 174, 236, 238, 239, 241, 242, 253, 263], but others failed to observe significant changes. The reason for these discrepancies may be found in the variable composition of fish lipids, especially the amounts of IPA, DHA and cholesterol. DHA has been reported to be more effective than IPA in increasing HDL-cholesterol in rats [181]. Also MaxEPA oil contains 3.6–6 mg cholesterol per gram [192, 253]. In trials in which the cholesterol intake was controlled, HDL-cholesterol did not change [115] or decreased [190, 192, 213] when volunteers ingested large amounts of fish lipids. Furthermore, the rise in HDL-cholesterol reported in some trials in which the cholesterol intake was not controlled, seems to be due to an increase in the HDL_3 fraction [234, 243] whose pathophysiology is uncertain, rather than to an increase in the HDL_2 fraction which is believed to protect against atherosclerosis.

VIII. ω3-FA and Platelet Function

Platelet aggregation is involved in the initial events leading to hemostasis and thrombosis, the one being a biologically useful process, while the other is life-threatening. Through their interaction with the vessel wall, platelets also play a role in atherogenesis [231]. Dietary modification of platelet function has, therefore, important health implications.

A. Epidemiologic Observations

As in the case of the hypolipidemic effects of ω3-FA, observations on seafood-eating populations played a dominant part in directing attention to the anti-aggregating properties of ω3-FA. The low incidence of thrombotic cardiovascular diseases in Eskimos, Japanese and other peoples in which seafood constitutes an important part of the diet was referred to in a previous section. The bruising or bleeding tendency of Greenland Eskimos has often been noted. Accounts dating back to as early as the 15th century mention delayed blood clotting among Eskimos [72, 75]. Measurements of bleeding times by the template technique in Greenland Eskimos and age- and sex-matched Danes yielded mean values of 8.1 and 4.8 min, respectively [74]. Also, the threshold concentration of ADP required for secondary platelet aggregation was considerably higher in Eskimos than in Danes, indicating a reduced platelet aggregability in the Greenlanders. A similar difference in platelet aggregability was found between residents of a fishing village and a farming community in Japan [122].

B. The Antithrombotic Hypothesis

Experiments undertaken by Dyerberg et al. [78] revealed three important properties of IPA: (a) it failed to induce aggregation in human platelet-rich plasma under conditions under which arachidonic acid was strongly pro-aggregatory; (b) it inhibited first-phase aggregation induced by ADP in human platelet-rich plasma, while arachidonic acid was not inhibitory, and (c) it was converted by rat arterial tissue to a potent anti-aggregating substance, assumed to be PGI_3. The authors pointed out that TXA_3, formed by rat platelets from IPA, was already known to be devoid of significant pro-aggregating activity. In view of these results, and against the background of the low incidence of thrombotic diseases and the elevated ratio of IPA to arachidonic acid in Eskimos, Dyerberg et al. [78] put forth the suggestion that IPA might have anti-thrombotic properties. The rationale was that the replacement of arachidonic acid by IPA, as seen in Eskimo plasma, would create a favorable balance of pro-aggregating and anti-aggregating factors, hence a decreased thrombotic tendency.

C. Experimental Studies

Following the publication of the paper by Dyerberg et al. [78], experimental evidence began to accumulate showing that ingestion of seafood and dietary supplements rich in IPA leads to changes in hemostasis and platelet function in volunteers, consistent with the observations made on Eskimos.

A one-man experiment was carried out by Sinclair who had previously joined Bang and Dyerberg on the fourth expedition to Northwest Greenland. As the expedition had to be cut short by the sudden onset of winter, Sinclair obtained a deep-frozen seal in March 1979 and went on a diet consisting solely of seal, fish, crustaceans, mollusks and water for 100 days

[257, 258]. Platelet IPA rose, while 20:4ω6 fell. Template bleeding times increased considerably and stabilized at 15 min. The platelet count dropped to a very low value of $83 \times 10^3/mm^3$.

In a study reported by Siess et al. [251], 7 volunteers consumed 500–800 g mackerel/day, which was estimated by the authors to supply 7–11 g IPA/day. At the end of a week, the levels of IPA and DHA in platelet microsomes increased at the expense of arachidonic acid. There was a reduction in platelet aggregation upon low-dose collagen stimulation of platelet-rich plasma. Both IPA and arachidonic acid were readily released from platelet phospholipids upon aggregation.

Thorngren and Gustafson [281] studied 10 healthy men who changed their habitual Swedish diet to one containing predominantly mackerel and salmon during a period of 11 weeks. ω3-FA in platelets rose and ω6-FA fell, except arachidonic acid. Bleeding times rose to a maximum (42% increase) after 6 weeks and tended to decrease thereafter. Platelet aggregability in the presence of adenosine 5′-diphosphate (ADP) and collagen decreased. Interestingly, the ADP threshold value for secondary aggregation continued to increase as late as 11 weeks after the discontinuation of the fish diet, long after normalization of the FA composition. Later reports by Thorngren et al. [283, 284] confirmed that the changes in bleeding times and platelet aggregation did not coincide in time with the alteration in FA composition.

Goodnight et al. [102] also studied the effect of large amounts of fish, under more strictly controlled conditions. Healthy subjects consumed a 1-lb salmon steak and 60–90 ml salmon oil/day (about 10 g ω3-FA/day) during a period of 4 weeks. A control group received a 'typical American diet' with virtually no ω3-FA, but of similar fat, protein, carbohydrate and cholesterol content. After a 3-week washout period, the diets were switched and the regimens continued for another 4 weeks. The fish diet resulted in the incorporation of IPA and DHA into platelet phospholipids, while the levels of linoleic and arachidonic acid fell. Bleeding times increased in all but one of the 11 subjects measured, with a mean increase of 48%, platelet retention on glass beads was reduced, and platelet aggregation in response to dilute ADP was inhibited by the fish diet. The platelet count decreased, severely so in some of the subjects, but reverted to normal one week after the end of the experiment.

A more moderate intake of fish (300–400 g/day of sardines, pilchard, herring and kabeljou, providing an estimated 1–4 g IPA/day) during 8–21 days, also caused an increase in the ratio of IPA to arachidonic acid in the platelets and a decrease in platelet aggregability in the presence of ADP, epinephrine and collagen, but not arachidonic acid [31].

Cod liver oil produced results similar to those reported for fish diets, i.e. an increased ratio of IPA to arachidonic acid in platelets, and either elevated bleeding times or reduced platelet aggregability or both [3, 239, 244], though the observed changes in platelet FA, aggregability and hemostasis did not always follow similar time patterns [37]. A crossover study showed that cod liver oil was more effective than corn oil in reducing platelet aggregability [36].

Encapsulated MaxEPA oil was used in several trials. A supplement of 10 g MaxEPA (1.8 g IPA) or 10 g olive-corn oil was supplied daily to healthy volunteers in a double-blind crossover study lasting 4 weeks for each of the oils [81, 182]. The fish oil caused an increase in the ratio of IPA to arachidonic acid and in bleeding time, but platelet aggregability was not significantly altered. Sanders and Hochland [236] used a similar design in a 2-week trial and found that platelet aggregation induced by the lowest dose of collagen was reduced by both oil supplements, while other aggregating agents failed to reveal any treatment effect.

An open trial [238] showed that 20 ml/day of MaxEPA over 2 weeks resulted in an elevated ratio of IPA to arachidonic acid and prolonged bleeding times but had no effect on platelet aggregability. A long-term trial with heart patients [243] revealed that after 12 months, bleeding times were increased with a daily supplement of 20 ml MaxEPA, but not with 10 ml. When platelet kinetics were examined in some of these patients after 5 weeks [117], it was found that platelet survival time was lengthened by 10%, the platelet count decreased by 15%, and the plasma levels of platelet factor 4 and thromboglobulin fell by 75 and 30%, respectively. A large dose of MaxEPA (50 ml, or 9 g IPA), given daily to atherosclerotic patients and healthy subjects for 4 weeks, resulted in the incorporation of IPA into platelet lipids, a rise in bleeding time and a fall in plasma thromboglobulin [153]. Platelet aggregation by arachidonic acid was not affected.

A concentrate containing 75% IPA as the ethyl ester in encapsulated form was tested during 4 weeks in healthy subjects ingesting 4.8 g/day, equivalent to 3.6 g IPA/day [274]. IPA in platelets rose, while aggregation induced by collagen, ADP and epinephrine decreased. Platelet aggregation stimulated by arachidonic acid remained unchanged, and whole-blood viscosity decreased. The same IPA concentrate in smaller doses (up to 3.6 g/day, or 2.7 g IPA/day) was given during 16 weeks to patients with diabetes mellitus, vascular diseases, various types of hyperlipidemia and hypertension [123], with essentially similar results. Decreased platelet aggregability was also reported in healthy volunteers receiving during 4 weeks an ethyl ester concentrate containing 67% IPA [186]. Platelet activity in diabetics was decreased by as little as 40 mg IPA/day [289].

Von Schacky and Weber [246] studied the metabolism and effects of purified IPA and DHA on platelet function. IPA appeared in plasma lipids 4 h after ingestion of IPA but was not incorporated into platelet phospholipids until day 6, which points to a role of megakaryocyte maturation in the establishment of the platelet PUFA pattern. Administration of DHA also resulted in a rise in plasma IPA, showing that retroconversion was likely to have occurred. Both IPA and DHA caused a reduction in platelet aggregation in response to collagen. It should be noted that in platelets, IPA is taken up specifically by phosphatidylcholine and phosphatidylethanolamine, with little or no incorporation into phosphatidylinositol and phosphatidylserine [3, 36, 245, 246]. That IPA and DHA enter different metabolic pathways is indicated by the preferential incorporation of IPA into plasma cholesteryl esters, while DHA appears mainly in triglycerides [261].

Compared to fish oils and long-chain ω3-FA, α-linolenic acid supplied by linseed oil is much less effective in raising the concentration of IPA in plasma lipids [20, 49, 76, 179, 240, 260] and in platelets [238]. Sanders and Younger [240] have pointed out that the large reserves of linoleic acid in body lipids will interfere with the conversion of α-linolenic acid to its long-chain metabolites. It is therefore unreasonable to expect marked changes in long-chain PUFA in plasma and membrane lipids of subjects ingesting linseed oil in trials lasting only weeks or months.

The results obtained with some animal models are relevant in this connection. A model used by Nørdoy [199, 200] consisted of rats rendered hypercholesterolemic by a diet rich in cholesterol and saturated fat. In these rats, a supplement of corn oil exacerbated the characteristic platelet adhesiveness and venous thrombosis, while linseed oil completely prevented venous thrombosis and brought platelet stickiness back to nearly normal values. In a different rat model [201], pulmonary thrombosis was induced by intravenous injection of ADP, after the animals had received a saturated fat diet. A dietary supplement of linseed oil was more effective than cottonseed oil in reducing the incidence of pulmonary thrombosis. Recently, Ishinaga et al. [138] showed that linseed oil reduced the collagen-induced aggregation of rat platelets under conditions under which dietary safflower oil and cocoa butter were ineffective. Kloeze et al. [152] failed to find differences between the effects of dietary supplements of safflower and linseed oil on platelet adhesiveness in rabbits, but later experiments showed that rabbit platelet aggregation induced by collagen and thrombin was reduced to a greater extent by dietary linseed oil than by safflower oil [288].

The evidence concerning changes in platelet function in humans by dietary α-linolenic acid is sparse. Early reports were contradictory or negative [28, 96, 209, 210]. More recently, a group of French farmers agreed to use rapeseed oil and margarine rich in rapeseed oil instead of butter over a one-year period [223]. This change resulted in a decreased intake of saturated FA and a slight rise (from 1.2 to 3.6% of total FA) in dietary α-linolenic acid. IPA in platelets increased slightly (up to 0.6%) and arachidonic acid dropped from 29.1 to 26.8%. In spite of these relatively minor alterations in platelet PUFA content, there was a marked decrease in platelet aggregability and platelet coagulant activity.

Platelet aggregability was measured in platelet-rich plasma of 2 healthy subjects who took a daily supplement of 60 ml linseed oil during 48–53 days [49]. There was a considerable rise in the concentration of collagen required for aggregation.

D. The Role of Prostanoids

The above results are remarkably consistent in showing that, except for occasional negative findings expected from variable experimental conditions, dietary ω3-FA cause increased ratios of IPA to arachidonic acid, accompanied by prolonged bleeding times and diminished platelet aggregability ex vivo. The role of prostanoids as mediators of the observed changes in platelet function has been intensively investigated.

A decreased formation of TXB_2 was first demonstrated in collagen-stimulated platelet-rich plasma from volunteers on a mackerel diet [251]. This was abundantly confirmed for platelets stimulated with a variety of agonists [31, 36, 37, 86, 123, 173, 236, 245]. A reduced production of TXB_2 after ingestion of ω3-FA was also found by assay of TXB_2 in serum [153, 244, 259] and by estimation of TXB_2 metabolites in urine [153, 244]. Thorngren et al. [284] also observed less TXB_2 in clotting blood after a fish diet but found no changes in the small amounts of TXB_2 in blood from incisions made in the course of bleeding time determinations. The authors expressed doubt on the role of local TXA_2 production on the delay in hemostasis caused by ω3-FA.

Ingestion of fish or fish oil supplements led to increased formation of TXB_3 by clotting blood or stimulated platelets [153, 173, 244]. Furthermore, the appearance of TXB_3 in urine shows that this IPA metabolite is actually formed in vivo [153, 244].

Platelet function may also be affected by ω3-FA via PGI production by the vessel wall. Dyerberg and Jørgensen [79] and Dyerberg et al. [80] reported that human umbilical vasculature was able to convert IPA to PGI_3 without interference with the conversion of arachidonic acid to PGI_2. In agreement with these results, obtained in vitro, urinary excretion data presented by Fischer and Weber [87] and von Schacky et al. [244] established that PGI_3 is formed in vivo after ingestion of ω3-FA, without decrease in excretion of PGI_2 metabolites. Only individuals with a high basal rate of PGI_2 excretion exhibited a lower urinary PGI_2 level after dietary ω3-FA [153]. According to Zuccato et al. [299], Eskimos excrete more total PGI metabolites than Danes, while the level of urinary total TX metabolites is lower in Eskimos than in Danes.

Urinary excretion of PGE metabolites in healthy volunteers was increased by supplemental linoleic acid and decreased by α-linolenic acid [2]. Thus, endogenous PG production is affected by α-linolenic acid in spite of the low levels of IPA induced by the ω3-FA precursor.

E. Mechanism of Action

The observations on the effects of ω3-FA on platelet aggregation and hemostasis, and the biochemical interactions outlined earlier, lead to the following picture: (a) Dietary IPA and DHA are incorporated into plasma and membrane lipids, the level of IPA being further increased by partial retroconversion of DHA to IPA. (b) The availability of arachidonic acid for TXA_2 formation is reduced by ω3-FA because of (1) inhibition by α-linolenic acid of the synthesis of archidonic acid from linoleic acid; (2) competition between long-chain ω3-FA and arachidonic acid for incorporation into the 2-position of the phosphoglyceride molecules where the cyclooxygenase substrates are located, and (3) competitive inhibition of cyclooxygenase by ω3-FA. (c) IPA is readily released from platelet phospholipids upon activation of phospholipase A_2 and becomes available for the synthesis of small amounts of TXA_3 [245, 251], while the vessel wall utilizes IPA for the synthesis of PGI_3, usually without impairment of PGI_2 formation.

The reduced production of pro-aggregating and vasoconstrictor TXA_2 and the formation of the weakly active TXA_3 by platelets, together with the arterial generation of anti-aggregating and vasodilatory PGI_2 and PGI_3, would be expected to result in a less thrombotic state, as postulated by Dyerberg et al. [78].

The actual mechanism by which ω3-FA attenuate platelet function is undoubtedly more complex than outlined here. Von Schacky et al. [245] suggested that the higher fluidity of platelet membranes induced by dietary ω3-FA might impair the coupling of the thrombin receptor with phospholipases C and A_2, and thus reduce the amount of arachidonic acid available for TXA_2 formation. Altered fluidity could also affect platelet function in other ways, e.g. by changes in membrane permeability and membrane-anchored enzyme activities.

IX. Hypotensive Effects

A drop in systolic and diastolic blood pressure (BP) was noted by Sanders et al. [239] in an open trial with healthy men taking 20 ml cod liver oil/day (4 g ω3-FA/day) during 6 weeks. The effect was still evident 5 weeks after the oil supplement had been stopped. Lorenz et al. [173] also reported a fall in systolic BP in healthy men receiving a daily dose of 40 ml cod liver oil during 25 days. Moreover, the fish oil supplement in this trial caused an attenuated BP response to infusions of norepinephrine and angiotensin II, the oil effect being significant in the case of norepinephrine. There were no changes in plasma norepinephrine and epinephrine during the supplementation, whereas plasma renin activity and urinary excretion of aldosterone, kallikrein, PGE_2 and $PGF_{2\alpha}$ all tended to decrease (effect not significant). There was a significant rise in urinary sodium excretion.

A fall in BP was found when healthy men received encapsulated MaxEPA oil (10 g/day, or 4 g ω3-FA/day) in a double-blind trial of 4 weeks duration, in which control capsules provided a vegetable oil mixture with a similar content of linoleic acid [182]. Systolic BP in both standing and recumbent position decreased by 5 mm Hg in the fish oil group, compared to the vegetable oil group. Plasma renin values remained unchanged. Hypotensive effects achieved with MaxEPA were also reported by Norris et al. [202] and Rogers and James [229].

A 2-week crossover experiment with mackerel and herring diets was undertaken with healthy volunteers by Singer et al. [261]. The mackerel regimen resulted in a marked drop in systolic and diastolic BP. Three months after the discontinuation of the experimental diet, the mean diastolic BP was still low, i.e. 7 mm Hg less than before the regimen. The plasma renin concentration also decreased. The herring diet produced no changes in BP and renin value. Similar hypotensive effects were obtained with the same mackerel diet in individuals with mild essential hypertension in short-term and long-term experiments [259, 263] and in patients with types IV and V hyperlipoproteinemia [262]. The latter study showed that in such patients, BP was lowered by a herring diet which provided only about half as much ω3-FA as mackerel and which was ineffective in normolipidemic subjects. The hypotensive effect was particularly pronounced in individuals with a high basal BP. Vegetable oils rich in either linoleic or α-linolenic acid had much weaker effects in short-term experiments [260].

Analytical data on the FA composition of adipose tissue from 399 free-living men in the USA revealed an inverse correlation between the α-linolenic acid content and blood pressure [23]: an absolute 1% increase in 18:3ω3 was associated with a fall of 5 mm Hg in the systolic and diastolic arterial BP. There was no correlation between BP and linoleic acid. The data suggest a long-term effect of dietary α-linolenic acid on BP.

The mechanism by which ω3-FA exert their hypotensive effect might involve the same alteration in prostanoid pattern discussed in relation to the attenuation of platelet function, i.e. a shift away from the pro-aggregatory and vasoconstrictor state dominated by TXA_2 to an antiaggregating and vasorelaxant situation in which PGI_2 and PGI_3 prevail. Also, altered rheological properties of erythrocytes, already referred to, could lead to an improved microcirculation and thus contribute to the lowering of BP. Other mechanisms suggested [173, 261] involve a reduction in neurotransmitter release, or altered cell membrane fluidity resulting in a weakened coupling of receptors with neurotransmitters and pressor hormones [99]. The possibility that increased membrane fluidity and other rheological changes are involved is suggested by observations on lower whole-blood viscosity and increased erythrocyte deformability in healthy subjects and in patients with peripheral vascular disease, after ingestion of ω3-FA [56, 154, 274, 295]. Neither plasma viscosity nor hematocrit values were altered by the oil treatment, so that the observed changes could be ascribed to the incorporation of ω3-FA into the erythrocyte membrane. These changes, induced by ω3-FA, would decrease the resistance of capillary blood vessels to the blood flow and would therefore be expected to exert a beneficial effect on BP. A more detailed discussion of these and other mechanisms, as suggested by animal models, is found in Land's book [163].

X. ω3-FA and Immune-Inflammatory Responses

Arachidonic acid-derived icosanoids are produced by different types of immunocompetent cells and play a role in the cell-mediated and humoral immune response [101, 104] and inflammation [119]. Because of the complex cellular interactions in the immune defense system, the intricate pattern of icosanoids produced by different cells and the diversity of effects exerted by icosanoids on immunocompetent cells, no clear picture has emerged concerning the relation between icosanoids and the immune response [142, 143]. What is clear, however, is that dietary ω6- and ω3-FA do affect the immune and inflammatory responses, that the two types of PUFA often exert opposing effects, and that their action takes place, at least in part, via alterations in the spectrum of icosanoids produced by the tissues and immunocompetent cells.

A. Systemic Lupus Erythematosus

Human systemic lupus erythematosus (SLE) is an autoimmune disease of unknown etiology, most often affecting women of child-bearing age and involving damge to kidneys and blood vessels. Inflammation is a characteristic feature of the pathology. Some mouse strains have been developed which serve as experimental models for the human disease [268, 278].

Female (NZBxNZW)F_1 mice are such a model. When given a beef tallow control diet, the mice developed proteinuria and mortality was high, but inclusion of 25% menhaden oil in the diet prevented the kidney damage and reduced the mortality of the animals [218, 219]. An oil rich in ω6-FA increased the renal pathology in this mouse strain [145].

Another useful model of fulminant SLE is the MRL/MP-lpr mouse, which also responds to fish oil with a less severe glomerulonephritis but exhibits an increased incidence of vasculitis [228]. Compared to safflower oil, fish oil decreased the massive lymphoproliferation in this model, prevented the increase in surface antigen expression of peritoneal macrophages, reduced the formation of circulating immune complexes, delayed the onset of renal disease and prolonged the survival of the mice [148]. These fish oil effects were accompanied by a reduced production of immunoreactive PGE and TX and the formation of PGE_3 in renal and lung tissues.

A third lupus strain, male BxSB mice, also responded to dietary menhaden oil by less severe renal disease, longer survival, reduced weights of spleen and lymph nodes and depressed production of arachidonic acid-derived cyclooxygenase products [228]. It was suggested [148, 228] that the attenuating effects of dietary fish oil on the immune and inflammatory responses in these mouse models were due to the reduced production of cyclooxygenase metabolites formed from arachidonic acid, together with the appearance of IPA-derived metabolites and possibly the partial substitution of LTB_5 for LTB_4.

Hamazaki et al. [108], in a brief letter, reported that patients with IgA nephropathy responded to dietary fish oil (2.6 g/day of ω3-FA) given over a period of one year, by a stabilization of renal function, as measured by creatinine excretion. Kidney function continued to deteriorate in patients not receiving fish oil. The oil did not repair the damage already present.

B. Rheumatoid Arthritis

A trial was recently carried out on patients with active rheumatoid arthritis [156]. The design was double-blind and randomized. The experimental group received a diet high in PUFA (P/S ratio of 1.4) with a supplement of 10 MaxEPA capsules/day, providing a daily dose of 1.8 g IPA. The control group consumed a diet with a P/S ratio of 0.25, made to resemble an 'experimental' diet by random dietary manipulation from different food groups. This was supplemented with 10 capsules/day containing liquid paraffin. The study lasted 12 weeks with a follow-up period of 1–2 months. Morning stiffness time increased in the control group but not in the experimental group and was significantly different in the two groups at the end of 12 weeks. The number of tender joints decreased in both groups, more so in the fish oil treatment than in the control patients, but at 12 weeks the difference between the treatment effects was not significant. Follow-up evaluation revealed that the slight improvement in some of the clinical manifestations of rheumatoid arthritis was transient. It is unfortunate that the two groups had a very different intake of PUFA and saturated FA, thus introducing a confounding element into the design. The results however seem to be sufficiently encouraging to warrant further controlled trials.

Some rat experiments support the conclusion that dietary IPA is able to reduce the severity of inflammatory reactions. For instance, IPA, supplied as the ethyl ester, significantly reduced the concentrations of PGE_2 and TXB_2 in inflammatory exudates after subcutaneous implantation of carrageenin-impregnated sponges in rats [277]. LTB_4 concentrations and the number of leukocytes also decreased, but not significantly. This IPA treatment also reduced the swelling induced by injection of carrageenin into the hind paws, probably via decreased synthesis of PGE_2 [277]. But other rat models, especially the collagen-induced arthritis model, yield results that raise serious questions of interpretation.

Inflammatory arthritis, induced in rats by intradermal injection of type II collagen, is widely used as a model for human rheumatoid arthritis. When such rats received a diet containing either menhaden oil or beef fat as the only source of fat, the severity of inflammation was similar in both dietary treatments, but the incidence of arthritis was significantly *higher* in the group receiving fish oil [220]. It was previously shown [217] that fish oil-fed rats, sensitized with egg albumin, developed greater immediate hypersensitivity reactions and increased titers of IgE and IgG than rats receiving beef fat.

The paradoxical effect of fish oil in rats is intriguing. Lands [163] suggested that in the absence of icosanoid production from arachidonic acid, ω3-FA might interfere in some way with T helper cell function and antibody production. There is also the possibility that ω3-FA mediated inhibition of PGE_2, a PG which has been shown to be immunosuppressive [215], leads to an increase in immune-inflammatory response, at least in this particular model.

C. Other Immune-Mediated Diseases

Little information is available on the effects of ω3-FA on other immune-related disorders. Bronchial asthma did not improve when patients took a daily supplement of 20 ml MaxEPA oil during 10 weeks [11], and a guinea pig model showed that the pulmonary responses to antigen challenge involved a *greater* bronchial constriction when the diet contained added menhaden oil [168]. Fish oil caused a modest improvement in patients with psoriasis [32, 298]. Diabetes and multiple sclerosis are also candidates for intervention studies with ω3-FA [163].

XI. ω3-FA, Heart Disease and Stroke

The antiplatelet and hypotriglyceridemic actions together lead to the expectation that marine foods and fish oils rich in ω3-FA will favorably affect the course of atherosclerotic and thrombotic diseases. Epidemiological observations, already discussed, point in this direction. Animal experiments and some retrospective data on fish consumption and heart disease strengthen the expectation.

A. Atherosclerosis

Weiner et al. [291] studied the effects of cod-liver oil in a hypercholesterolemic swine model in which atherosclerosis is pathologically similar to the human disease. The animals received during 8 months a diet rich in lard, with added cholesterol and sodium cholate, with and without supplementary cod-liver oil. After the first 3 weeks the animals were subjected to coronary balloon abrasion in order to accelerate coronary atherosclerosis. The disease was significantly less in swine fed cod-liver oil than in controls, according to various morphometric criteria: mean lesion area/vessel, mean luminal encroachment/vessel, and mean maximal luminal encroachment/vessel. Both groups developed severe hyperlipidemia, and there was extensive replacement of arachidonic acid by IPA in platelet total FA. The serum TXB_2 content was considerably lowered by the cod-liver oil treatment. The authors concluded that marine oil or its components might be useful in the prevention or slowing of progression of atherosclerosis in humans.

B. Myocardial Infarction

The effect of dietary menhaden oil (10% of the diet) on experimental myocardial infarction in dogs was investigated by Culp et al. [64]. In this model, myocardial infarction was induced by electric stimulation of the left circumflex artery. Compared to the unsupplemented diet, the fish oil regimen caused a better coronary circulation and smaller infarct size, and there were fewer ECG patterns with ectopic beats. Platelet aggregation ex vivo was not affected by the fish oil.

In a different dog model, myocardial infarction was produced by occlusion of the left coronary artery [183]. Upon reperfusion, massive migration of neutrophils into the myocardium was observed. Nonsteroidal anti-inflammatory drugs failed to reduce infarct size, but drugs that inhibited both the cyclooxygenase and lipoxygenase pathways were effective. This experiment highlights the importance of leukocytes in experimentally induced myocardial damage and, together with the negative platelet aggregation test ex vivo in fish oil-fed dogs [64], indicates that platelets may not play a primary role in this type of experimental myocardial infarction.

Although beneficial effects of fish oil are usually ascribed to IPA, DHA may be an active participant in the process. Talesnik and Hsia [270] reported that coronary flow reactions to arachidonic acid were inhibited by infusion of DHA.

An early study of the relation between fish consumption and heart disease [189] became generally known only after Stansby [266] drew attention to it. Nelson [189] recorded the survival rates of 206 of his patients who had previously suffered at least one heart attack. He asked 80 of the patients to adhere to a fish diet every day of the week but one, on which they were allowed free choice of food. The other 126 patients continued to eat their usual diet. The results were impressive: only 8% of the subjects on the ordinary diet survived during the observation period which lasted 16–19 years, while the survival rate of those on the fish diet reached 36%. In older patients (56–70 years old), survival rates were 5 and 32%, respectively.

Kromhout et al. [158] collected information about fish consumption in 852 middle-aged men free of coronary heart disease (CHD) in 1960 and recorded all death from the disease among these men during the following 20 years. The mortality was inversely related to fish consumption in 1960 and was over twice as high among those not consuming any fish as for those eating at least 30 g fish/day or one or two fish dishes/week. Kromhout et al. [158] estimated that two thirds of the 1960 fish consumption consisted of lean fish and one third of fatty fish, so that the estimated intake of IPA in the group with the highest consumption (> 45 g fish/day) was only about 0.4 g/day. The inverse relation between fish consumption and deaths from CHD was confirmed by Shekelle et al. [250] but not by others [66, 290].

A surprising finding in the studies by Kromhout et al. [158] and Shekelle et al. [250] was that the risk of mortality from CHD was decreased by IPA intakes far less than the 2 or 3 g/day reported to decrease platelet aggregability and plasma triglyceride levels in most human intervention trials. Fish protein does not seem to differ from casein in its effect on plasma cholesterol in rabbits [54]. Does the consumption of very small amounts of ω3-FA over many years have beneficial effects on human health not revealed by trials lasting only weeks or months?

The large-scale Norwegian vegetable oil trial [187] failed to reveal any beneficial effects of linseed oil over sunflower oil in the incidence of heart disease in men aged 50–59 years, after one year of observation. The small amount of supplemental oils, 10 ml/day, did not affect the serum cholesterol levels, when compared to control subjects not taking any oil supplement. Under these conditions, an effect on heart disease could hardly be expected.

A daily dose of 10 ml encapsulated MaxEPA oil relieved anginal pain in each of 12 heart patients [243]. This was seen from the number of glyceryl trinitrate tablets required by the subjects. The mean weekly consumption of tablets was 25 (range: 3–70) before the oil, and 2 (range: 0–6) after 9 months of oil supplement.

C. Stroke

Black et al. [26] induced ischemic stroke in cats by ligation of the middle cerebral artery. In this model, the size of the infarcted brain area in cats kept on a diet supplemented with menhaden oil (8 cal%) was about one third that seen in animals receiving the unsupplemented diet. This experimental aproach did not involve thrombosis, unlike stroke induced in rats by carotid injection of sodium arachidonate [91]. Again, it appears that ω3-FA may act by modification of leukocyte function, possibly via inhibition of the lipoxygenase pathway.

Temporary arterial occlusion in gerbils resulted in edema and reduction of blood flow in brain [27]. Dietary menhaden oil prevented these effects but did not affect arachidonic acid-derived brain prostanoids. Again, ω3-FA appear to prevent brain damage by mechanisms not involving their antithrombotic action.

XII. ω3-FA and Cancer

Interest in possible beneficial effects of ω3-FA on certain kinds of human cancer stems from two sets of observations: (a) epidemiological data on malignancies, especially breast cancer, in Japanese and Greenlanders whose traditional diets are rich in ω3-FA of marine origin, and (b) animal experiments and observations on human cancers pointing to the involvement of prostanoids in tumor development.

A. Epidemiological Observations

Japanese have an extremely low mortality from cancer of the breast and prostate. According to data collected from 21 countries of the Organization of Economic Cooperation and Development during 1975–1979, Japan was at the bottom of the list with figures far below those of the other countries [248].

Cancer used to be virtually unknown among Eskimos in Alaska, Canada and Greenland, according to several explorers, including the great authority V. Stefansson, who lived with the Eskimos for extended periods of time [160]. A case of cancer in an Eskimo became the subject of a paper published in 1952 [160]. Recent surveys have revealed that cancer nowadays is not unusual among Eskimos, but that the distribution of cancer types greatly differs from that in Western populations [157, 160]. In a detailed survey of breast cancer among indigenous Greenlandic women between 1950 and 1974 [197], the number of cases was found to be half that of Danish women. There appeared to be an upward trend from low-risk to medium-risk during that time, in parallel with increasing urbanization and Westernization. Nielsen and Hansen [197] also stated that prostate cancer was almost nonexistent in Greenlandic men.

B. Role of Prostanoids

The involvement of PG in tumor development was suspected ever since high PG concentrations were found in human thyroid carcinoma [294]. The suspicion was strengthened by numerous observations on rats and mice according to which the growth of mammary tumors was related to the dietary level of linoleate intake [129]. The subject was reviewed by Welsh and Aylsworth [292] and further investigated by Kollmorgen et al. [155] and Ip et al. [135]. Evidence implicating PG in tumorigenesis was provided by observations showing that indomethacin retarded tumor growth, as first reported by Plescia et al. [215], and abolished the enhancing effect of dietary linoleic acid on tumor development [55, 121, 155]. It has been suggested that an elevated PG production may be used as a marker for the metastatic potential of breast cancer cells [230]. Karmali et al. [146] mentioned that TXB_2 production was related to tumor size and extent of metastasis of human breast cancer.

The mode of action of prostanoids in tumorigenesis is not clear. According to Plescia et al. [215], PG produced in large amounts by tumor cells 'subvert' the immune system of the host. A potent inhibitory effect of PG on murine natural killer cell activity in vitro and in vivo was demonstrated by Brunda et al. [38]. According to Honn et al. [127], TXA_2 and PGI_2 exert pro- and antimetastatic actions, respectively. Bennett [21] suggested that tumor cells in transit, i.e. in the circulation, are protected by platelets that aggregate around them, which would make the metastatic invasiveness dependent on the balance of proaggregating and antiaggregating factors, such as TXA_2 and PGI_2.

C. Animal Experiments

The restraining action of ω3-FA on the metabolism of arachidonic acid provides the rationale for the expectation that these FA may be beneficial in the prevention and management of some types of tumors.

Animal experiments have given encouraging results. Much of the recent research concentrated on mammary tumors for which murine models are available. A fish oil concentrate rich in 20:5ω3 and 22:6ω3 reduced the growth of transplanted mammary adenocarcinomas in female rats, depressed the synthesis and tumor content of arachidonic acid-derived PG and TX, and increased the ratio of linoleic to arachidonic acid in tumor tissue [146]. Menhaden oil also reduced the growth of the same type of tumor transplanted into mice [92]. Chemically induced tumors as well are affected by dietary fish oil. Oils rich in ω3-FA caused a decrease in the number of mammary tumors in DMBA-treated rats [30, 146]. The yield of mammary tumors induced in rats by N-methyl-N-nitrosourea was lowered by increasing dietary intakes of menhaden oil, whereas corn oil had the opposite effect [144].

Not only mammary tumors are inhibited by fish oils. Menhaden oil at 20% of the diet reduced the preneoplastic lesions induced in rat pancreas by *L*-azaserine, compared to 20% corn oil [206]. Mice bearing the PG-producing HSDM fibrosarcoma had greatly increased circulating PG metabolite levels [272]. Inclusion of menhaden oil in the diet resulted in a threefold decrease in plasma PG metabolites in tumor-bearing mice. Immunoreactive circulating levels of 12-HETE and LT were not elevated in tumor-bearing mice and remained unaffected by the fish oil treatment.

D. Mechanisms of Action of ω3-FA

There is little doubt that a reduction of the excessively high prostanoid production in tumors plays an important role in the way in which ω3-FA affect tumorigenesis. By reducing the level of PG and TXA_2 produced by tumor cells, ω3-FA may partially restore the host's immune defenses against invading cells; or by virtue of their antiplatelet properties, ω3-FA may prevent the protection of tumor cells in transit by platelet aggregates forming around the cells.

XIII. Implications of the Dietary Balance of ω3- and ω6-FA

The view taken here is that an absolute ω3-FA deficiency is very unlikely to occur in humans (except perhaps on prolonged intravenous feeding), but that an imbalance in the ratio of ω3-FA to ω6-FA may have far-reaching implications. Several authors looking at this question from different angles have expressed the same opinion [40, 41, 44, 162, 163, 233, 273]. The evidence supporting this thesis is as follows:

A. Restraining Action of ω3-FA on Arachidonate Metabolism

Unrestrained arachidonate metabolism can have detrimental consequences. Intravenous sodium arachidonate caused pulmonary platelet aggregation and sudden death in rabbits [252] and stroke in rats [91]. Ingestion of ethyl arachidonate by volunteers led to increased platelet aggregability [249]. In this connection, it should be noted that human stroke patients have an increased plasma pool of arachidonic acid [130]. Overproduction of prostanoids is undoubtedly involved in these cases.

Dietary linoleic acid provided by corn or cottonseed oil exacerbated platelet thrombosis in certain rat models, as discussed in section VIII [199–201], while linseed oil had an attenuating effect on these models. The level of linoleate in corn and cottonseed oils exceeds that of α-linolenate by some two orders of magnitude.

Chick nutritional encephalomalacia (NE) is another example of excessive arachidonate metabolism. This is a classical syndrome of vitamin E deficiency [211] which can be induced in young chicks by diets low in tocopherol and containing a source of linoleic or arachidonic acid [67, 68]. The target organ is the cerebellum which exhibits occlusions of the microvessels, edema and hemorrhages [69]. Chicks showing signs of NE have a lower bleeding time than symptomless chicks or vitamin-E-sufficient controls [46]. The blood coagulation system appears to be involved in the pathogenesis of NE, as shown by the protective effect of dicoumarol [43]. Chicks are most susceptible to experimental NE during the third week of life; this is when a spurt of PUFA accumulation occurs in the brain [45, 47]. NE is a particularly useful model because of the rapid onset, easy recognition and fatal outcome of the disease. α-Linolenic acid not only fails to induce the disease when included in the diet instead of linoleic acid [67], but it also protects the chicks against the cerebellar lesion and mortality in the presence of dietary linoleic acid [46, 57]. Cod-liver oil FA appeared to be less protective than linseed oil FA, in spite of more extreme changes in the ω3/ω6-FA ratios in liver and brain brought about by the fish oil [46]. Although the mode of action of linoleic and α-linolenic acid in NE is not known, it is likely that they exert opposing effects on icosanoid production [47].

These examples, together with the metabolic interactions discussed in section V and the effects of ω3-FA on platelet function and some of the modern diseases (sections IX–XII), lend support to the thesis that ω3-FA play an important role in the modulation of arachidonic acid metabolism and in preventing the overproduction of icosanoids.

B. The Present PUFA Imbalance

It has been argued [273] that the modern epidemic of CHD is associated more with a rise in thrombotic properties of blood than with an increase in atherosclerosis, as witnessed by a sevenfold increase in deaths from CHD in London during the first half of this century, without substantial increase in the extent or severity of atherosclerosis. The authors thought that the PUFA balance during that period had shifted toward a higher consumption of linoleic acid and a greater thrombotic tendency. Figures quoted by the authors show that the food supply levels of linoleic acid rose by 65% between 1934–1938 and 1975, while those of α-linolenic acid remained virtually unchanged during that period. The rise in the ratio of ω6- to ω3-FA was attributed to the increasing consumption of vegetable margarines and cooking oils rich in linoleic acid and, to a small degree, to the drop in fish consumption. According to estimates quoted by Rice [224], consumption of fatty fish in 1848 was six times as high as in 1978, and the intake of ω3-FA from fish was seven times as high then as it is now. James [141] gives more recent statistics showing that the availability of PUFA for consumption in British households increased by one third between 1959 and 1982. Although no data are given for ω6- and ω3-FA, it is likely that the PUFA increase is due to a growing consumption of linoleic-rich vegetable oils.

According to Rizek et al. [227], food supply levels of linoleic acid in the USA almost tripled between 1909–1913 and 1980, mainly because of a 15-fold rise in the consumption of salad and cooking oils rich in linoleic acid, and a compensatory drop in consumption of butter and lard which contain little linoleic acid. The huge expansion of the vegetable-oil industry and the beginnings of the modern imbalance of dietary PUFA have been traced to important innovations in oil extraction and refining that occurred at the turn of the century [41]. Anderson's 'Expeller' press and Wesson's steam-vacuum deodorization process were patented at that time. Later, large-scale application of solvent extraction contributed to the expansion of the production of vegetable oils, as did the 'cholesterol scare' of the 1950s and 1960s. These developments affected most of all oils rich in linoleic acid. On the other hand, strenuous efforts are continually being made to reduce the level of α-linolenic acid in oils such as soybean oil, because of flavor problems. Selective partial hydrogenation is commonly used to this end, and new strains of soybeans are being developed which have an especially low content of α-linolenic acid [7]. These technological and agrotechnical developments are at the root of the modern PUFA imbalance.

The value of 10, estimated by Taylor et al. [273] for the ω6/ω3-FA ratio in Britain is probably typical of Western countries, though values as low as 6 have been reported for urban households in Britain [50] and a ratio of 14 was found in a French farming community [223].

The food available to prehistoric man from noncultivated plants, wild animals, fish and crustaceans was, on the whole, low in fat, and the lipids were rich in PUFA, with a fairly evenly balanced ω6/ω3-FA ratio [41, 44]. The present imbalance in dietary PUFA, like the high fat intake in the Western world, is a late consequence of the industrial revolution.

XIV. Possible Problems Related to Fish Oil Consumption

Several questions have been raised regarding the consumption of fish oils in large amounts. The questions are related to the long-chain ω3-FA in the oils, as well as to some other constituents.

A. Long-Chain Monoenoic FA

Gadoleic and cetoleic acids (20:1ω9 and 22:1ω11, respectively) are found in marine oils in variable amounts, totalling as much as 35% in some herring oils [1]. Additional monoene isomers are formed during partial hydrogenation of fish oils for the margarine industry. Cetoleic acid is an isomer of erucic acid, the major FA or rapeseed oil. Both are known to cause transient cardiac lipidosis, necrosis and fibrosis in different animal species, including monkeys. The metabolism and nutritional effects of 22:1 have been reviewed recently [59] and need not be detailed here.

There is no evidence that long-chain monoenes from fish oils affect human heart muscle. It should be noted, however, that concern about possible effects of erucic acid in humans has led to the development of low-erucic acid rapeseed (LEAR) cultivars. Volunteers consuming very large amounts of fish oils have on occasion shown severe thrombocytopenia, an effect that could have been caused by the high level of long-chain monoenes ingested [102, 257]. The experimental conditions in these cases were extreme and involved, in the case of Sinclair [257], a diet consisting entirely of seal, fish and shellfish during 100 days, and in the experiment by Goodnight et al. [102], a diet that included a daily consumption of 60–90 ml salmon oil and 1-lb salmon steak. A slight decrease in platelet count was reported in several of the fish oil experiments on human subjects mentioned in previous sections. For instance, in the 25-day long trial in which healthy volunteers received 40 ml/day of cod-liver oil [173], the daily consumption of 20:1 and 22:1, computed from Ackman's data [1], was 3 and 2 g, respectively. In that trial, the average platelet count decreased from 217 to 193 $\times$ $10^3/\mu l$, remaining well within the normal range. Some additional data may be useful: herring, a fatty fish, provides 1–4 g 20:1 and 2–6 g 22:1/100 g fish, while menhaden oil contains only 2 and 0.5% 20:1 and 22:1, respectively [1]. Christophersen et al. [59] calculated that the average daily intake of 22:1 in Norway, mainly from partially hydrogenated capelin oil, was 2.5 g per capita.

It would appear that long-chain monoenes from fish oil supplements such as menhaden oil should not cause undue concern. However, with refined fish oils and partially hydrogenated fish oils becoming without doubt freely available in the near future, it may be advisable to have some indication of the long-chain monoene content on the label.

B. Excess Vitamins A and D

Cod-liver oil has been used traditionally to supplement the intake of vitamins A and D in children for prophylactic and curative purposes. Cases of poisoning, due to hypervitaminosis A or D, have been the result of excessive doses of pharmaceutical vitamin preparations, rather than cod-liver oil. The problem does not exist at all in the case of fish body oils, e.g. menhaden oil, in which only insignificant quantities of these fat-soluble vitamins are found. Since the origin of the oil is not specified in some of the commercially available oils, it may be advisable to declare the contents of vitamins A and D.

C. Autoxidation and Vitamin E

ω3-FA in marine oils are the most unsaturated FA known. As such, they are highly susceptible to autoxidation. There are two aspects to this problem. One concerns the flavor deterioration that occurs on exposure of freshly refined fish oil to air. This is a technological problem, rather than a health-threatening one, since the repulsive odor and flavor will make the oil unacceptable for human consumption. Encapsulated oil is protected from contact with air and will be quite stable, but strict quality control is necessary to ensure that the oil is not spoiled before encapsulation. The other aspect pertaining to the high degree of unsaturation of ω3-FA concerns their presence in cell membrane lipids *after* their absorption. These FA are extremely susceptible to free-radical attack which causes damage to the structure and function of the membranes. α-Tocopherol acts as a free-radical scavenger and biological antioxidant [48], hence it is prudent to increase the vitamin E supply when fish oils are consumed. Some of the commercial preparations contain added α-tocopherol in ample amounts, e.g. 1 mg/g oil in the case of MaxEPA capsules.

D. Digestibility and Absorption

Long-chain ω3-FA occur in fish oils as glyceryl esters. But ω3-FA have also been prepared and tested in a more concentrated form as the ethyl esters. Thomasson and Gottenbos [280] compared the EFA activity of linoleic acid as the triglyceride and as methyl and ethyl esters in the rat growth test under conditions of restricted water supply. They reported that the triglyceride form was about 50% more active than the methyl and ethyl esters. This points to a more efficient digestion of the triglyceride. It is not known whether a similar difference between the two chemical forms exists for IPA and DHA.

There is a different digestibility question, arising from the observation [29] that IPA and DHA in whale oil, in which these FA are attached to the glyceride molecule in positions 1 and 3, are resistant to pancreatic hydrolysis in vitro. The authors used molecular models to show that the twisted shape of the IPA and DHA molecules places the terminal methyl group in close proximity to the carboxyl group, and they suggested that steric hindrance might interfere with the hydrolysis of the ester bonds. 22:5ω3, with a more open shape, was readily split off from the glyceride by pancreatic lipase. Opstvedt's [208] summary of the digestibility data for fish oil FA in different animal species shows that the long-chain ω3-FA are efficiently digested and absorbed. Chen et al. [58] reported that free IPA was absorbed and transported in the rat like other unsaturated FA. Therefore, the digestion and absorption of long-chain ω3-FA from fish oils in humans would be expected to present no special problems. Whale blubber used to be a traditional food for Eskimos. Whether whale oil, and perhaps oil from other marine mammals, is well digested by people not used to this type of fat is a question that requires clarification, as new sources of marine ω3-FA will become available.

XV. Concluding Remarks

Epidemiologic observations and recent experimental work have focussed attention on ω3-FA. Important advances have been made in our understanding of how these FA affect health and disease. Most of the studies were done with fish diets or marine oils which are a rich source of long-chain in ω3-FA.

The most striking and best documented property of these FA is their hypotriglyceridemic activity which far exceeds that of linoleic acid in vegetable oils. Long-chain ω3-FA in fish oils have been shown to result in a dramatic decrease in plasma triglyceride levels in patients suffering from different types of hyperlipoproteinemia. This opens up a new avenue of approach to the management of these disorders.

ω3-FA causes a decrease in the production of icosanoids derived from ω6-FA, which play important roles in several thrombotic and immune-inflammatory disorders. Encouraging results have been obtained by dietary ω3-FA in the attentuation of platelet and leukocyte function, decrease of blood pressure, and in animal models of atherogenesis and myocardial and cerebral infarction. A requirement for ω3-FA in vision has been demonstrated in nonhuman primates and is likely to exist also in brain development.

From a nutritional point of view, it appears that the PUFA intake has been thrown out of balance by modern technological developments which have resulted in a low consumption of α-linolenic acid relative to the linoleic acid intake. With long-chain ω3-FA in the limelight, too little attention is being given to α-linolenic acid from vegetable sources.

Careful evaluation of ω3-FA in health and disease is being carried out in many laboratories throughout the world. Unbased or premature claims and high-pressure salesmanship [267] could do much damage to an exciting new development.

Note Added in Proof

Recent books in which ω3-FA are given extensive treatment are the proceedings of the Biloxi short course on polyunsaturated fatty acids and eicosanoids [9], edited by W.E.M. Lands, American Oil Chemists Society, Champaign 1987, and a monograph by J.E. Kinsella entitled 'Seafoods and fish oils in human health and disease' (Dekker, New York 1987). A one-day symposium 'Health effects of omega-3 fatty acids: fish oil and other sources' took place in October 1987 at the Massachusetts Institute of Technology,

Boston (proceedings to be published in book form by Dekker, New York). Meetings on ω3-FA planned for 1988 include a NATO Workshop on 'Dietary omega-3 and omega-6 fatty acids: nutritional essentiality' at Belgirate, Italy, proceedings to be published by Plenum Press (Co-Directors: C. Galli and A. Simopoulos); an international conference 'Health effects of fish and fish oils' in Newfoundland, Canada (Chairman: A.K. Chandra), and the Acta Medica Scandinavica International Symposium on n-3 fatty acids/fish oils (Chairmen: J. Dyerberg and A. Nordøy).

References

1 Ackman, R.G.: Fatty acid composition of fish oils; in Barlow, Stansby, Nutritional evaluation of long-chain fatty acids in fish oil, pp. 25–88 (Academic Press, London 1982).

2 Adam, O.; Wolfram, G.; Zöllner, N.: Wirkung der Linol- und Linolensäure auf die Prostaglandinbildung und die Nierenfunktion beim Menschen. Fette Seifen Anstr-Mittel *86:* 180–183 (1984).

3 Ahmed, A.A.; Holub, B.J.: Alteration and recovery of bleeding times, platelet aggregation and fatty acid composition of individual phospholipids in platelets of human subjects receiving a supplement of cod-liver oil. Lipids *19:* 617–624 (1984).

4 Ahrens, E.M.; Hirsch, J.; Peterson, M.C.; Insull, W.; Stoffel, W.; Farquhar, J.W.; Miller, T.; Thomasson, H.J.: The effect on human serum lipids of a dietary fat, highly unsaturated but poor in essential fatty acids. Lancet *i:* 115–119 (1959).

5 AIN-FASEB: Symposium related to n-3 fatty acids, St. Louis 1986.

6 Anderson, R.E.: Lipids of ocular tissues. IV. Comparison of the phospholipids from the retina of six mammalian species. Expl Eye Res. *10:* 339–344 (1970).

7 Anon: Researchers report gains in hunt for low-linolenic soybeans. J. Am. Oil Chem. Soc. *59:* 882A–884A (1982).

8 AOCS: Short course on marine lipids and EPA, Oahu 1986.

9 AOCS: Short course on eicosanoids and dietary polyunsaturated fatty acids, Biloxi 1987.

10 Appleman, D.; Fulco, A.J.; Shugarman, P.M.: Correlation of linolenate to photosynthetic O_2 production in chlorella. Plant Physiol. *41:* 136–142 (1966).

11 Aro, A.; Stenius-Aarniala, B.; Hakulinen, A.; Kostiainen, E.; Seppälä, E.; Vapaatalo, H.: Symptomatic and metabolic effects of evening primrose oil, fish oil and olive oil in patients with bronchial asthma (Abstract). 13th Int. Congr. on Nutrition, Brighton 1985. Book of abstracts, p. 103.

12 Arthaud, B.: Cause of death in 339 Alaskan natives as determined by autopsy. Archs Path. *90:* 433–438 (1970).

13 Balasubranamiam, S.; Simons, L.A.; Chang, S.; Hickie, J.B.: Reduction in plasma cholesterol and increase in biliary cholesterol by a diet rich in n-3 fatty acids in the rat. J. Lipid Res. *26:* 684–689 (1985).

14 Bang, H.O.; Dyerberg, J.: Plasma lipids and lipoproteins in Greenlandic West Coast Eskimos. Acta med. scand. *192:* 85–94 (1972).

15 Bang, H.O.; Dyerberg, J.; Brøndum-Nielsen, A.: Plasma lipid and lipoprotein pattern in Greenlandic West Coast Eskimos. Lancet *i:* 1143–1146 (1971).

16 Bang, H.O.; Dyerberg, J.; Hjørne, N.: The composition of food consumed by Greenland Eskimos. Acta med. scand. *200:* 69–73 (1976).
17 Bang, H.O.; Dyerberg, J.; Sinclair, H.M.: The composition of Eskimo food in Western Greenland. Am. J. clin. Nutr. *33:* 2657–2661 (1980).
18 Barlow, S.M.; Stansby, M.E.: Nutritional evaluation of long-chain fatty acids in fish oil (Academic Press, London 1982).
19 Basnayake, V.; Sinclair, H.M.: The effect of deficiency of essential fatty acids upon the skin; in Popjak, LeBreton, Biochemical problems of lipids, pp. 476–484 (Butterworth, London 1956).
20 Beitz, J.; Mest, H.-J.; Förster, W.: Influence of linseed oil diet on the pattern of serum phospholipids in man. Acta biol. med. germ. *40:* K31–K35 (1981).
21 Bennett, A.: The production of prostanoids in human cancers and their implications for tumor progression. Prog. Lipid Res. *25:* 539–542 (1986).
22 Bernsohn, J.; Spitz, F.J.: Linoleic- and linolenic acid dependency of some brain membrane-bound enzymes after lipid deprivation in rats. Biochem. biophys. Res. Commun. *57:* 293–298 (1974).
23 Berry, E.M.; Hirsch, J.: Does dietary linolenic acid influence blood pressure? Am. J. clin. Nutr. *44:* 336–340 (1986).
24 Beynen, A.C.; Katan, M.B.: Why do polyunsaturated fatty acids lower serum cholesterol? Am. J. clin. Nutr. *42:* 560–563 (1985).
25 Bimbo, A.P.: The emerging marine oil industry. J. Am. Oil Chem. Soc. *64:* 706–715 (1987).
26 Black, K.L.; Culp, B.R.; Madison, D.; Randall, O.S.; Lands, W.E.M.: The protective effects of dietary fish oil on cerebral infarction. Prostaglandins Med. *5:* 257–268 (1979).
27 Black, K.L.; Hoff, J.T.; Radin, N.S.; Deshmukh, G.D.: Eicosapentaenoic acid: effect on brain prostaglandins, cerebral blood flow and edema in ischemic gerbils *(Meriones unguiculatus).* Stroke *15:* 65–69 (1984).
28 Borchgrevink, C.F.; Berg, K.J.; Skaga, E.; Skjaeggestad, Ö.; Stormorken, H.: Effect of linseed oil on platelet adhesiveness and bleeding time in patients with coronary heart disease. Lancet *ii:* 980–982 (1965).
29 Bottino, R.N.; Vandenburg, G.A.; Reiser, R.: Resistance of certain long-chain polyunsaturated fatty acids of marine oils to pancreatic lipase hydrolysis. Lipids *2:* 489–493 (1967).
30 Braden, L.M.; Carroll, K.K.: Dietary polyunsaturated fatty acids in relation to mammary carcinogenesis in the rat. Lipids *21:* 285–288 (1986).
31 Bradlow, B.A.; Chetty, N.; Westhuyzen, J. van der; Mendelsohn, D.; Gibson, J.E.: The effects of a mixed fish diet on platelet function, fatty acids and serum lipids. Thromb. Res. *29:* 561–568 (1983).
32 Bradlow, B.A.; Fretzin, D.F.; Rubenstein, D.; Newmark, J.; Cotter, R.; Matlin, M.: A double-blind trial of n-3 fatty acids from fish oil in psoriasis (abstract). Int. Conf. on Leukotrienes and Prostaglandins in Health and Disease, Tel-Aviv and Rehovot 1985, p. 35.
33 Brenner, R.; Peluffo, R.O.: Effect of saturated and unsaturated fatty acids on the desaturation in vitro of palmitic, stearic, oleic, linoleic and linolenic acids. J. biol. Chem. *241:* 5213–5219 (1966).
34 Bronsgeest-Shoute, H.C.; Van Gent, C.M.; Luten, J.B.; Ruiter, A.: The effect of

various ω3 fatty acids on the blood lipid composition in healthy human subjects. Am. J. clin. Nutr. *34:* 1752–1757 (1981).
35 Bronte-Stewart, B.A.; Antonis, A.; Eales, L.; Brock, J.F.: Effects of feeding different fats on serum cholesterol levels. Lancet *i:* 521–526 (1956).
36 Brox, J.H.; Killie, J.-E.; Gunnes, S.; Nordøy, A.: The effect of cod liver oil and corn oil on platelets and vessel wall in man. Thromb. Haemostasis *46:* 604–611 (1981).
37 Brox, J.H.; Killie, J.A.; Osternd, B.; Holme, S.; Nordøy, A.: Effects of cod liver oil on platelets and coagulation in familial hypercholesterolemia (type IIa). Acta med. scand. *213:* 137–144 (1984).
38 Brunda, M.J.; Herberman, R.B.; Holden, H.T.: Inhibition of murine natural killer cell activity by prostaglandins. J. Immun. *124:* 2682–2687 (1980).
39 Brussard, J.H.; Katan, M.B.; Hautvast, J.G.A.J.: Faecal excretion of bile acids and neutral steroids on diets differing in type and amount of dietary fat in young healthy persons. Eur. J. clin. Invest. *13:* 115–122 (1983).
40 Budowski, P.: Review: nutritional effects of ω3-polyunsaturated fatty acids. Israel J. med. Scis *17:* 223–231 (1981).
41 Budowski, P.: Dietary linoleic acid should be balanced by alpha-linolenic acid; a discussion of the nutritional implications of the dietary ratio of polyunsaturated fatty acids. Int. Conf. on Diet and Nutrition, Tel-Aviv 1983; in Horwitz, Advances in diet and nutrition, pp. 199–206 (Libbey, London 1985).
42 Budowski, P.: Why do polyunsaturated fatty acids lower serum cholesterol? (letter) Am. J. clin. Nutr. *44:* 155–156 (1986).
43 Budowski, P.; Bartov, I.; Dror, Y.; Frankel, E.N.: Lipid oxidation products and chick nutritional encephalopathy. Lipids *14:* 768–772 (1979).
44 Budowski, P.; Crawford, M.A.: α-Linolenic acid as a regulator of the metabolism of arachidonic acid: dietary implications of the ratio, n-6:n-3 fatty acids. Proc. Nutr. Soc. *44:* 221–229 (1985).
45 Budowski, P.; Crawford, M.A.: Effect of dietary linoleic and α-linolenic acid on the fatty acid composition of brain lipids in the young chick. Prog. Lipid Res. *25:* 615–618 (1986).
46 Budowski, P.; Hawkey, C.M.; Crawford, M.A.: L'effet protecteur de l'acide α-linolénique sur l'encephalomalacie chez le poulet. Annls Nutr. Aliment. *34:* 389–400 (1980).
47 Budowski, P.; Leighfield, M.J.; Crawford, M.A.: Nutritional encephalomalacia in the chick: an exposure of the vulnerable period for cerebellar development and the possible need for both ω6- and ω3-fatty acids. Br. J. Nutr. *58:* 511–520 (1987).
48 Budowski, P.; Sklan, D.: Vitamins E and A; in Vergroesen, Crawford, The role of fats in human nutrition; 2nd ed. (Academic Press, London, in press).
49 Budowski, P.; Trostler, N.; Lupo, M.; Vaisman, N.; Eldor, A.: Effect of linseed oil ingestion on plasma lipid fatty acid composition and platelet aggregation in healthy volunteeers. Nutr. Res. *4:* 343–346 (1984).
50 Bull, N.L.; Day, M.J.L.; Buss, D.H.: Individual fatty acids in the British household food supply. Human Nutr. appl. Nutr. *37A:* 373–377 (1983).
51 Burr, G.O.; Burr, M.M.: A new deficiency disease produced by the rigid exclusion of fat from the diet. J. biol. Chem. *82:* 345–367 (1929).
52 Burr, G.O.; Burr, M.M.: On the nature and role of fatty acids in nutrition. J. biol. Chem. *86:* 587–621 (1930).

53 Carlson, S.E.; Rhodes, P.G.; Ferguson, M.G.: Docosahexaenoic acid status of preterm infants at birth and following feeding with human milk or formula. Am. J. clin. Nutr. *44:* 798–804 (1986).

54 Carroll, K.K.: The role of dietary protein in hypercholesterolemia and atherosclerosis. Lipids *13:* 360–365 (1978).

55 Carter, C.A.; Milholland, R.J.; Shea, W.; Ip, M.M.: Effect of the prostaglandin synthetase inhibitor indomethacin on 7,12-dimethylbenz(a)anthracene-induced mammary tumorigenesis in rats fed different levels of fat. Cancer Res. *43:* 3559–3562 (1983).

56 Cartwright, I.J.; Pockley, A.G.; Galloway, J.H.; Greaves, M.; Preston, F.E.: The effects of dietary ω3-polyunsaturated fatty acids on erythrocyte membrane phospholipids, erythrocyte deformability and blood viscosity in healthy volunteers. Atherosclerosis *55:* 267–281 (1985).

57 Century, B.; Horwitt, M.K.: Effect of fatty acids on chick encephalomalacia. Proc. Soc. exp. Biol. Med. *102:* 375–377 (1959).

58 Chen, I.S.; Subranamiam, S.; Cassidy, M.M.; Sheppard, A.J.; Vahouny, G.V.: Intestinal absorption and lipoprotein transport of ω3-eicosapentaenoic acid. J. Nutr. *115:* 219–225 (1985).

59 Christophersen, B.O.; Norseth, J.; Thomassen, M.S.; Christiansen, E.N.; Norum, K.R.; Osmundsen, H.; Bremer, J.: Metabolism and metabolic effects of C22:1 fatty acids with special reference to cardiac lipids; in Barlow, Stansby, Nutritional evaluation of long-chain fatty acids in fish oil, pp. 89–139 (Academic Press, London 1982).

60 Clandinin, M.T.; Chappell, J.E.; Heim, T.: Do low-weight infants require nutrition with chain elongation-desaturation products of essential fatty acids? Prog. Lipid Res. *21:* 901–904 (1982).

61 Corey, E.J.; Shih, C.; Cashman, J.R.: Docosahexaenoic acid is a strong inhibitor of PG but not LT biosynthesis. Proc. natn. Acad. Sci. USA *80:* 3581–3584 (1983).

62 Coscina, D.V.; Yehuda, S.; Dixon, L.M.; Kish, S.J.: Leprohon-Greenwood, C.E.: Learning is improved by a soybean oil diet in rats. Life Sci. *38:* 1789–1794 (1986).

63 Crawford, M.A.; Casperd, N.M.; Sinclair, A.J.: The long-chain metabolites of linoleic and linolenic acids in liver and brain in herbivores and carnivores. Compar. Biochem. Physiol. *54B:* 395–401 (1976).

64 Culp, B.R.; Lands, W.E.M.; Lucchesi, B.R.; Pi, H.R.; Romson, J.: The effect of dietary supplementation of fish oil on experimental myocardial infarction. Prostaglandins *20:* 1021–1031 (1980).

65 Culp, B.R.; Titus, B.G.; Lands, W.E.M.: Inhibition of prostaglandin biosynthesis by eicosapentaenoic acid. Prostaglandins Med. *3:* 269–278 (1979).

66 Curb, J.D.; Reed, D.M.: Fish consumption and mortality from coronary heart disease. New Engl J. Med. *313:* 821 (1985).

67 Dam, H.; Nielsen, G.K.; Prange, I.; Søndergaard, E.: Influence of linoleic and linolenic acids on symptoms of vitamin E deficiency in chicks. Nature *182:* 802–803 (1958).

68 Dam, H.; Søndergaard, E.: The encephalomalacia-producing effect of arachidonic and linoleic acids. Z. ErnährWiss. *2:* 217–222 (1962).

69 Dror, Y.; Budowski, P.; Bubis, J.J.; Sandbank, U.; Wolman, M.: Chick nutritional

encephalopathy induced by diet rich in oxidized oil and deficient in tocopherol; in Zimmerman, Progress in neuropathology, vol. 3, pp. 343–357 (Grune & Stratton, New York 1976).
70 Drury, B.: Proceedings of the second MaxEPA Research Conference, Hull, July 20–22, 1983. Br. J. clin. Pract. *38:* symp. suppl. 31 (1984).
71 Dyerberg, J.: The influence of the diet on the interaction of the platelets and the vessel walls. Phil. Trans. R. Soc. ser. B *294:* 373–381 (1981).
72 Dyerberg, J.: Observations on populations in Greenland and Denmark; in Barlow, Stansby, Nutritional evaluation of long-chain fatty acids in fish oil, pp. 245–261 (Academic Press, London 1982).
73 Dyerberg, J.: Linolenate-derived polyunsaturated fatty acids and prevention of atherosclerosis. Nutr. Rev. *44:* 125–133 (1986).
74 Dyerberg, J.; Bang, H.O.: Lipid metabolism, atherogenesis and haemostasis in Eskimos: the role of the prostaglandin-3 family. Haemostasis *8:* 227–233 (1979).
75 Dyerberg, J.; Bang, H.O.: Effect on hemostasis by feeding eicosapentaenoic acid; in Beers, Bassett, Nutritional factors modulating effects and metabolic processes, pp. 511–521 (Raven Press, New York 1981).
76 Dyerberg, J.; Bang, H.O.; Aagard, O.: α-Linolenic acid and eicosapentaenoic acid. Lancet *i:* 199 (1980).
77 Dyerberg, J.; Bang, H.O.; Hjørne, N.: Fatty acid composition of the plasma lipids in Greenland Eskimos. Am. J. clin. Nutr. *28:* 958–966 (1975).
78 Dyerberg, J.; Bang, H.O.; Stoffersen, E.; Moncada, S.; Vane, J.R.: Eicosapentaenoic acid and prevention of thrombosis and atherosclerosis? Lancet *ii:* 117–119 (1978).
79 Dyerberg, J.; Jørgensen, K.A.: The effect of arachidonic and eicosapentaenoic acid on the synthesis of prostacyclin-like material in human umbilical vasculature. Artery *8:* 12–17 (1980).
80 Dyerberg, J.; Jørgensen, K.A.; Arnfred, T.: Human umbilical cord converts all cis-5,8,11,14,17-eicosapentaenoic acid to prostaglandin I_3. Prostaglandins *22:* 857–862 (1981).
81 Dyerberg, J.; Mortensen, J.Z.; Nielsen, A.H.; Schmidt, E.B.: n-3 Polyunsaturated fatty acids and ischaemic heart disease. Lancet *ii:* 614 (1982).
82 Eggstein, M.; Schettler, G.: The effect of feeding various fats on the level of blood lipids; in Sinclair, Essential fatty acids, pp. 111–121 (Butterworth, London 1958).
83 Federal Register: Petition to the Food and Drug Administration requesting affirmation of menhaden oil and partially hydrogenated menhaden oil as Generally Recognized as Safe for Use in Foods. Fed. Reg. *51:* 27461 (1986).
84 Fehili, A.M.; Burr, M.L.; Phillips, K.M.; Deadman, N.M.: The effect of fatty fish on plasma lipid and lipoprotein concentrations. Am. J. clin. Nutr. *38:* 349–351 (1983).
85 Fiennes, R.N.T.-W.; Sinclair, A.J.; Crawford, M.A.: Essential fatty acid studies in primates – linolenic acid requirements of capuchins. J. med. Primatol. *2:* 155–169 (1973).
86 Fischer, S.; Weber, P.C.: (TXA_3) is formed in human platelets after dietary eicosapentaenoic acid (C20:5ω3). Biochem. biophys. Res. Commun. *116:* 1091–1099 (1983).
87 Fischer, S.; Weber, P.C.: Prostacyclin I_3 is formed in vivo in man after dietary eicosapentaenoic acid. Nature *307:* 165–168 (1984).

88 Fogerty, A.C.; Evans, A.J.; Ford, G.L.; Kennett, B.H.: Distribution of ω6 and ω3 fatty acids in lipid classes in Australian fish. Nutr. Rep. int. *33:* 777–786 (1986).

89 François, M.; Pascal, G.; Durant, G.: Effets de la carence alimentaire en acide α-linolénique chez le rat. Annls Nutr. Aliment. *34:* 443–450 (1980).

90 Fulco, A.J.; Mead, J.F.: Metabolism of essential fatty acids. 8. Origin of 5,8,11 – 20:3 formed from 18:1 in fat-deficient rats. J. biol. Chem. *234:* 1411–1416 (1959).

91 Furlow, T.; Bass, N.: Stroke in rats produced by carotid injection of sodium arachidonate. Science *187:* 658 (1975).

92 Gabor, H.; Abraham, S.: Effect of dietary menhaden oil on tumor cell loss and the accumulation of mass of a transplantable mammary adenocarcinoma in BALB/c mice. J. natn. Cancer Inst. *76:* 1223–1229 (1986).

93 Galli, C.: Dietary influences on prostaglandin synthesis; in Draper, Advances in nutritional research, vol. 3, pp 95–125 (Plenum Press, New York 1980).

94 Galli, C.; Spagnuolo, C.; Bosisio, E.; Tosi, L.; Folco, G.C.; Galli, G.: Dietary essential fatty acids, polyunsaturated fatty acids and prostaglandins in the central nervous system; in Coceani, Olley, Advances in prostaglandin and thromboxane research, vol. 14, pp. 181–189 (Raven Press, New York 1978).

95 Galli, C.; Trzeciak, H.I.; Paoletti, R.: Effects of dietary fatty acids on the fatty acid composition of brain ethanolamine phosphoglyceride: reciprocal replacement of n-6 and n-3 polyunsaturated fatty acids. Biochim. biophys. Acta *248:* 449–454 (1971).

96 Geill, T.; Dybkaer, R.: The effect of linolenic acid orally on platelet adhesiveness and fibrinogen concentration. Scand. J. clin. Lab. Invest. *23:* 255–258 (1969).

97 German, B.; Bruckner, G.; Kinsella, J.: Evidence against $PGF_{4\alpha}$ prostaglandin structure in trout tissue – a correction. Prostaglandins *26:* 207–211 (1983).

98 Gibson, R.A.: Australian fish – an excellent source of both arachidonic acid and w3-polyunsaturated fatty acids. Lipids *18:* 743–752 (1983).

99 Ginsberg, B.H.; Jabour, J.; Spector, A.A.: Effect of alterations in membrane lipid unsaturation on the properties of the insulin receptor of Ehrlich ascites cells. Biochim. biophys. Acta *690:* 157–164 (1982).

100 Goldmann, D.W.; Pickett, W.C.; Goetzl, E.J.: Human neutrophil chemotactic and degranulating activities of leukotriene B_5 derived from eicosapentaenoic acid. Biochem. biophys. Res. Commun. *117:* 282–288 (1983).

101 Goldyne, M.E.; Stobo, J.D.: Immunoregulatory role of prostaglandins and related lipids; in CRC Crit. Rev. Immunol., pp. 189–223 (CRC Press, Boca Raton 1981).

102 Goodnight, S.H., Jr.; Harris, W.S.; Connor, W.E.: The effects of dietary ω3-fatty acids on platelet composition and function in man: a prospective, controlled study. Blood *58:* 880–885 (1981).

103 Goodnight, S.H., Jr.; Harris, W.S.; Connor, W.E.; Illingworth, D.R.: Polyunsaturated fatty acids, hyperlipidemia, and thrombosis. Arteriosclerosis *2:* 87–113 (1982).

104 Goodwin, J.S.; Webb, D.R.: Regulation of the immune response by prostaglandins. Clin. Immunol. Immunopathol. *15:* 106–122 (1980).

105 Green, J.; Tsiong, B.K.; Kamminga, E.; Willerbrands, A.F.: The influence of nutrition, individuality and some other factors, including various forms of stress, on serum cholesterol and phospholipid levels. Voeding *13:* 556–587 (1952).

106 Gudbjarnason, S.; Doell, B.; Oskardottir, G.; Hallgrimsson, J.: Modification of cardiac phospholipids and catecholamine stress tolerance; in De Duve, Hayaishi, Tocopherol, oxygen and biomembranes, pp. 297–310 (Elsevier/North-Holland Biomedical Press, Amsterdam 1978).

107 Guesnet, P.; Pascal, G.; Durand, G.: Effects of α-linolenic acid deficiency on reproduction and growth in rats. Prog. Lipid Res. *25:* 391–394 (1986).
108 Hamazaki, T.; Tateno, S.; Shishido, H.: Eicosapentaenoic acid and IgA nephropathy. Lancet *i:* 1017–1018 (1984).
109 Hammarström, S.: Leukotriene C_5: a slow-reacting substance derived from eicosapentaenoic acid. J. biol. Chem. *255:* 7093–7094 (1980).
110 Hansen, H.S.: Dietary essential fatty acids and in vivo prostaglandin production in mammals. Wld Rev. Nutr. Diet., vol. 42, pp. 102–134 (Karger, Basel 1983).
111 Hansen, H.S.; Jensen, B.: Essential function of linoleic acid esterified in acylglucosylceramide and acylceramide in maintaining the epidermal water permeability barrier. Evidence from feeding studies with oleate, linoleate, arachidonate, columbinate and α-linolenate. Biochim. biophys. Acta *834:* 357–363 (1985).
112 Hansen, H.S.; Jensen, B.; Wettstein-Knowles, P. von: Apparent in vivo retroconversion of dietary arachidonic to linoleic acid in essential fatty acid-deficient rats. Biochim. biophys. Acta *878:* 284–287 (1986).
113 Harris, W.S.; Connor, W.E.: The effects of salmon oil upon plasma lipids, lipoproteins and triglyceride clearance. Trans. Ass. Am. Physns *93:* 148–155 (1980).
114 Harris, W.S.; Connor, W.E.; Inkeles, S.B.; Illingworth, D.R.: Dietary n-3 fatty acids prevent carbohydrate-induced hypertrigliceridemia. Metabolism *33:* 1016–1019 (1984).
115 Harris, W.S.; Connor, W.E.; McMurry, M.P.: The comparative reductions of plasma lipids and lipoproteins by dietary polyunsaturated fats: salmon oil versus vegetable oils. Metabolism *32:* 179–184 (1983).
116 Hassam, A.G.; Rivers, J.P.W.; Crawford, M.A.: The failure of the cat to desaturate linoleic acid; its nutritional implications. Nutr. Metab. *21:* 321–328 (1977).
117 Hay, C.R.M.; Durber, A.P.; Saynor, R.: Effect of fish oil on platelet kinetics in patients with ischaemic heart disease. Lancet *i:* 1269–1272 (1982).
118 Herold, P.M.; Kinsella, J.E.: Fish oil consumption and decreased risk of cardiovascular disease: a comparison of findings from animal and human feeding trials. Am. J. clin. Nutr. *43:* 566–598 (1986).
119 Higgs, E.A.: The role of eicosanoids in inflammation. Prog. Lipid Res. *25:* 555–561 (1986).
120 Higgs, E.A.; Moncada, S.; Vane, J.R.: The biological importance and therapeutic potential of prostacyclin; in Conn, Felice, Kuo, Prostaglandins, platelets, lipids, pp. 1–202 (Elsevier/North-Holland, New York 1981).
121 Hillyard, L.A.; Abraham, S.: Effect of dietary polyunsaturated fatty acids on growth of mammary adenocarcinomas in mice and rats. Cancer Res. *39:* 4430–4437 (1979).
122 Hirai, A.; Hamazaki, T.; Terano, T.; Nishikawa, T.; Tamura, Y.; Kumagai, A.; Sajiki, J.: Eicosapentaenoic acid and platelet function in Japanese. Lancet *ii:* 1132 (1980).
123 Hirai, A.; Terano, T.; Tamura, Y.; Yoshida, S.; Kumagai, A.: Eicosapentaenoic acid and thrombotic disorders – epidemiological and clinical approach. Conf. on n-3 fatty acids, Reading 1984.
124 Holman, R.T.: The ratio of trienoic:tetraenoic acids in tissue lipids as a measure of essential fatty acid requirement. J. Nutr. *70:* 405–410 (1960).
125 Holman, R.T.: Essential fatty acid deficiency; in Holman, Progress in the chemistry of fats and other lipids, vol. 9, pp. 274–348 (Pergamon Press, Oxford 1968).

126 Holman, R.T.; Johnson, S.B.; Hatch, T.F.: A case of human linolenic acid deficiency involving neurological abnormalities. Am. J. clin. Nutr. *35:* 617–623 (1982).
127 Honn, K.V.; Busse, W.D.; Sesane, B.F.: Prostacyclin and thromboxanes: implications for their role in tumor cell metastasis. Biochem. Pharmacol. *32:* 1–11 (1983).
128 ten Hoor, F.; Deckere, E.A.M. de; Haddeman, E.; Hornstra, G.; Quadt, J.F.A.: Dietary manipulation of prostaglandin and thromboxane synthesis in heart, aorta and blood platelets of the rat; in Samuelsson, Ramwell, Paoletti, Advances in prostaglandin and thromboxane research, vol. 8, pp. 1771–1781 (Raven Press, New York 1980).
129 Hopkins, G.J.; West, C.E.: Possible roles of dietary fats in carcinogenesis. Life Sci. *19:* 1103–1116 (1976).
130 Horning, E.C.; Lin, S.-N.: Analytical studies of human plasma lecithins, cholesteryl esters, free fatty acids and α-tocopherol; in de Duve, Hayaishi, Tocopherol, oxygen and biomembranes, pp. 273–282 (Elsevier/North-Holland Biomedical Press, Amsterdam 1978).
131 Houtsmuller, U.M.T.; Beek, A. van der: Effects of topical application of fatty acids. Prog. Lipid Res. *20:* 219–224 (1981).
132 Hwang, D.H.; Carroll, A.E.: Decreased formation of prostaglandins derived from arachidonic acid by dietary linolenate in rats. Am. J. clin. Nutr. *33:* 590–597 (1980).
133 IAFMM: Conference on n-3 fatty acids, Reading 1984.
134 Illingworth, D.R.; Harris, W.S.; Connor, W.E.: Inhibition of low-density-lipoprotein synthesis by dietary ω3 fatty acids in humans. Arteriosclerosis *4:* 270–275 (1984).
135 Ip, C.; Carter, C.A.; Ip, M.M.: Requirement of essential fatty acid for mammary tumorigenesis in the rat. Cancer Res. *45:* 1997–2001 (1985).
136 Iritani, N.; Fujikawa, S.: Competitive incorporation of dietary ω-3 and ω-6 polyunsaturated fatty acids into the tissue phospholipids in rats. J. Nutr. Sci. Vitaminol. *28:* 621–629 (1982).
137 Iritani, N.; Inoguchi, K.; Endo, M.; Fukudu, E.; Moreta, M.: Identification of shellfish fatty acids and their effects on lipogenic enzymes. Biochim. biophys. Acta *618:* 378–392 (1980).
138 Ishinaga, M.; Kakuta, M.; Narita, H.; Kito, M.: Inhibition of platelet aggregation by dietary linseed oil. Agr. Biol. Chem. *47:* 903–906 (1983).
139 IUPAC-IUB: The nomenclature of lipids. Eur. J. Biochem. *79:* 11–21 (1977).
140 Jakschik, B.A.; Sams, A.R.; Sprecher, H.; Needleman, P.: Fatty acid structural requirement for leukotriene biosynthesis. Prostaglandins *20:* 401–410 (1980).
141 James, W.P.T.: Dietary trends in Britain; in Padley, Podmore, The role of fats in human nutrition, pp. 9–22 (Ellis Horwood, Chichester 1985).
142 Johnston, P.V.: Dietary fat, eicosanoids, and immunity. Adv. Lipid Res. *21:* 103–141 (1985).
143 Johnston, P.V.; Marshall, L.A.: Dietary fat, prostaglandins and the immune response. Prog. Food Nutr. Sci. *8:* 3–25 (1984).
144 Jurkowski, J.J.; Cave, W.T., Jr.: Dietary effects of menhaden oil on the growth and membrane lipid composition of rat mammary tumors. J. natn. Cancer Inst. *74:* 1145–1150 (1985).
145 Karmali, R.A.; Hanrahan, R.; Volkman, A.; Smith, N.: Prostaglandins and essential fatty acids in regulation of autoimmunity and development of antibodies of DNA in NZBxNZW F_1 mice. Prog. Lipid Res. *20:* 655–661 (1982).

146 Karmali, R.A.; Marsh, J.; Fuchs, C.: Effect of omega-3 fatty acids on growth of a rat mammary tumor. J. natn. Cancer Inst. *73:* 457–461 (1984).
147 Kato, M.; Tillotson, J.; Nichaman, M.Z.; Rhoads, G.G.; Hamilton, H.B.: Epidemiological studies of coronary heart disease and stroke in Japanese men living in Japan, Hawaii and California – serum lipids and diet. Am. J. Epidem. *97:* 372 –385 (1973).
148 Kelley, V.E.; Ferretti, A.; Izni, S.; Strom, T.B.: A fish oil diet rich in eicosapentaenoic acid reduces cyclooxygenase metabolites and suppresses lupus in MRL-lpr mice. J. Immun. *134:* 1914–1919 (1985).
149 Keys, A.; Kimura, N.: Diet of middle-aged farmers in Japan. Am. J. clin. Nutr. *23:* 212–223 (1970).
150 Kinsell, L.W.; Partridge, G.; Boling, L.; Margen, S.; Michaels, G.D.: Dietary modification of serum cholesterol and phospholipid levels. J. clin. Endocrinol. *12:* 909–913 (1952).
151 Kinsella, J.E.; Shimp, J.L.; Mai, J.: The proximate and lipid composition of several species of freshwater fishes. N.Y. Food Life Sci. Bull. *69:* 1–19 (1978).
152 Kloeze, J.; Houtsmuller, U.M.T.; Vles, R.O.: Influences of dietary fat mixtures on platelet adhesiveness, atherosclerosis and plasma cholesterol content of rabbits. J. Atheroscler. Res. *9:* 319–334 (1969).
153 Knapp, H.R.; Reilly, I.A.G.; Allessandrini, P.; Fitzgerald, G.A.: In vivo indexes of platelet and vascular function during fish-oil administration in patients with atherosclerosis. New Engl. J. Med. *314:* 937–942 (1986).
154 Kobayashi, S.; Hirai, A.; Terano, T.; Hamazaki, T.; Tamura, Y.; Kumagai, A.: Reduction in blood viscosity by eicosapentaenoic acid. Lancet *ii:* 197 (1981).
155 Kollmorgen, G.M.; King, M.M.; Kosanke, S.D.; Do, C.: Influence of dietary fat and indomethacin on the growth of transplantable mammary tumors in rats. Cancer Res. *43:* 4714–4719 (1983).
156 Kremer, J.M.; Michalek, A.V.; Lininger, L.; Huyek, C.; Biganoette, J.; Timchalk, M.A.; Rynes, R.I.; Zieminski, J.; Bartholomew, L.E.: Effects of manipulation of dietary fatty acids on clinical manifestations of rheumatoid arthritis. Lancet *i:* 184–187 (1985).
157 Kromann, N.; Green, A.: Epidemiological studies in the Upernavik district, Greenland. Acta med. scand. *208:* 401–406 (1980).
158 Kromhout, D.; Bosschieter, E.B.; Lezenne Coulander, C. de: The inverse relation between fish consumption and 20-year mortality from coronary heart disease. New Engl. J. Med. *312:* 1205–1209 (1985).
159 Lamptey, M.S.; Walker, B.L.: A possible essential role for dietary linolenic acid in the development of the young rat. J. Nutr. *106:* 86–93 (1976).
160 Editorial: Eskimo diets and diseases. Lancet *i:* 1139–1141 (1983).
161 Lands, W.E.M.: The biosynthesis and role of prostaglandins. A. Rev. Physiol. *41:* 633–652 (1979).
162 Lands, W.E.M.: Biochemical observations on dietary long-chain fatty acids from fish oil and their effect on prostaglandin synthesis in animals and humans; in Barlow, Stansby, Nutritional evaluation of long-chain fatty acids in fish oil, pp. 267–282 (Academic Press, London 1982).
163 Lands, W.E.M.: Fish and human health (Academic Press, Orlando 1986).
164 Lands, W.E.M.; LeTellier, P.R.; Rome, L.H.; Vanderhoek, J.Y.: Inhibition of pros-

taglandin biosynthesis; in Bergstrom, Advances in the biosciences, vol. 9, pp. 15–28 (Pergamon Press, Oxford 1973).
165 Laserre, M.; Mendy, F.; Spielmann, D.; Jacotot, B.: Effects of different dietary intake of essential fatty acids on C20:3ω6 and C20:4ω6 serum levels in human adults. Lipids *20:* 227–233 (1985).
166 Leat, W.M.F.; Northrop, C.A.: Effect of dietary linoleic and linolenic acids on gestation and parturition in the rat. Q. Jl exp. Physiol. *66:* 99–103 (1981).
167 Lee, T.H.; Hoover, R.L.; Williams, J.D.; Sperling, R.I.; Ravalese, J., III; Sour, B.W.; Robinson, D.R.; Corey, E.J.; Lewis, R.A.; Austen, K.F.: Effect of dietary enrichment with eicosapentaenoic and docosahexaenoic acids on in vitro neutrophil and monocyte leukotriene generation and neutrophil function. New Engl. J. Med. *312:* 1217–1224 (1985).
168 Lee, T.H.; Lewis, R.A.; Robinson, D.; Drazen, J.M.; Austen, K.F.: The effects of a diet enriched in menhaden fish oil on the pulmonary response to antigen challenge. J. Allergy clin. Immunol. *73:* 150 (1984).
169 Lee, T.H.; Mencia-Huerta, J.M.; Shih, C.; Corey, E.J.; Lewis, R.A.; Austen, K.F.: Characterization and biologic properties of 5,12-dihydroxy derivatives of eicosapentaenoic acid, including leukotriene B_5 and the lipoxygenase product. J. biol. Chem. *259:* 2383–2389 (1984).
170 Leitch, A.G.; Lee, T.H.; Ringel, E.W.; Pricket, J.D.; Robinson, D.R.; Pym, S.G.; Corey, E.J.; Drazen, J.M.; Austen, K.F.; Lewis, R.S.: Immunologically induced generation of tetraene and pentaene leukotrienes in the peritoneal cavities of menhaden-fed rats. J. Immun. *132:* 2559–2565 (1984).
171 Lemarchal, P.: Rôle biologique de l'acide linolénique. Revue fr. Corps gras *25:* 303–308 (1978).
172 Lewis, R.A.; Austen, K.F.: The biologically active leukotrienes: biosynthesis, metabolism, receptors, functions, and pharmacology. J. clin. Invest. *73:* 889–897 (1984).
173 Lorenz, R.; Spengler, U.; Fischer, S.; Duhm, J.; Weber, P.C.: Platelet function, thromboxane formation and blood pressure control during supplementation of the Western diet with codliver oil. Circulation *67:* 504–511 (1983).
174 Lossonczy, T.O. von; Ruiter, A.; Bronsgeest-Schoute, H.C.; Gent, C.M. van; Hermus, R.J.J.: The effect of a fish diet on serum lipids in healthy human subjects. Am. J. clin. Nutr. *31:* 1340–1346 (1978).
175 Machlin, L.J.: Effect of dietary linolenate on the proportion of linoleate and arachidonate in liver fat. Nature *194:* 868–869 (1962).
176 Magrum, L.J.; Johnston, P.V.: Modulation of prostaglandin synthesis in rat peritoneal macrophages with ω-3 fatty acids. Lipids *18:* 514–521 (1983).
177 Mai, G.; Goswami, S.K.; Bruckner, C.; Kinsella, J.E.: A new prostaglandin, C_{22}-$PGF_{4\alpha}$, synthesized from docosahexaenoic acid $C_{22:6n3}$ by trout gill. Prostaglandins *24:* 691–698 (1981).
178 Marshall, L.A.; Johnston, P.V.: Modulation of tissue prostaglandin synthesizing capacity by increased ratio of dietary alpha-linolenic acid to linoleic acid. Lipids *17:* 905–913 (1982).
179 Mest, H.J.; Beitz, J.; Heinroth, H.U.; Förster, W.: The influences of linseed oil on fatty acid pattern in phospholipids and thromboxane formation in platelets in man. Klin. Wschr. *61:* 187–191 (1983).
180 Mohrhauer, H.; Holman, R.T.: Effect of linolenic acid upon the metabolism of linoleic acid. J. Nutr. *81:* 67–74 (1963).

181 Morisaki, N.; Shinomya, M.; Matsuoka, N.; Saito, Y.; Kumagai, A.: In vivo effects of cis-5,8,11,14,17–20:5(n-3) and cis-4,7,10,13,16,19–22:6(n-3) on serum lipoprotein, platelet aggregation and lipid metabolism in the aorta of rats. Tohoku J. exp. Med. *141:* 397–405 (1983).
182 Mortensen, J.Z.; Schmidt, E.B.; Nielsen, A.H.; Dyerberg, J.: The effect of n-6 and n-3 polyunsaturated fatty acids on hemostasis, blood lipids and blood pressure. Thromb. Haemostasis *50:* 543–546 (1983).
183 Mullane, K.M.; Read, N.; Salmon, J.A.; Moncada, S.: Role of leukocytes in acute myocardial infarction in anesthetized dogs: relationship to myocardial salvage by antiinflammatory drugs. J. Pharmac. exp. Ther. *228:* 510–522 (1984).
184 Murphy, R.C.; Picket, W.C.; Culp, B.R.; Lands, W.E.M.: Tetraene and pentaene leukotrienes: selective production from murine mastocytoma cells after dietary manipulation. Prostaglandins *22:* 613–622 (1981).
185 n-3 News: Department of Preventive Medicine, Massachussetts General Hospital, Boston, Mass., USA (first issue: January, 1986).
186 Nagakawa, Y.; Orimo, H.; Harasawa, M.; Morita, I.; Yashiro, K.; Murota, S.: Effect of eicosapentaenoic acid on the platelet aggregation and composition of fatty acids in man. Atherosclerosis *47:* 71–75 (1983).
187 Natvig, H.; Borchgrevink, C.F.; Dedichen, J.; Owren, P.A.; Schiøtz, E.H.; Westlund, K.: A controlled trial of the effect of linolenic acid on incidence of coronary heart disease. Scand. J. clin. Lab. Invest. *22:* suppl. 105, pp. 1–20 (1968).
188 Needleman, P.; Raz, A.; Minkes, M.S.; Ferrendelli, J.A.; Sprecher, H.: Triene prostaglandins: prostacyclin and thromboxane biosynthesis and unique biological properties. Proc. natn. Acad. Sci. USA *76:* 944–948 (1979).
189 Nelson, A.M.: Diet therapy in coronary disease – effect on mortality of high-protein high-seafood, fat-controlled diet. Geriatrics *27:* 103–116 (1972).
190 Nestel, P.J.: Fish oil attenuates the cholesterol-induced rise in lipoprotein cholesterol. Am. J. clin. Nutr. *43:* 752–757 (1986).
191 Nestel, P.; Connor, W.E.; Reardon, M.F.; Connor, S.: Suppression by dietary fish oil of lipoprotein synthesis. Circulation *68:* 111–118 (1983).
192 Nestel, P.J.; Connor, W.E.; Reardon, M.F.; Connor, S.; Wong, S.; Boston, R.: Suppression by diets rich in fish oil of very low density lipoprotein production in man. J. clin. Invest. *74:* 82–89 (1984).
193 Nettleton, J.A.: Seafood nutrition: facts, issues and marketing of nutrition in fish and shellfish (Osprey Books, Huntington 1986).
194 Neuringer, M.; Connor, W.E.: n-3 Fatty acids in the brain and retina: evidence for their essentiality. Nutr. Rev. *44:* 285–294 (1986).
195 Neuringer, M.; Connor, W.E.; Lin, D.S.; Barstad, L.; Luck, S.J.: Biochemical and functional effects of prenatal and postnatal ω3 fatty acid deficiency in retina and brain in rhesus monkey. Proc. natn. Acad. Sci. USA *83:* 4021–4025 (1986).
196 Neuringer, M.; Connor, W.E.; Van Petten, C.; Barstad, L.: Dietary omega-3 fatty acid deficiency and visual loss in infant Rhesus monkeys. J. clin. Invest. *73:* 272–276 (1984).
197 Nielsen, N.H.; Hansen, J.P.H.: Breast cancer in Greenland – selected epidemiological, clinical and histological features. J. Cancer Res. clin. Oncol. *98:* 287–299 (1980).
198 Noelle, H.: Nahrung aus dem Meer (Springer, Berlin 1981).

199 Nordøy, A.: The influence of saturated fats, cholesterol, corn oil and linseed oil on experimental venous thrombosis in rats. Thromb. Diath. haemorrh. *13:* 244–256 (1965).
200 Nordøy, A.: The influence of saturated fat, cholesterol, corn oil and linseed oil on the ADP-induced platelet adhesiveness in the rat. Thromb. Diath. haemorrh. *13:* 543–549 (1965).
201 Nordøy, A.; Hamlin, J.T.; Chandler, A.B.; Newland, H.: The influence of dietary fats on plasma and platelet lipids and ADP-induced platelet thrombosis in the rat. Scand. J. Haemat. *5:* 458–473 (1968).
202 Norris, P.G.; Jones, C.J.H.; Weston, M.J.: Beneficial effect of MaxEPA on systolic blood pressure of patients with mild hypertension. Br. med. J. *293:* 104–105 (1986).
203 Norum, K.R.; Drevon, C.A.: Dietary n-3 fatty acids and cardiovascular diseases. Arteriosclerosis *6:* 352–355 (1986).
204 Nouvelot, A.; Bourre, J.M.; Sezille, G.; Dewailly, P.; Jaillard, J.: Changes in the fatty acid patterns of brain prostaglandins during development of rats fed peanut or rapeseen oil, taking into account differences between milk and maternal food. Annls Nutr. Metab. *27:* 173–181 (1983).
205 Ochi, K.; Yoshimoto, T.; Yamamoto, S.; Taniguchi, K.; Myamoto, T.: Arachidonate 5-lipoxygenase of guinea pig peritoneal polymorphonuclear leukocytes: activation by adenosine 5′-triphosphate. J. biol. Chem. *258:* 5754–5758 (1983).
206 O'Connor, T.P.; Roebuck, B.C.; Peterson, F.; Campbell, T.C.: Effect of dietary intake of fish oil and fish protein on the development of *L*-azaserine induced preneoplastic lesions in rat pancreas (Abstract). Fed. Proc. *44:* 769 (1985).
207 O'Dea, K.; Sinclair, A.J.: High arachidonic acid content in Australian fish caught off the coast at 17 °S. Am. J. clin. Nutr. *36:* 868–872 (1982).
208 Opstvedt, J.: Fish fats; in Wiseman, Fats in animal nutrition, pp. 53–82 (Butterworth, London 1984).
209 Owren, P.A.; Hellem, A.J.; Ödergaard, A.: Linolenic acid for the prevention of thrombosis and myocardial infarction. Lancet *ii:* 975–978 (1964).
210 Owren, P.A.; Hellem, A.J.; Ödergaard, A.: Linolenic acid and platelet adhesiveness. Lancet *ii:* 849–850 (1965).
211 Pappenheimer, A.M.; Goettsch, M.: A cerebellar disorder in chicks, apparently of nutritional origin. J. exp. Med. *53:* 11–26 (1931).
212 Peifer, J.J.: Hypocholesterolemic effects of marine oils; in Stansby, Fish oils; their chemistry, technology, stability, nutritional properties, and uses, pp. 322–361 (Avi Publishing, Westport 1967).
213 Phillipson, B.E.; Rothrock, D.W.; Connor, W.E.; Harris, W.W.; Illingworth, D.R.: Reduction of plasma lipids, lipoproteins and apoproteins by dietary fish oils in patients with hypertriglyceridemia. New Engl. J. Med. *312:* 1210–1216 (1985).
214 Piper, P.J.: The evolution and future horizons of research on the metabolism of arachidonic acid by 5-lipoxygenase. J. Allergy clin. Immunol. *74:* 441–444 (1984).
215 Plescia, O.J.; Smith, A.H.; Grinwich, K.: Subversion of immune system by tumor cells and role of prostaglandins. Proc. natn. Acad. Sci. USA *72:* 1848–1851 (1975).
216 Prescott, S.M.: The effect of eicosapentaenoic acid on leukotriene B production by human neutrophils. J. biol. Chem. *259:* 7615–7621 (1984).

217 Prickett, J.D.; Robinson, D.R.; Bloch, K.J.: Enhanced production of IgE and IgG antibodies associated with a diet enriched in eicosapentaenoic acid. Immunology *46:* 819–826 (1982).
218 Prickett, J.D.; Robinson, D.R.; Steinberg, A.D.: Dietary enrichment with the polyunsaturated fatty acid eicosapentaenoic acid prevents proteinuria and prolongs survival in NZBxNZW/F_1 mice. J. clin. Invest. *68:* 556–559 (1981).
219 Prickett, J.D.; Robinson, D.R.; Steinberg, A.D.: Effects of dietary enrichment with eicosapentaenoic acid upon autoimmune nephritis in female NZBxNZW F/F_1 mice. Arthritis Rheum. *26:* 131–139 (1983).
220 Prickett, J.D.; Trentham, D.E.; Robinson, D.R.: Dietary fish oil augments the induction of arthritis in rats immunized with type II collagen. J. Immun. *132:* 725–729 (1984).
221 Pudelkewicz, C.; Seufert, J.; Holman, R.T.: Requirements of the female rat for linoleic and linolenic acids. J. Nutr. *94:* 138–146 (1968).
222 Rahm, J.R.; Holman, R.T.: Effect of linoleic acid upon the metabolism of linolenic acid. J. Nutr. *84:* 15–19 (1964).
223 Renaud, S.; Nordøy, A.: 'Small is beautiful': α-linolenic acid and eicosapentaenoic acid in man. Lancet *i:* 1169 (1983).
224 Rice, R.D.: The effects of low doses of MaxEPA for long periods. Br. J. clin. Pract. *38:* symp. suppl. 31, pp. 85–88 (1984).
225 Rivers, J.P.W.; Hassam, A.G.; Crawford, M.A.; Brambell, M.R.: The inability of the lion, *Panthera leo,* to desaturate linoleic acid. FEBS Lett. *67:* 269–270 (1976).
226 Rivers, J.P.W.; Sinclair, A.J.; Crawford, M.A.: Inability of the cat to desaturate essential fatty acids. Nature *285:* 171–173 (1975).
227 Rizek, R.L.; Welsh, S.O.; Marston, R.M.; Jackson, E.M.: Levels and sources of fat in the US food supply and in diets of individuals; in Perkins, Visek, Dietary fats and health, pp. 13–43 (Am. Oil Chemists Society, Champaign 1983).
228 Robinson, D.; Prickett, J.; Makoul, G.; Colvin, R.; Levine, L.; Steinberg, A.: Dietary marine lipids and immunologic inflammation. Conf. on n-3 Fatty Acids, Reading 1984.
229 Rogers, S.; James, K.S.: Blood pressure-lowering effect of MaxEPA on normal volunteers compared to olive oil. Br. med. J. *293:* 454 (1986).
230 Rolland, P.H.; Martin, D.M.; Jacquemier, J.; Rolland, A.M.; Toga, M.: Prostaglandin in human breast cancer: evidence suggesting that an elevated prostaglandin production is a marker of high metastatic potential for neoplastic cells. J. natn. Cancer Inst. *64:* 1061–1070 (1980).
231 Ross, R.; Glomset, J.A.: The pathogenesis of atherosclerosis. New Engl. J. Med. *295:* 369–377, 420–425 (1976).
232 Rotstein, N.P.; Llincheta de Boschero, M.G.; Giusto, N.M.; Aveldaño, M.I.: Effects of aging on the composition and metabolism of docosahexaenoate-containing lipids of retina. Lipids *22:* 253–260 (1987).
233 Rudin, D.O.: The dominant diseases of modernized societies as omega-3 essential fatty acid syndrome: substrate beriberi. Med. Hypotheses *8:* 17–47 (1982).
234 Sanders, R.A.B.: The importance of eicosapentaenoic and docosahexaenoic acids; in Padley, Podmore, The role of fats in human nutrition, pp. 101–116 (Ellis Horwood, Chichester 1985).
235 Sanders, T.A.B.: Influence of fish-oil supplements on man. Proc. Nutr. Soc. *44:* 391–397 (1985).

236 Sanders, T.A.B.; Hochland, M.: A comparison of the influence on plasma lipids and platelet function of supplements of ω3 and ω6 polyunsaturated fatty acids. Br. J. Nutr. *50:* 521–529 (1983).

237 Sanders, T.A.B.; Mistry, M.: Controlled trials of fish oil supplements on plasma lipid concentrations. Br. J. clin. Pract. *38:* symp. suppl. 31, pp. 78–81 (1984).

238 Sanders, T.A.B.; Roshanai, F.: The influence of different types of ω3 polyunsaturated fatty acids on blood lipids and platelet function in healthy volunteers. Clin. Sci. *64:* 91–99 (1983).

239 Sanders, T.A.B.; Vickers, M.; Haines, A.P.: Effect on blood lipids and haemostasis of a supplement of cod-liver oil, rich in eicosapentaenoic and docosahexaenoic acids, in healthy young men. Clin. Sci. *61:* 317–324 (1981).

240 Sanders, T.A.B.; Younger, K.M.: The effect of dietary supplements of ω3 polyunsaturated fatty acids on the fatty acid composition of platelets and plasma choline phosphoglycerides. Br. J. Nutr. *45:* 613–616 (1981).

241 Saynor, R.: Effects of ω3 fatty acids on serum lipids. Lancet *ii:* 696–697 (1984).

242 Saynor, R.; Verel, D.: Effect of a marine oil high in eicosapentaenoic acid on blood lipids and coagulation. IRCS med. Sci. Metab. Nutr. *8:* 378–379 (1980).

243 Saynor, R.; Verel, D.; Gillot, T.: The long-term effect of dietary supplementation with fish lipid concentrate on serum lipids, bleeding time, platelets and angina. Atherosclerosis *50:* 3–10 (1984).

244 Schacky, C. von; Fischer, S.; Weber, P.C.: Long-term effects of dietary marine ω-3 fatty acids upon plasma and cellular lipids, platelet function, and eicosanoid formation in humans. J. clin. Invest. *76:* 1626–1631 (1985).

245 Schacky, C. von; Siess, W.; Fischer, S.; Weber, P.C.: A comparative study of eicosapentaenoic acid metabolism by human platelets in vivo and in vitro. J. Lipid Res. *26:* 457–464 (1985).

246 Schacky, C. von; Weber, P.C.: Metabolism and effects on platelet function of the purified eicosapentaenoic and docosahexaenoic acids in humans. J. clin. Invest. *76:* 2446–2450 (1985).

247 Schaefer, O.: Medical observation and problems in the Canadian Artic. Can. med. J. *81:* 386–393 (1959).

248 Seely, S.: Cancers of the breast and prostate; in Seely, Freed, Silverstone, Rippere, Diet-related diseases, pp. 190–205 (Avi, Westport 1985).

249 Seyberth, M.D.; Oelz, O.; Kennedy, T.; Sweetman, B.J.; Frölich, J.C.; Heimberg, M.; Oates, J.A.: Increased arachidonate in lipids after administration to man: effects on prostaglandin synthesis. Clin. Pharmacol. Ther. *18:* 521 (1975).

250 Shekelle, R.B.; Missell, L.; Paul, O.; Shyrock, A.M.; Stamler, J.: Fish consumption and mortality from coronary heart disease. New Engl. J. Med. *313:* 820 (1985).

251 Siess, W.; Scherer, B.; Böhling, B.; Roth, O.; Kurzman, I.; Weber, P.C.: Platelet-membrane fatty acids, platelet aggregation, and thromboxane formation during a mackerel diet. Lancet *i:* 441–444 (1980).

252 Silver, M.J.; Hoch, W.; Kocsis, J.J.; Ingerman, C.M.; Smith, J.B.: Arachidonic acid causes sudden death in rabbits. Science *183:* 1085 (1974).

253 Simons, L.A.; Hickie, J.B.; Balasubramaniam, S.: On the effects of dietary n-3 fatty acids (MaxEPA) on plasma lipids and lipoproteins in patients with hyperlipidaemia. Atherosclerosis *54:* 75–88 (1985).

254 Simopoulos, A.; Kifer, R.R.; Martin, R.E.: Health effects of polyunsaturated fatty acids in seafoods (Academic Press, Orlando 1986).

255 Sinclair, A.J.; O'Dea, K.; Naughton, J.M.: Elevated levels of arachidonic acid in fish from Northern Australian coastal waters. Lipids *18:* 877–881 (1983).
256 Sinclair, H.M.: The diet of Canadian Indians and Eskimos. Proc. Nutr. Soc. *12:* 69–82 (1953).
257 Sinclair, H.M.: Advantages and disadvantages of an Eskimo diet; in Fumagelli, Kritchevsky, Paoletti, Drugs affecting lipid metabolism, pp. 363–370 (Elsevier/North-Holland, Amsterdam 1980).
258 Sinclair, H.M.: The relative importance of essential fatty acids of the linoleic and linolenic acid families: studies with an Eskimo diet. Prog. Lipid Res. *20:* 897–899 (1982).
259 Singer, P.; Berger, I.; Lück, K.; Taube, C.; Naumann, E.; Gödicke, W.: Long-term effect of mackerel diet on blood pressure, serum lipids and thromboxane formation in patients with mild essential hypertension. Atherosclerosis *62:* 259–265 (1986).
260 Singer, P.; Jaeger, W.; Voigt, S.; Thiel, H.: Defective desaturation and elongation of n-6 and n-3 fatty acids in hypertensive patients. Prostaglandins Leukotrienes Med. *15:* 159–162 (1984).
261 Singer, P.; Jaeger, W.; Wirth, M.; Voigt, S.; Naumann, E.; Zimontkowski, S.; Hajdu, I.; Goedicke, W.: Lipid and blood pressure-lowering effect of mackerel diet in man. Atherosclerosis *49:* 99–108 (1983).
262 Singer, P.; Wirth, M.; Berger, I.; Voigt, S.; Gerike, U.; Goedicke, W.; Koberle, U.; Heine, H.: Influence on serum lipids, lipoproteins and blood pressure of mackerel and herring diet in patients with type IV and V hyperlipoproteinemia. Atherosclerosis *51:* 111–118 (1985).
263 Singer, P.; Wirth, M.; Voigt, S.; Richter-Heinrich, E.; Gödicke, W.; Berger, I.; Naumann, E.; Listing, J.; Hardrodt, W.; Taube, C.: Blood pressure- and lipid-lowering effect of mackerel and herring diet in patients with mild essential hypertension. Atherosclerosis *56:* 223–235 (1985).
264 Stamler, J.: Population studies; in Levy, Rifkind, Dennis, Ernst, Nutrition, lipids, and coronary heart disease, pp. 25–88 (Raven Press, New York 1979).
265 Stansby, M.E.: Nutritional properties of fish oils. Wld Rev. Nutr. Diet., vol. 11, pp. 46–105 (Karger, Basel 1969).
266 Stansby, M.E.: A clinical study on the role of fish oil in alleviating human heart disease; in Barlow, Stansby, Nutritional evaluation of long-chain fatty acids in fish oil, pp. 263–266 (Academic Press, London 1982).
267 Stare, F.J.: Marketing a nutritional 'revolutionary breakthrough'. New Engl. J. Med. *315:* 971–973 (1986).
268 Steinberg, A.D.; Huston, D.P.; Taurog, J.D.; Cowdery, J.S.; Raveche, E.S.: The cellular and genetic basis of murine lupus. Immunol. Rev. *55:* 121–154 (1981).
269 Strasser, S.; Fischer, S.; Weber, P.C.: Leukotriene B_5 is formed in human neutrophils after dietary supplementation with icosapentaenoic acid. Proc. natn. Acad. Sci. USA *82:* 1540–1543 (1985).
270 Talesnik, J.; Hsia, J.C.: Coronary flow reactions to arachidonic acid are inhibited by docosahexaenoic acid. J. Pharmacol. *80:* 255–258 (1982).
271 Tamura, Y.; Hirai, A.; Terano, T.; Takenaga, M.; Saitoh, H.; Tahara, K.; Yoshita, S.: Clinical and epidemiological studies of eicosapentaenoic acid (EPA) in Japan. Prog. Lipid Res. *25:* 461–466 (1986).
272 Tashjian, A.H., Jr.; Voelkel, E.F.; Robinson, D.R.; Levine, L.: Dietary menhaden oil

lowers plasma prostaglandins and calcium in mice bearing the prostaglandin-producing $HSDM_1$ fibrosarcoma. J. clin. Invest. *74:* 2042–2048 (1984).
273 Taylor, T.G.; Gibney, M.J.; Morgan, J.B.: Haemostatic function and polyunsaturated fatty acids. Lancet *ii:* 1378 (1979).
274 Terano, T.; Hirai, A.; Hamazaki, T.; Kobayashi, S.; Fujita, T.; Tamura, Y.; Kumagai, A.: Effect of oral administration of highly purified eicosapentaenoic acid on platelet function, blood viscosity and red cell deformability in healthy human subjects. Atherosclerosis *46:* 321–331 (1983).
275 Terano, T.; Hirai, A.; Tamura, Y.; Yoshida, S.; Salmon, J.A.; Moncada, S.: Effect of eicosapentaenoic acid on eicosanoids formation by stimulated human polymorphonuclear leukocytes. Prog. Lipid Res. *25:* 129–137 (1986).
276 Terano, T.; Salmon, J.A.; Moncada, S.: Biosynthesis and biological activity of leukotriene B_5. Prostaglandins *27:* 217–232 (1984).
277 Terano, T.; Salmon, J.A.; Moncada, S.: Biosynthesis and biological activity of LTB_5. Prostaglandins *28:* 668 (1984).
278 Theophilopoulos, A.N.; Dixon, F.J.: Etiopathogenesis of murine SLE. Immunol. Rev. *55:* 179–216 (1981).
279 Thomasson, H.J.: Biological standardization of essential fatty acids (a new method). Int. Z. VitamForsch. *25:* 62–82 (1953).
280 Thomasson, H.J.; Gottenbos, J.J.: Bioassay of essential fatty acids. Comparison of effect of triglycerides, methyl and ethyl esters. Proc. Soc. exp. Biol. Med. *111:* 261–262 (1962).
281 Thorngren, M.; Gustafson, A.: Effects of 11-week increase in dietary eicosapentaenoic acid on bleeding time, lipids, and platelet aggregation. Lancet *ii:* 1190–1192 (1981).
282 Thorngren, M.; Nilsson, E.; Gustafson, A.: Plasma lipoproteins and fatty acid composition during a moderate EPA (eicosapentaenoic acid) diet. Acta med. scand. *219:* 23–28 (1986).
283 Thorngren, M.; Shafi, S.; Born, G.V.R.: Quantification of blood from skin bleeding-time determinations. Effects of fish diet or acetylsalicylic acid. Haemostasis *13:* 282–287 (1983).
284 Thorngren, M.; Shafi, S.; Born, G.V.R.: Non-involvement of thromboxane A_2 in the delay of primary haemostasis induced by a fish diet. Br. J. Haemat. *58:* 567–578 (1984).
285 Tinoco, J.: Dietary requirements and functions of α-linolenic acid in animals. Prog. Lipid Res. *21:* 1–45 (1982).
286 Tinoco, J.; Babcock, R.; Hincenbergs, I.; Medwadowski, B.; Miljanich, P.: Linolenic acid deficiency: changes in fatty acid patterns in female and male rats raised on a linolenic acid-deficient diet for two generations. Lipids *13:* 6–17 (1978).
287 Tinoco, J.; Babcock, R.; Hincenbergs, I.; Medwadowski, B.; Miljanich, P.; Williams, M.A.: Linolenic acid deficiency. Lipids *14:* 166–173 (1979).
288 Vas Dias, F.W.; Gibney, M.J.; Taylor, T.G.: The effect of polyunsaturated fatty acids of the n-3 and n-6 series on platelet aggregation and platelet and aorta fatty acid composition in rabbits. Atherosclerosis *43:* 245–257 (1982).
289 Velardo, B.; Lagarde, M.; Guichardant, M.; Dechavanne, M.; Beylot, M.; Sautant, G.; Berthezène, F.: Decrease of platelet activity after intake of small amounts of eicosapentaenoic acid in diabetics. Thromb. Haemostasis. *48:* 344 (1982).

290 Vollset, S.E.; Hench, I.; Bjelke, E.: Fish consumption and mortality from coronary heart disease. New Engl. J. Med. *313:* 820–821 (1985).
291 Weiner, B.H.; Ockene, I.S.; Levine, P.H.; Cuénoud, H.F.; Fisher, M.; Johnson, B.F.; Daoud, A.S.; Jarmolych, J.; Hosmer, D.; Johnson, M.H.; Natale, A.; Vaudreuil, C.; Hoogesian, J.J.: Inhibition of atherosclerosis by cod-liver oil in a hyperlipidemic swine model. New Engl. J. Med. *315:* 841–846 (1986).
292 Welsch, C.W.; Aylsworth, C.F.: The interrelationship between dietary lipids, endocrine activity, and the development of mammary tumors in experimental animals; in Perkins, Visek, Dietary fats and health, pp. 790–816 (Am. Oil Chemists Society, Champaign 1983).
293 Wheeler, T.G.; Benolken, R.M.; Anderson, R.E.: Visual membranes: specificity of fatty acid precursors for the electrical response to illumination. Science *188:* 1312–1314 (1975).
294 Williams, E.D.; Karim, S.M.; Sandler, M.: Prostaglandin secretion by medullary carcinoma of the thyroid. Lancet *i:* 22 (1968).
295 Woodcock, B.E.; Smith, E.; Lambert, W.H.; Jones, W.M.; Galloway, J.H.; Greaves, M.; Preston, F.E.: Beneficial effects of fish oil on blood viscosity in peripheral vascular disease. Br. med. J. *288:* 591–594 (1984).
296 Yang, Y.-T.; Williams, M.A.: Comparison of C_{18}-, C_{20}-, and C_{22}-polyunsaturated fatty acids in reducing fatty acid synthesis in isolated rat hepatocytes. Biochim. biophys. Acta *531:* 133–140 (1978).
297 Yokoyama, C.; Mizuno, K.; Mitachi, H.; Yoshimoto, T.; Yamamoto, S.; Pace-Asciak, C.R.: Partial purification and characterization of arachidonate 12-lipoxygenase from rat lung. Biochim. biophys. Acta *750:* 237–243 (1983).
298 Ziboh, V.A.; Miller, C.; Kragballe, K.; Cohen, K.; Ellis, C.N.; Voorhees, J.J.: Significance of dietary intake of polyunsaturated fatty acids in the clinical management of psoriasis. II. Int. Congr. on Essential Fatty Acids, Prostaglandins and Leukotrienes, London 1985, abstract, pp. 135–136.
299 Zuccato, E.; Hornstra, G.; Dyerberg, J.: Life-long 'marine diet' in Eskimos is not associated with altered urinary excretion of total tetranor prostaglandin metabolites. Prostaglandins *30:* 465–478 (1985).

Prof. P. Budowski, Faculty of Agriculture, The Hebrew University of Jerusalem, Rehovot 76100 (Israel)

Wld Rev. Nutr. Diet., vol. 57, pp. 275–329 (Karger, Basel 1988)

Dietary Regulation of Small Intestinal Disaccharidases[1]

Toshinao Goda, Otakar Koldovský

Section of Neonatology and Nutritional Sciences, Department of Pediatrics and Physiology, University of Arizona College of Medicine, Tucson, Ariz., USA

Contents

Introduction

The final stage of carbohydrate digestion occurs on the luminal surface of small intestinal epithelial cells called brush border membrane or microvillar membrane. In this membrane, several glycosidases which hydrolyze di- and oligosaccharides originating from ingested nutrients are present. These glycosidases are referred to as disaccharidases. The activity of disaccharidases is known to be modified by various factors such as age,

[1] This work was supported by National Institutes of Health Grant AM27624.

nutritional status, hormones, pancreatic secretions and dietary composition. This review will deal with the variation of disaccharidase activities which occurs in response to dietary composition. For a comprehensive coverage of other factors, readers are referred to the previous review [Koldovský, 1981].

Metabolism of Disaccharidases in Small Intestinal Epithelial Cells

To understand the mechanisms of the dietary related variation of disaccharidase activities, a brief review of the characteristics of disaccharidases and their metabolic processes in small intestinal epithelial cells will be helpful. Knowledge of biosynthetic processing of microvillar glycoproteins, including disaccharidases and peptidases, has increased considerably during the last several years [Semenza, 1986]. In most mammals, including man, four disaccharidases complexes have been identified (and purified from various species; see table I). The *sucrase-isomaltase complex* consists of two subunits, sucrase and isomaltase. Sucrase is responsible for all the sucrase activity present in the small intestine while isomaltase is responsible for nearly all (greater than 95%) isomaltase activity. Since both sucrase and isomaltase hydrolyze maltose, some maltase activity in the small intestine, estimated as 30% in rat [Goda, unpublished] and 80–85% in man [Semenza, 1981], is derived from sucrase-isomaltase complex. Thus, sucrase-isomaltase is responsible for the hydrolysis of sucrose and also for the digestion of starch in its final stage. The *glucoamylase-maltase complex* (referred to as glucoamylase in this review) also consists of two heterogeneous subunits. Each of the two catalytic sites hydrolyze glucose oligomers of various length and structures which result from the process of starch digestion. This α-glucosidase complex possesses maltase activity as well as a slight isomaltase activity; *trehalase* hydrolyzes trehalose, a disaccharide which consists of two glucose molecules with α-1,1-glucosidic linkage. The potential significance of trehalose depends on its presence in meals (major source of trehalose in meals is mushrooms and insects). Since trehalase is not readily solubilized from the brush border membrane by the action of proteases such as papain, it is possible that this disaccharidase is embedded deeper in the membrane than other disaccharidases. Trehalase has been purified only in a detergent solubilized form [Sasajima et al., 1975; Nakano et al., 1977; Galand, 1984; Riby and Galand, 1985]. All three glycosidase complexes as mentioned above are α-glucosidases, i.e. they

Table I. Substrate specificities of small intestinal disaccharidases

Enzyme complex	Catalytic activity	Enzyme category	Major substrate	Ref.
1 Sucrase-isomaltase	sucrase	α-glucosidase	sucrose	1
			maltose	1
	isomaltase	α-glucosidase	isomaltose	1
			maltose	1
			dextrin (palatinose[1])	
2 Maltase-glucoamylase	maltase and/or glucoamylase	α-glucosidase	1,4-α-glucans (maltose, maltotriose, etc.)	2
3 Trehalase	trehalase	α-glucosidase	trehalose	3
4 Lactase-phlorizin hydrolase	lactase	β-galactosidase	lactose	4
	phlorizin hydrolase	β-glycosidase	phlorizin	4
			glycosyl ceramides	

[1] Palatinose is not present in large quantity in average meal, but it is often used as substitute for isomaltose for enzyme assay.
References: 1 = Gray et al. [1979]; 2 = Kelly and Alpers [1973]; 3 = Semenza [1981]; 4 = Leese and Semenza [1973].

recognize α-configurated glucose molecule (of nonreducing end in case of oligosaccharide) and hydrolyze the α-glucosidic linkage, producing a glucose as a product. These disaccharidases are, therefore, referred to as α-disaccharidases. In this regard, the *β-glycosidase complex* is distinguishable from other disaccharidases. This β-glycosidase complex is composed of two subunits. Two distinct catalytic sites are known to be present in this β-glycosidase complex. One catalytic site hydrolyzes lactose, the other hydrolyzes phlorizin and various glycosylceramides which are naturally present in milk [Leese and Semenza, 1973], but whether each catalytic site is located in different subunits is not known. This β-glycosidase complex will be referred to as lactase.

It should be noted that sucrase, lactase and trehalase activities in the small intestine originate from specific enzymes; sucrase, lactase and trehalase, respectively (table I). Maltase activity, however, is derived from glucoamylase and sucrase-isomaltase. Therefore, the interpretation of this change in maltase activity in the small intestine is complicated. Since changes in maltase activity are usually parallel to that of sucrase activity,

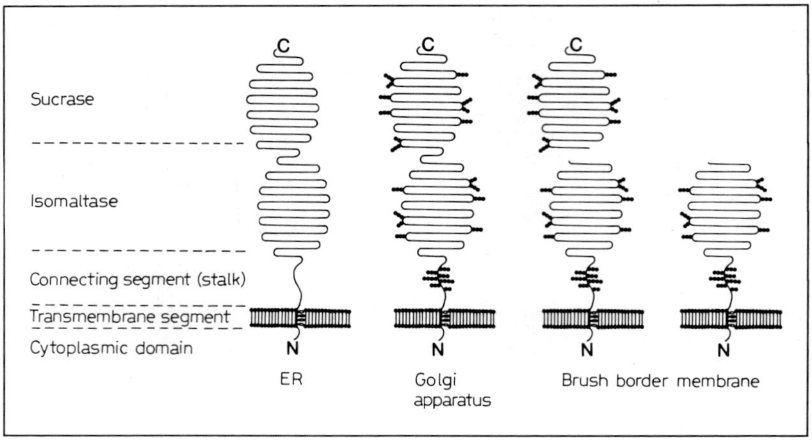

Fig. 1. Model of biosynthesis, positioning, processing and degradation of sucrase-isomaltase. The five suggested domains are shown in relation to the lipid bylayer. The isomaltase and sucrase subunits are marked with their amino-(N) and carboxy-(C) termini. Potential N-linked and O-linked sugars are indicated. ER = Endoplasmic reticulum. Modified from Hunziker et al. [1986].

the dietary related change of sucrase and maltase activity will be discussed simultaneously.

Biosynthesis and positioning in the brush border membrane of sucrase-isomaltase has been extensively characterized. The sucrase-isomaltase complex is synthesized as a single, large polypeptide chain (fig. 1) in intracellular membrane fractions, i.e. endoplasmic reticulum [Sjöström et al., 1980]. Recently, the primary structure of this pro-sucrase-isomaltase was reported by Hunziker et al. [1986]. While sucrase-isomaltase is being transferred from intracellular membrane to the brush border membrane, glycosylation occurs. On the brush border membrane, pro-sucrase-isomaltase is split into two mature subunits (sucrase and isomaltase) by pancreatic protease action present in the lumen. Pro-sucrase-isomaltase was thought to be fully catalytically active [Sjöström et al., 1980], but a partially inactive form of sucrase-isomaltase has been found in intracellular membrane fractions of pig small intestine [Sjöström et al., 1985]. Since these intracellular membrane fractions contain a high mannose form of sucrase-isomaltase (i.e. with incomplete glycosylation), this suggests that subsequent glycosylation process is required for activation *or* stabilization of this enzyme. It was demonstrated that glucoamylase-maltase complex

[Danielsen et al., 1981] and lactase-phlorizin hydrolase complex [Danielsen et al., 1984] are synthesized as single large precursor proteins and are processed similarly; there is only a slight difference in the processing step of lactase-phlorizin hydrolase which is proteolytically cleaved by intracellular protease(s). Kinetic studies of intracellular transfer of disaccharidases revealed that intracellular processing and transfer of disaccharidases is relatively slow (from 60 min to several hours) as compared to 20–40 min for microvillar peptidases [Hauri, 1986].

Degradation processes of disaccharidases are not as well defined as those for biosynthetic processes. Alpers and Tedesco [1975] first demonstrated that pancreatic proteases play a significant role in degradation of disaccharidases. Although the earlier studies implicated a solubilization of disaccharidases by the action of proteases, a sequential degradation of sucrase-isomaltase on the membrane has been reported [Goda and Koldovský, 1985]. Sucrase subunit is more susceptible to proteolysis than isomaltase subunit in the brush border membrane [Goda and Koldovský, 1985]. As a consequence, a considerable amount of isomaltase is present as isomaltase monomer (48–68% of total isomaltase) in the lower portion of jejunum of adult rats [Goda et al., 1988a]. Lactase appears to be susceptible to pancreatic protease(s) to a similar extent with the isomaltase subunit of sucrase-isomaltase [Goda and Koldovský, 1986]. The half-life of disaccharidases (in rats fed a standard laboratory chow diet ad libitum) was estimated to be 11.5 h [James et al., 1971]. However, the half-life of disaccharidases might exhibit diurnal variation as demonstrated in the case of sucrase (6–38 h) [Kaufman et al., 1980]. Since the estimated rate of synthesis of sucrase at the time of peak activity is similar to that of nadir activity, degradation seems to be a major factor responsible for diurnal variations of disaccharidase activities [Kaufman et al., 1980]. The turnover of disaccharidases is faster than the half-life of villus cells which was reported to be approximately 2 days in adult rats [Leblond and Stevens, 1948; Loran and Althausen, 1960; Koldovský et al., 1966]. Thus, it is reasonable to consider that degradation of disaccharidases occurs while the small intestinal epithelial cells migrate toward the tip of the villi.

Taking the above basic information into consideration, we posed the following question: Which process of the metabolism of disaccharidases is regulated by dietary nutrients? The possible sites of regulation are present in the following six steps: (1) transcription of specific genes and production of primary transcripts; (2) post-transcriptional modification (including splicing) of RNA to produce mature mRNA in nucleus; (3) translocation of mRNA to endoplasmic reticulum; (4) translation of mRNA to specific proteins; (5) post-translational modifications of synthesized polypeptides, including glycosylation, and (6) degradation of glycosylated disaccharidases in intracellular organelles (e.g. lysosomes) and on the brush border membrane.

The first four processes are referred to as 'synthesis process'. A few recent studies have reported the rates of synthesis of disaccharidases in animals fed various diets [Cézard et al., 1983; Riby and Kretchmer, 1984; Tsuboi et al., 1985b]. These studies are important in exploring the mechanisms of dietary regulation of disaccharidases and will be discussed later.

Basic Variations of Disaccharidase Activities

There are three important aspects concerning the expression of disaccharidases in a single small intestinal epithelial cell of adult mammals; (a) maturation levels of the cell, (b) diurnal rhythm, and (c) dietary adaptation. Although little is known about the cellular mechanisms involved, these occur within the life span of the cell and may be mutually related. Before discussing dietary adaptation, the other two basic variations of disaccharidase activities will be discussed.

Variation during Life Span of Cells

In crypt cells, disaccharidase activities are not detected, but with their migration toward the villus tip, activity gradually increases [Nördström et al., 1967, 1969; Nördström and Dahlqvist, 1973]. The site of maximal expression of lactase activity is located in the upper villus (fig. 2) which is more apical than the locus of maximal expression of sucrase activity [Boyle et al., 1980]. Studies in piglets suggest that increased cell migration rates of the intestinal epithelium during and after viral invasions leads to an increased proportion of undifferentiated crypt-like cells [Kerzner et al., 1979]. This expression of lactase activity in apical villus cells might explain the limited lactose hydrolysis exhibited during and after a bout of viral gastroenteritis [Kerzner et al., 1979]. The synthesis rate of sucrase, estimated by an accumulation of incorporated ^{3}H-leucine injected intraperitoneally into sucrase-isomaltase, was reported to be maximal in the lower half of the villus [Riby and Kretchmer, 1984]. The degradation of sucrase and lactase appeared to occur along the entire height of the villus since

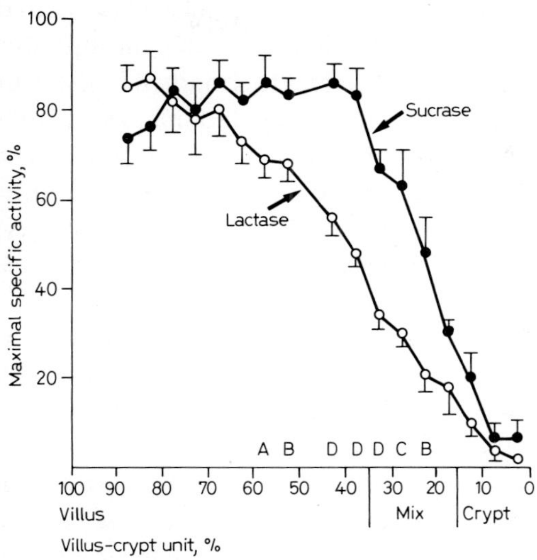

Fig. 2. Relative activity expressed as mean percent maximal specific activity of sucrase (closed circles) and lactase (open circles) along the villus-crypt unit. The highest specific activity in each tissue block was set at 100% and activities in all other homogenates expressed as a percent of that highest activity. Letters denote level of statistical significance between lactase and sucrase activities at any point along the villus-crypt unit (*A* $p < 0.05$; *B* $p < 0.02$; *C* $p < 0.01$; *D* $p < 0.001$). Absence of letter indicates no significant differences between maximal activities at a given height. Data reproduced with permission [Boyle et al., 1980].

occlusion of pancreatic ducts in adult rats led to an increase of these enzyme activities along the entire height of the villus [Riby and Kretchmer, 1985].

Diurnal Variation

Activities of small intestinal sucrase, maltase, trehalase and lactase activities exhibit rhythmical changes during the 24-hour cycle [Saito, 1972; Stevenson et al., 1975]. This rhythm has been extensively studied in rats. In rats fed a standard nonpurified diet ad libitum, under 'normal' night-day (12–14 h of light per day) conditions, disaccharidase activities showed a monophasic pattern with a peak around midnight [Saito, 1972; Saito et al., 1975] which appeared similar to diurnal pattern of food intake [Siegel, 1961]. Although a circadian variation of disaccharidase activities was reported along the entire length of the small intestine, the amplitude of the fluctuation was greatest in the jejunum and less marked in the ileum [Saito et al., 1975]. Diurnal variation of sucrase and maltase activities was observed in brush border membrane fraction as well as in the mucosal homogenate of rat small intestine [Saito and Suda, 1978]. Diurnal variation of disaccharidase activities appeared shortly after weaning was completed [Beam and Henning, 1978; Saito et al., 1978b]. Appearance of nocturnal feeding behavior appeared to play a major role.

In order to identify the factor(s) responsible for the diurnal variation of small intestinal disaccharidase activities, diurnal variation of these activities was studied under various experimental conditions, i.e. restriction of food intake and altered lighting conditions. Whenever food intake was restricted to 4 or 6 h a day, whether 'normal' lighting or continuous illumination was provided, the peak of disaccharidase activities was shifted accordingly [Saito, 1972; Saito et al., 1976b; Stevenson et al., 1975; Stevenson and Fierstein, 1976; Nishida et al., 1978]. Under continuous illumination, nocturnal eating and drinking patterns were abolished within 6–10 days [Siegel, 1961; Zucker, 1971]. After 4 weeks on a constant lighting and ad libitum feeding regime, there was no daily rhythmicity of food intake, sucrase activity or maltase activity observed [Nishida et al., 1978]. However, after 4 weeks of continuous darkness with free access to food, both food intake and disaccharidase activities maintained diurnal variations similar to those in rats kept under a 'normal' lighting condition [Nishida et al., 1978]. Thus, considerable evidence points to the timing of food intake rather than lighting conditions as the primary synchronizer.

However, the following evidence demonstrates that the diurnal variation of disaccharidase activities is not a mere consequence of each meal. First, rats starved for one or 2 days continue to exhibit rhythmicity of sucrase and maltase activities [Saito et al., 1976a, b) which disappears after several subsequent days of starvation (fig. 3). It is noteworthy that the nadir of activity does not change (starvation causes a decrease in peak activity only). Secondly, a considerable increase in disaccharidase activities occurs prior to the start of the feeding period [Saito et al., 1976a, b; Stevenson and Fierstein, 1976]. Therefore, some investigators [Saito et al., 1976a, b; Stevenson et al., 1975] have suggested the possibility of 'anticipation mechanism) which cues the rise in disaccharidase activity. The anticipation of periodical feeding has been observed in rats where diet was

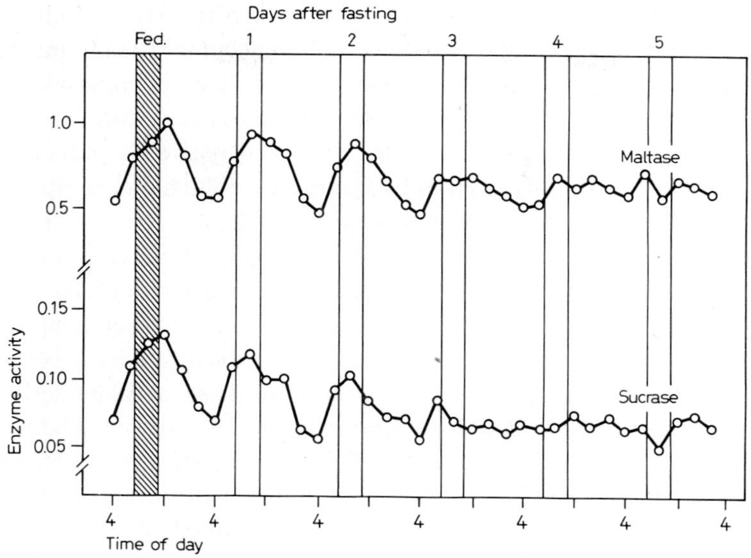

Fig. 3. Effect of fasting on the circadian rhythms of maltase and sucrase of the small intestine of rats fed from 09.00 to 15.00 hours for 2 weeks. The activities are expressed as μmol product formed per min per mg homogenate protein. Each point represents the mean value for 5 rats [reproduced with permission, Saito et al., 1976b].

offered every 24 h; rats failed to anticipate adiurnal feeding periods, i.e. every 19 or 29 h [Bolles and Stokes, 1965]. There is some evidence which demonstrates that adiurnal cycle of disaccharidase activities can be induced by restricted feeding [Furuya et al., 1979; Saito et al., 1980].

In rats fed for 3 h (every 12 h) under a constant lighting condition, a 12-hour cycle of sucrase, isomaltase, maltase and trehalase activities was induced [Furuya et al., 1979]. A diurnal variation, which is similar to that in rats fed once every 24 h, was observed when rats were fed for 12 h, once every 48 h. When rats had access (once every 32 h) to food for 8 h, sucrase and maltase activities exhibited rhythmic changes of 32-hour cycle, but the level of activity was observed to be lowest during the feeding period. The rhythmic period of 32 h was replaced by a 24-hour diurnal rhythm as soon as the rats were starved [Saito et al., 1980].

Thus, it appears that there is a basic diurnal oscillator, supposedly a neural or hormonal signal (unidentified), which affects the rhythmic pattern of disaccharidase activities. This intrinsic rhythm may be hindered or replaced by an extrinsic rhythm of feeding (which is a strong inducer of rhythmicity of disaccharidases). Neither adrenalectomy [Beam and Henning, 1978] nor insulin deficiency induced by streptozotocin [Sasaki et al., 1980] affects the rhythmic change of disaccharidase activities.

The following two questions were examined regarding induction of rhythm of disaccharidase activities by feeding. (1) Which diet composition is responsible for diurnal variation of disaccharidase activities? (2) Is it necessary to stimulate small intestinal cells by orally delivered nutrients to maintain the diurnal variation of disaccharidase activities? To answer these questions, various synthetic diets were fed to rats. When high carbohydrate, protein-free diet and high protein, carbohydrate-free diet were given alternately every 12 h, a 24-hour cycle of disaccharidase activities (which peak during feeding of high protein diet) was observed. The results suggested that protein content in the diet has a stronger cuing effect on rhythmic variations of disaccharidase activities than does carbohydrate [Furuya et al., 1979]. In contrast, rats which consumed either one type of protein-free or carbohydrate-free diet ad libitum exhibited similar diurnal variations of disaccharidase activities regardless of the type of diet [Saito et al., 1978a]. Thus, neither dietary protein nor dietary carbohydrate is essential for maintaining diurnal rhythm of disaccharidase activities. Moreover, diurnal rhythm of disaccharidase activities is observed in isolated jejunum [Saito et al., 1978a] and in small intestine of rats which received continuous intravenous infusion of a liquid diet [Stevenson et al., 1980].

It is apparent that direct contact of orally delivered nutrients to small intestinal epithelial cells is not essential to maintain diurnal variation of disaccharidase activities. However, it is noteworthy that the pattern of diurnal rhythm of disaccharidase activities in intravenously infused rats was dissimilar to that in orally fed rats [Stevenson et al., 1980].

It is unclear what mechanism in diurnal rhythm is involved in the increase or decrease of disaccharidase activities. Two possibilities that have been considered are: (1) Changes in cell populations (e.g. villus cells vs crypt cells) by either alteration of cell migration rate or alteration of the rate of slanting of upper villus cells. The number of cells lining villus and villus height in a middle portion of small intestine has been demonstrated to exhibit diurnal variation [Stevenson et al., 1979]. However, this observation requires further study as the total protein content in the small intestine does not exhibit diurnal variation [Saito and Suda, 1978; Yamada et al., 1985], and the rate of cell migration during a 24-hour cycle has not

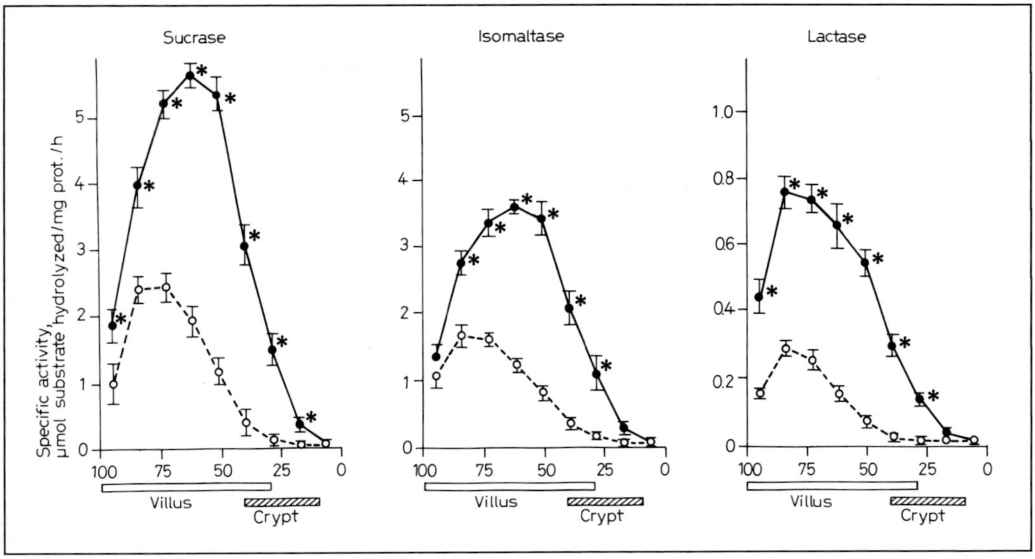

Fig. 4. Diurnal rhythm of sucrase, isomaltase and lactase specific activities of serial sections along the villus-crypt axis in rat jejunum. Abscissa denotes total height of jejunal wall with 100% representing top part of the villus and 0% bottom of serosal side. Activities are shown by specific activities expressed per protein. Values are expressed as means ± SE. Villus and crypt portions are depicted with horizontal bars, overlapping area is crypt-villus transition (mix) zone: open circles = light; closed circles = dark. * Significantly different from light group at the corresponding location ($p < 0.05$). Reproduced with permission [Yamada et al., 1985].

been studied. The other possibility to consider is (2) the change in the amount of enzyme protein per (mature) cell. Diurnal variation of sucrase, isomaltase and lactase activities (fig. 4) is observed along the entire villus [Yamada et al., 1985]. Since the diurnal variation of enzyme activity and the immunoreactive amount is parallel for sucrase-isomaltase [Kaufman et al., 1980; Yamada et al., 1985] and for lactase [Goda et al., unpublished], changes should have occurred in rate of synthesis and/or degradation of these disaccharidases.

Kaufman et al. [1980] studied the rate of degradation of sucrase-isomaltase using ^{14}C-labeled sodium carbonate as precursor of protein synthesis (fig. 5) and found a remarkable change of degradation rate from pre-meal ($t½ = 38$ h) to post-meal period ($t½ = 6$ h). In contrast, no difference was observed in rate of ^{14}C-leucine incorporation into sucrase-isomal-

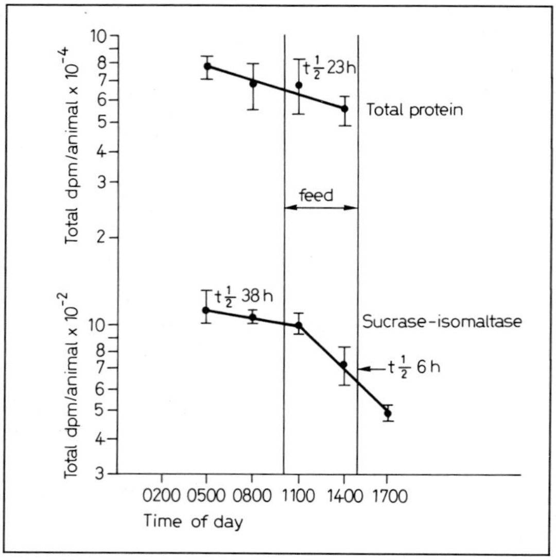

Fig. 5. Degradation of sucrase-isomaltase and papain solubilized total protein between 05.00 and 17.00 hours. Mean values for 4 animals ± SEM are given. Regression lines were calculated by the least squares method using individual values. The difference between the two slopes for sucrase-isomaltase degradation was statistically significant ($p < 0.001$). Reproduced with permission [Kaufman et al., 1980].

tase between the period of high sucrase activity and the period of low sucrase activity [Kaufman et al., 1980]. This result suggests that the change in degradation rate of disaccharidases might be the primary mechanism involved in diurnal variation of these enzymes. Since pancreatic proteases have been implicated as a factor in the degradation of disaccharidases [Alpers and Tedesco 1975; Riby and Kretchmer, 1985], information of cyclic pattern of secretion of pancreatic proteases is required. At present, there is no literature regarding diurnal rhythm of rate of pancreatic secretion. Partial information of pancreatic secretion may be obtained from rate of synthesis of total pancreatic protein and pancreatic enzyme contents [Girard-Globa et al., 1980]. There was no cyclic pattern of pancreatic trypsinogen content observed [Girard-Globa et al., 1980; George et al., 1985], but pancreatic chymotrypsinogen content does follow a daily cyclic pattern with two peaks just prior to and at the end of the meal [Girard-Globa et al., 1980]. Synthesis of total pancreatic protein also exhibits a cyclic pattern with a single peak during the feeding period. Since chymotrypsin content decreases at the time of the start of feeding, while synthesis of total pancreatic protein peaks, pancreatic secretion of proteases appears to be increased by the start of the feeding period (decreasing after the meal). Thus, it is possible that diurnal variation of small intestinal disaccharidase activities is secondary to cyclic variation of secretion of pancreatic protease(s). However, it is not clear which protease is responsible; and the candidate does not appear to be trypsin since no diurnal variation of luminal trypsin activity is observed [Samulitis, 1986]. Further study is required to delineate the involvement of pancreatic protease(s) in diurnal variation of small intestinal disaccharidases.

It is unknown whether there is diurnal variation of disaccharidase activities in human small intestine. However, diurnal variation of another microvillar enzyme, alkaline phosphatase, has been demonstrated in human duodenal biopsy using a histochemical staining of enzyme activity [Markiewicz et al., 1983].

Effect of Variation of Carbohydrate Intake on Disaccharidase Activities

For many years it has been thought that small intestinal disaccharidases might be adaptational enzymes, and if this is the case, intake of substrates (carbohydrates) should play a certain role in the regulation of the amount of these enzymes. In fact, many investigators have shown that carbohydrate intake is the major factor involved in variations of small intestinal disaccharidase activities.

The variation of carbohydrate intake in experimental animals has been carried out by two different methods. The first method involves refeeding of carbohydrate-containing diets after short-term starvation. Since starvation is not only carbohydrate deprivation but also caloric deprivation, the effect of refeeding of carbohydrate-containing diet is complicated by the concomitant administration of caloric intake in the diet. Therefore, the intrinsic effect of starvation on activities of disaccharidases should be characterized.

The second method of variation of carbohydrate intake deals with feeding of isocaloric diets which contain various amounts of carbohydrate. This method insures a regular caloric intake, but it inevitably involves the concomitant change in fat or protein intake. Thus, it is difficult to exclude the possibility that change in fat or protein content might also affect the levels of activity of disaccharidases. Recent studies revealed that these two methods of variation of carbohydrate intake resulted in different responses of the small intestinal epithelial cells (see below). In order to characterize the mechanism of dietary regulation of disaccharidases, the following short-term experiments of 3 days or less were conducted.

Effect of Starvation

Starvation is a simple method used for the deprivation of dietary carbohydrate. However, due to concomitant caloric deprivation, a remarkable change occurs in morphological and biochemical parameters of the small intestinal mucosa. After 3–5 days of induced starvation in rats, the height of the villus decreases [Yamada et al., 1983, 1986] and the size of epithelial cells, e.g. height and surface area of cells, decreases [Yamada et al., 1986]; correspondingly, protein and DNA content in small intestinal segments decreased remarkably in rats starved for 2–3 days [Yamada et al., 1983]. It has been corroborated in many laboratories that in studied jejunum of adult rats (activity expressed per intestinal segment), sucrase and maltase activities were decreased (fig. 6b) by a few days' starvation [Blair et al., 1963; McNeill and Hamilton, 1971; Powell and McElveen, 1974; Soares et al., 1976; Saito et al., 1976a, b; Ecknauer, 1978; Raul et al., 1982a; Yamada et al., 1983, 1986]. Some investigators have reported that specific activity of sucrase (per protein of DNA) in jejunum is decreased in starved rats [Raul et al., 1982a; Yamada et al., 1983, 1986] although others found no significant change [McNeill and Hamilton, 1971; Powell and McElveen, 1974; Ecknauer, 1978]. This discrepancy is apparently due to the lack of a reliable reference system which could be used to compare specific activity when the denominator is considerably changed. To obtain information regarding cellular events following starvation, an ideal reference system might be specific activity expressed per unit DNA in designated cell fractions (e.g. villus cells and crypt cells). Unfortunately, this information is unavailable, but in spite of this limitation, there is some evidence supporting the hypothesis that sucrase activity in individual epithelial cells is decreased in starved rats. First, sucrase activity per unit DNA in intestinal homogenates is decreased [Yamada et al., 1983], and secondly, brush border membranes isolated from jejunal mucosa of starved rats have a decreased level of specific activity (per mg of total protein) of sucrase [Kim et al., 1973; Yamada et al., 1986] and the volume of microvilli per cell is decreased (by 40%) after 5 days' starvation [Yamada et al., 1986].

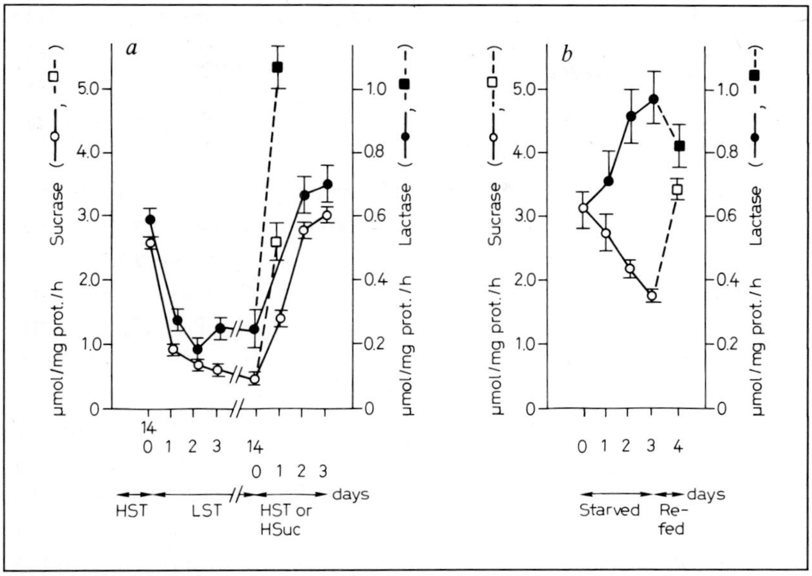

Fig. 6. Effect of variation of carbohydrate intake on the specific activity of sucrase and lactase in adult rat jejunum. *a* Rats fed for 2 weeks a high starch diet. Animals were then fed 1 to 14 days a low starch, high fat diet (LST), following which they were fed a high starch, low fat diet (HST) or a high sucrose low fat diet (HSuc). Solid line represents high starch diet; broken lines, sucrose diet. *b* Rats fed laboratory chow (Lab Blox) were starved for 3 days and then fed for 24 h a high sucrose, low fat diet. Mean (5–6 animals) and 2 SEM are given. Constructed from data of Yamada et al. [1981a, b; 1983].

Analysis of sucrase activity along the villus-crypt column in jejunum of starved rats revealed that sucrase activity decreased in the middle and lower villus with no significant change in upper villus [Yamada et al., 1983]. This finding is in agreement with the fact that the decrease of sucrase activity following starvation is not a rapid event, but a gradual decrease, taking 2–3 days to reach the lower plateau. This time period appears to coincide with that required for immature crypt cells to migrate up to the villus tip. It is possible that the primary effect of starvation on the metabolism of sucrase-isomaltase occurs during some process of synthesis in immature cells, presumably transcription activity and synthesis of mRNA. However, the extent of 'caloric' deprivation on the decrease of sucrase activity in starved animals is not clear. It should be noted that even after a prolonged starvation, a basal level of sucrase activity is maintained

[Saito et al., 1976a, b]. A similar effect of starvation on sucrase and maltase activities was reported in human subjects (obese volunteers); fasting of long duration led to a decrease of activity of sucrase, isomaltase and maltase [Knudsen et al., 1968a]. The effect of starvation on trehalase activity has not been reported.

In contrast to sucrase and maltase activities (which exhibit a decrease), lactase activity in the small intestine (expressed per protein as well as per segment) increases [Raul et al., 1982a; Nsi-Emvo and Raul, 1984; Yamada et al., 1983] (fig. 6b). The increase of lactase specific activity occurs also in the brush border membranes [Raul et al., 1982a]. The increase of lactase activity is due to an increase of the corresponding enzyme protein [Nsi-Emvo et al., 1986]. Total lactase activity in whole jejunoileum appears to be unaffected [Yamada et al., 1983]; thus, starvation leads to a differential effect on α-glucosidases and lactase. The mechanism of this effect is unclear although Raul et al. [1983] have demonstrated that the increase of lactase activity following starvation coincides with the decrease of serum thyroid hormone level, and that thyroidectomy prevents this increase of lactase activity [Raul et al., 1983] which suggests that lactase activity might be regulated by thyroid hormone as suggested in studies in adult rats injected with thyroxine [Celano et al., 1977; Boyle et al., 1982].

Effect of Intake of Low Carbohydrate Diet

Major human populations consume carbohydrates as a predominant energy source. In this aspect, the average meal is considered to be a carbohydrate-rich diet. The standard laboratory rat chow diet also contains 50–60 (w/w) percent carbohydrate. The significance of carbohydrate intake in maintaining a sufficient level of disaccharidase activities in small intestinal epithelial cells was demonstrated in studies where animals were fed isocaloric low carbohydrate diet. The low carbohydrate diet is rich in either fat or protein.

When carbohydrate-free, high casein diet was fed to adult rats for 7 days, Blair et al. [1963] observed that sucrase activity in jejunum decreased by 50%. This observation was confirmed by McCarthy et al. [1980] who fed rats for 7 days isocaloric amounts of three powdered diets, i.e. high carbohydrate (72 cal%) diet, low carbohydrate (18 cal%), high fat (72 cal%) diet or low carbohydrate (22 cal%) high protein (65 cal%) diet. Feeding of low carbohydrate diets with either high fat or high protein content led to a significant decrease of sucrase and maltase activities in both jejunum and ileum. A similar decreasing effect of low carbohydrate diets was seen in lactase activity, but it was significant only in jejunum of animals fed low carbohydrate, high fat diet as compared to animals fed high carbohydrate diet. The decrease of disaccharidase activities in rats fed low carbohydrate, high fat diet was further investigated in detail [Goda et al., 1983]. Three characteristic points which are distinct from starvation effect were delineated (fig. 6a). First, the decrease in disaccharidase activities following the low carbohydrate diet occurs more rapidly than the decrease following starvation. Feeding of low carbohydrate, high fat diet leads to a decrease in disaccharidase activities within 24 h [Blair et al., 1963; Goda et al., 1983] or even within 12 h [Goda et al., unpublished], whereas a significant decrease of sucrase activity is observed as long as 2–3 days after the start of starvation [Raul et al., 1982a; Yamada et al., 1983]. The rapid decrease of disaccharidase activities in rats fed low carbohydrate, high fat diet is attained by the concomitant decrease of disaccharidases (sucrase and lactase) activities along the entire height of the villus [Goda et al., 1983]. Secondly, the decreased level of sucrase specific activity observed in rats fed the low carbohydrate diet for 3 days is lower than the level found in starved rats [Yamada et al., 1983; Goda et al., 1983]. Thirdly, the feeding of low carbohydrate diet leads to a decrease in activities of both α-glucosidases (e.g. sucrase, glucoamylase) and lactase, whereas starvation decreases only the activities of α-glucosidases; starvation increases lactase specific activity.

Mechanisms of Short-Term Adaptation of Disaccharidases

The short-term adaptation of disaccharidases responding to the increase of carbohydrate intake has been investigated using animals in which disaccharidase activities were decreased either by starvation (except for lactase) or by feeding a low carbohydrate diet. As described above, these two dietary manipulations, qualitatively and quantitatively, had different effects on small intestinal disaccharidases. Thus, it is not surprising that the nature of the short-term adaptation following these two dietary manipulations are possibly different.

Investigators have attempted to solve the following questions regarding the mechanisms of dietary adaptation of disaccharidases.

(1) Which molecule of carbohydrates is responsible for the change in the activities of disaccharidases? To answer this question, rats with lowered disaccharidase activities were given diets containing various carbohydrates.

(2) Is the effect of variation of intake of carbohydrate specific to a single enzyme? To examine this, the effect on various microvillar enzymes was examined.

(3) At which metabolic process(es) of disaccharidases is the activity or amount of enzyme protein regulated? This question concerns cellular events: How does a stimulus transfer the information to the site of regulation of metabolic process? The site of regulation is possibly the process of (a) transcription, (b) post-transcriptional modification of primary transcripts, (c) translation, or (d) degradation.

(4) In which maturational level of cell populations does the adaptive response occur? This question is related to the capacity of villus cells to respond to dietary challenge and further examines how promptly the dietary adaptation may occur.

Refeeding of Carbohydrate-Containing Diet after Starvation. Nearly all animal experiments exploring the effect of refeeding of carbohydrate-containing diet on disaccharidase activities were performed in rats. There have been very few studies involving human subjects in this area of research [Knudsen et al., 1968a; Rosensweig and Herman, 1969a]. Blair et al. [1963] were the first to demonstrate that when starved rats were fed a high sucrose (70%) diet, sucrase activity increased 100% within 24 h. However, when the starved rats were fed a carbohydrate-free (high casein or high fat) diet, no effect was observed on sucrase activity. They further investigated the nature of carbohydrate-evoked increase of sucrase activity. The effect of fructose was comparable to that of sucrose. Refeeding of maltose, a mixture of fructose and glucose, galactose, α-methyl-*D*-glucoside or melizitose (glucose-[1→2]fructose-[3→1]glucose) also produced a significant increase of sucrase activity within 24 h.

Interestingly, the effect of a maltose diet was smaller than that of a sucrose diet. It should be noted also that the effect of a diet with a mixture of fructose and glucose was smaller than that of a sucrose diet. The absence of any effect, as in the case of a mannose diet, could possibly be explained by the low intake of this diet. A glucose diet (well consumed) and a lactose diet (low intake) produced only insignificant increases. A diet containing raffinose (galactose-[1→6]glucose-[1→6]glucose-[1→2]fructose), which does not appear to be hydrolyzed in the small intestine, even evoked a decrease of sucrase activity.

Deren et al. [1967] confirmed an increase of sucrase activity in previously starved rats as a result of a 24-hour feeding of carbohydrate-containing diet, except for the effect of glucose. As opposed to the studies of Blair et al. [1963], the feeding of a glucose diet (a comparable amount; 68% glucose in diet) evoked a significant increase of sucrase activity; the level reached was equal to that of rats fed sucrose or fructose [Deren et al., 1967]. Refeeding of sucrose diet to starved rats also led to an increase in maltase activity [Deren et al., 1967; Kimura et al., 1978; Yamada et al., 1983], but it did not affect the activity of lactase [Deren et al., 1967; Ulshen and Grand, 1979; Raul et al., 1980; Yamada et al., 1983], and even decreased aminopeptidase activity [Raul et al., 1980]. It is interesting to note that maltase activity in maltose-fed rats was higher than that in sucrose-fed rats [Deren et al., 1967].

The mechanisms of sucrose-mediated change of sucrase activity in refed rats have been explored. Determination of K_m for sucrase in intestinal homogenate demonstrated similar values in rats with induced activity when compared with those in starved rats, suggesting that an increase in the amount of sucrase-isomaltase occurs [Deren et al., 1967]. Analysis of the time course of change in sucrase activity after refeeding of starved rats revealed that an increase of sucrase-specific activity (per total protein) is not observed within the first 15–18 h after the start of refeeding, but it is clearly visible after 24–25 h [Kimura et al., 1978; Ulshen and Grand, 1979]. As enterocytes migrate from crypt base to upper villus, they differentiate and express disaccharidase activities.

At which maturational level of enterocytes (or at which height of the villus-crypt column) does the initial increase of sucrase activity occur? This question was explored by the determination of sucrase activity along the various heights of the villus-crypt column using a technique of cryostat slicing [Ulshen and Grand, 1979]. After radioactive-labeled thymidine is injected at the start of the sucrose diet, the leading region of radioactivity along the villus-crypt columns determined several hours later should indicate the location of cells which are proliferating in crypts at the start of refeeding. Ulshen and Grand [1979] demonstrated that the major region of increased sucrase activity coincided with the leading region of radioactivity determined at 12, 18, 24, and 36 h after the start of refeeding of the sucrose diet (fig. 7). This study suggests that the site of initial stimulation by refeeding of sucrose diet is the immature crypt cells. The time lag (18–24 h) observed prior to the appearance of the increase of sucrase activity may be explained by the lack of response in matured villus cells. A selective response of lower villus cells to sucrose diet in starved rats was confirmed by other investigators [Yamada et al., 1983; Gorostiza et al., 1984]. How-

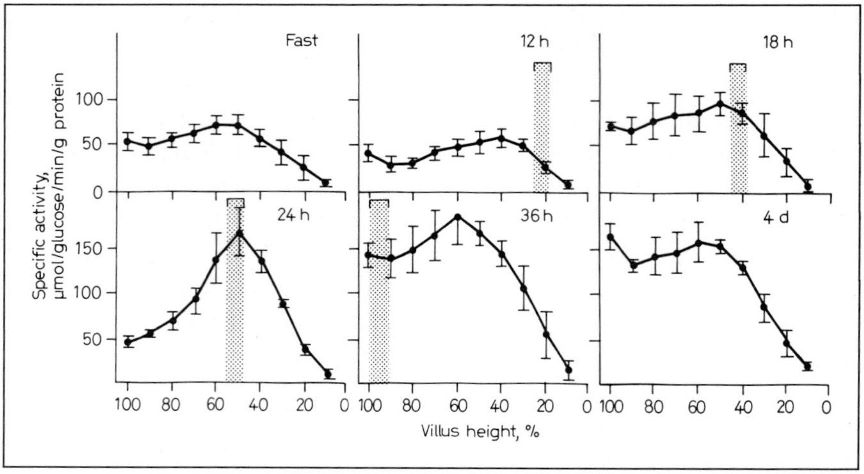

Fig. 7. Effect of sucrose feeding after a 3-day fast on jejunal sucrase-specific activity gradients. Each panel shows the gradient of sucrase activity plotted against location on the villus. The data shown are mean ± SE; n = 7 (24 h), n = 6 (fasted and 12 h), n = 3 (18, 36 h, 4 days). The stippled bar represents the leading edge of migrating cells at 12 h (22 ± 3%), 18 h (43 ± 3%), 24 h (53 ± 2%), 36 h (96 ± 4%). Reproduced with permission [Ulshen and Grand, 1979].

ever, it should be noted that sucrase activity was expressed as specific activity (per protein) in these studies, and that total activity of sucrase and maltase per intestinal segment (15 cm) increased within 15 h due to concomitant increase of total protein [Kimura et al., 1978]. In starved rats that were allowed to consume small amounts of sucrose diet (10 kcal/animal), sucrase activity (per protein and per segment) increased within 12 h [Kimura et al., 1978]; there was no increase in maltase activity. Thus, it appears that the increase of sucrase activity occurs with a small amount of sucrose intake with the effect being selective to sucrase-isomaltase.

Feeding of sucrose solution instead of a complete diet increased sucrase specific activity (per protein) in jejunal homogenate in starved rats as early as 5 h after feeding [Raul et al., 1982b]. Furthermore, at 15 h after a single feeding of sucrose solution, sucrase activity (per protein) in isolated cells was 2–3 times higher along the entire villus height than was found in starved rats [Raul et al., 1982a]. Therefore, it is possible that not only immature, but also mature enterocytes can react to dietary sucrose in starved rats. The apparent discrepancy regarding time response and site of stimulation between the studies of Ulshen and Grand [1979] and Raul et al. [1982b] appear to be due to differences in the nature of sucrose carrying vehicles, simple solution or complete diet. However, this possibility needs to be clarified in future studies.

The cellular or molecular mechanisms of sucrose-mediated change of sucrase activity in starved rats are not clear. The amount of sucrase-isomaltase in small intestinal epithelial cells is determined by the balance of synthesis and degradation rates, both of which occur relatively fast; with a half-life as rapid as 6 h [Kaufman et al., 1980]. Indirect evidence supporting that synthesis rate is affected by refeeding of sucrose was obtained by studies which employed protein synthesis inhibitors, cycloheximide and actinomycin D. These antibiotics inhibit the translation process or transcription process, respectively.

Kimura et al. [1978] reported that administration of cycloheximide at 15 h after the start of refeeding of sucrose diet completely abolished the increase in sucrase and maltase activities in jejunum of rats when observed at 25 and 30 h after start of refeeding.

Aminopeptidase activity was similarly decreased by the administration of cycloheximide. Kimura et al. [1978] also reported that administration of actinomycin D at 15 h after refeeding of sucrose diet produced a significant decrease in sucrase and maltase activities at 25 h after refeeding, but sucrase activity in actinomycin D treated rats at 25 h after the start of refeeding was higher than that at 15 h after start of refeeding. Thus, inhibition of sucrose-mediated increase of sucrase activity by actinomycin D was not complete. Raul et al. [1982b] reported that when actinomycin D was injected in rats at 30 min before a single gavage feeding of sucrose solution, sucrose-mediated increase of sucrase activity (determined at 15 h after refeeding) was eliminated in isolated enterocytes along the entire villus height. A complete inhibition of sucrase and maltase activities by administration of actinomycin D was also observed in brush border membrane of jejunal mucosa; in contrast, actinomycin D did not affect lactase and aminopeptidase activities [Raul et al., 1982b]. These studies suggest that sucrose feeding in starved rats affects the synthesis process of sucrase-isomaltase, presumably the transcription of genes encoding for sucrase-isomaltase. However, studies employing protein synthesis inhibitors are difficult to interpret because many side effects are known. First, stomach emptying is inhibited by actinomycin D administration [Yatvin, 1971] which would result in limited access of small intestinal epithelial cells to the dietary carbohydrate of interest. Secondly, actinomycin D was reported to arrest cell migration in rats [Grand et al., 1972]; thus, normal maturation process of cells might be inhibited. Thirdly, injection of actinomycin D decreases sucrase activity in brush border membranes, whereas sucrase activity increases in intestinal homogenate by injection of actinomycin D in rats [Grand et al., 1972]. Therefore, actinomycin D could affect not only RNA synthesis (transcription), but also intracellular transport of brush border digestive enzymes. Furthermore, actinomycin D administration would result in a decrease in the amount of mRNA (e.g. encoding for sucrase-isomaltase) which in turn diminishes the capacity of change in post-transcriptional modification, translation and degradation. Thus, the possibility of modification of other synthesis and degradation processes cannot be excluded. On the other hand, cycloheximide is known to cause premature exfoliation of upper villus cells and a shortening of microvilli and the height of epithelial cells in lower villus cells within 3–4 h [Attmann, 1975; Bernard and Carlier, 1985]. Therefore, in order to determine at which process the synthesis and/or degradation of sucrase-isomaltase is regulated by dietary sucrose, it is indispensable to determine the rates of synthesis and degradation of sucrase-isomaltase and the amount of mRNA encoding for sucrase-isomaltase. Information for this is not available at the present time. The increase of radioactivity in sucrase-isomaltase in sucrose refed rats as compared with starved rats has been reported [Raul et al., 1980]. However, in this report, (^{3}H)-valine was injected 12 h prior to killing, but this time period is considered to be too long to evaluate the rate of synthesis if rate of turnover of this enzyme protein is taken into consideration. Therefore, it is not clear whether the increased accumulation of labeled sucrase-isomaltase occurred because of an increase in the rate of incorporation of precursor amino acid into sucrase-isomaltase, or a decrease in the rate of degradation of sucrase-isomaltase in brush border membrane.

If an alteration of transcription activity of specific DNA (e.g. encoding for sucrase-isomaltase mRNA) is involved in sucrose-mediated increase of sucrase activity, a modification of structural chromatin and transcription-related activity in nucleus would be expected. Raul and Launay [1983] reported that refeeding of sucrose solution after 72 h starvation in rats led to an abrupt increase (within 1 h) of small intestinal chromatin template activity. This was determined in vitro by measuring the rate of incorporation of (^{3}H)-labeled uridine monophosphate (UMP) into RNA using nuclei isolated from jejunal mucosa as template and in the presence of *E. coli* RNA polymerase. Interestingly, a similar stimulatory effect was observed with fructose, whereas glucose exhibited only a weaker (but significant)

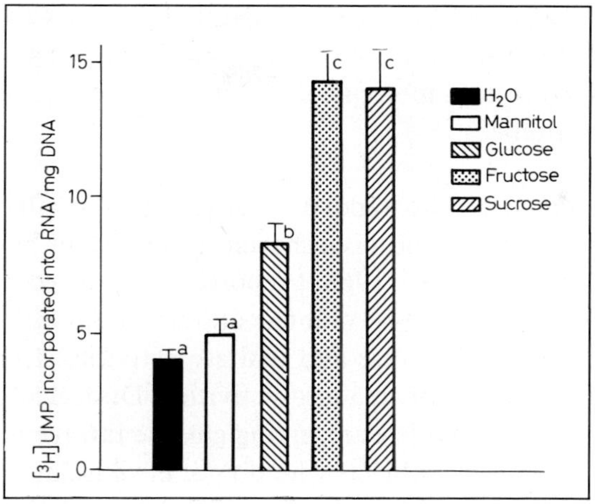

Fig. 8. Intestinal chromatin template activity measured 1 h after oral administration of 5 ml of water or of a 70% solution of mannitol, glucose, fructose or sucrose to rats previously starved for 72 h. The results are expressed relative to the DNA concentration as determined on identical chromatin aliquots. Each column represents the mean value ± SE of 5 animals. For each condition, columns not sharing a common superscript letter differ significantly ($p < 0.01$, Student's t-test). Reproduced with permission [Raul and Launay, 1983].

effect (fig. 8). Raul and von der Decken [1983, 1984] further demonstrated that in rats refed sucrose solution for 15 h after 48 h of starvation, chromatin-bound RNA polymerase activity of both α-amanitin-insensitive, i.e. I plus III, and α-amanitin-sensitive, i.e. II was increased by 60% in jejunal mucosa. The increase of chromatin-bound RNA polymerase activity was observed in both upper villus and lower villus-crypt cell fractions [Raul and von der Decken, 1985]. The change in chromatin-bound RNA polymerase activity appeared to coincide with changes in sedimentation profiles of chromatin [Raul and von der Decken, 1983, 1985]. These studies indicated that refeeding of a single carbohydrate (sucrose) is capable of altering transcription activity in rat intestinal epithelial cells. However, it is not clear if sucrose specifically affects transcription of the gene encoding for sucrase-isomaltase mRNA. Since activity of RNA polymerase II (mainly responsible for mRNA polymerization) as well as the activity of RNA polymerase I plus III (responsible for the production of ribosomal and transfer RNA) are increased in sucrose-refed rats, refeeding of sucrose apparently affects expression of genes other than that encoding for sucrase-isomaltase mRNA. Refeeding of a sugar solution provides energy to small intestinal epithelial cells; the role of this energy, distinguished from the signal transducted from a molecule derived from sucrose, needs to be evaluated in future studies.

Studies in Human Subjects. Two reports dealing with the effect of refeeding of carbohydrate on intestinal disaccharidase activity in human subjects are available. Knudsen et al. [1968a] reported that refeeding of lactose and glucose for 10 days in obese volunteers (after 14 days of starvation) resulted in an increase of sucrase and maltase activities; feeding of corn oil did not affect sucrase and maltase activities. Disaccharidase activity increase was also seen in subjects receiving glucose intravenously after starvation. Lactase activity of subjects who do not have isolated lactase deficiency was slightly increased by refeeding of lactose and glucose. Rosensweig and Herman [1969a] confirmed the results of Knudsen et al. [1968a]. When two individuals were fed a 2,000-kcal in carbohydrate-free diet for 1 week after 27 days of starvation, there was no increase in disaccharidase activities, whereas feeding of a 2000-kcal in 84% glucose diet for one additional week produced an increase of sucrase and maltase activities. Calories by themselves are insufficient to evoke an increase of sucrase and maltase activities in refed human subjects. Carbohydrate provided either orally or intravenously is required. Refeeding of sucrose-containing diet has not been reported in experiments with human subjects.

Increase of Carbohydrate Intake. In rats fed a synthetic diet rich in starch or sucrose (65 cal% or more) for 3 days or longer, not only the activity of sucrase [McCarthy et al., 1980; Bustamante et al., 1981; Riby and Kretchmer, 1984; Bustamante et al., 1986], maltase [Saito and Suda, 1975; McCarthy et al., 1980; Bustamante et al., 1981, 1986] and glucoamylase [Goda et al., 1983; Bustamante et al., 1986], but also the activity of lactase [McCarthy et al., 1980; Bustamante et al., 1981] is higher than that of rats fed an isocaloric carbohydrate-free or low carbohydrate diet. As discussed previously, digestion of starch does not produce substrates for lactase (a β-galactosidase). In this sense, dietary mediated change in lactase activity in rats is not substrate-specific. Trehalase activity is unaffected by variation of carbohydrate intake [Shinohara et al., 1986].

The mechanisms of dietary induced increase of disaccharidase activities were investigated in rats where disaccharidase activities were decreased by feeding a low carbohydrate diet. Changing isocaloric diets, either from low to high carbohydrate or high to low carbohydrate diets, did not affect the amount of total protein in small intestine [McCarthy et al., 1980; Bustamante et al., 1981; Yamada et al., 1981a, b; Goda et al., 1983], villus height [Goda et al., 1983; Gorostiza et al., 1984], height of enterocyte [Gorostiza et al., 1984], or cell migration rate [Yamada et al., 1981a, b; Goda et al., 1983, 1985a]. In these studies, change in specific activity (per mg protein) of disaccharidases was always accompanied by the change in total activity of disaccharidases in small intestinal segments.

Feeding of sucrose diet to rats previously fed a carbohydrate-free, high protein diet for 7 days led to a significant increase of sucrase, maltase and lactase activities in homogenate as well as in brush borders of jejunal mucosa within 24 h [Grand and Jaksina, 1973].

Administration of actinomycin D at the beginning of the feeding of sucrose diets [Grand and Jaksina, 1973] did not prevent the increase of disaccharidase activities, thus suggesting that modification of either the degradation process or synthesis process subsequent to the transcription process of disaccharidases might be involved. This is in contrast to the observation obtained in refed rats. In rats previously fed a low carbohydrate, high fat diet, the feeding of high carbohydrate (either starch or sucrose) produced similar increases of sucrase, maltase and lactase activities in jejunum within 18–24 h [Bustamante et al., 1981; Yamada et al., 1981a, b]. Bustamante et al. [1981] and Yamada et al. [1981a] demonstrated in two independent experiments, significant linear regression (fig. 9) between increased levels of sucrase and lactase activities. A linear dose dependency of the increase in sucrase and lactase activities on the amount of starch in diets (fig. 10) was observed [Yamada et al., 1981a]. Yamada et al. [1981b] further demonstrated that the increase of sucrase and lactase activities can be seen along the entire villus height at 18 h after the start of a sucrose diet (fig. 11). When a low carbohydrate diet was fed to rats previously given a high carbohydrate diet, a decrease of sucrase and lactase activities was observed along the entire villus height at 24 h (fig. 12) after the change of the diets [Goda et al., 1983]. These studies suggested that not only immature (crypt) enterocytes but also mature villus cells are capable of responding to an increase/decrease of carbohydrate intake. This is an explanation for the faster response of disaccharidase activities seen in intestinal mucosa of rats previously fed low carbohydrate diets than that observed in starved rats.

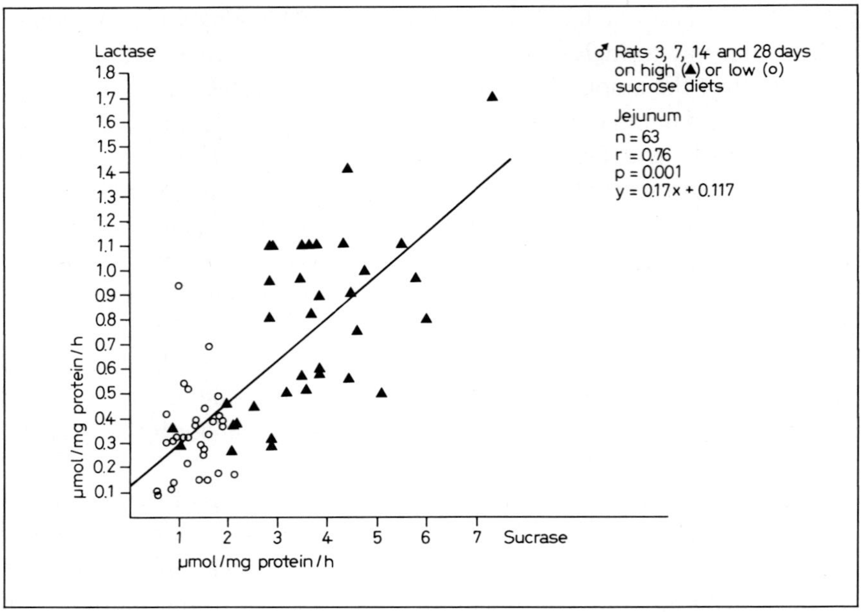

Fig. 9. Linear regression between sucrase and lactase specific activity in proximal segment of rats fed sucrose diets. Closed triangle = HS; open circle = LS; n = 63; r = 0.76; p = 0.001. Reproduced with permission [Bustamante et al., 1981].

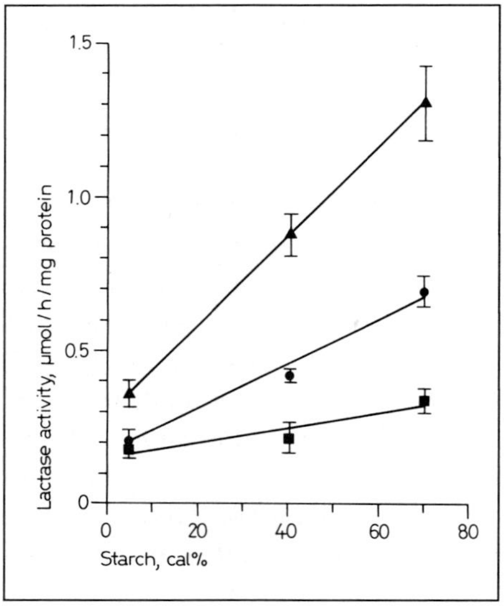

Fig. 10. Linear regression between the starch content of diet and lactase activity in various intestinal segments at 72 h after changing the diet from low (5%) to middle (40%) or high (70%) starch diet. Lines were calculated from individual values (n = 22). Mean values for each individual diet group are denoted by different symbols; short vertical lines denote 2 SE; closed triangles = middle (r = 0.93); closed circles = proximal (r = 0.92); closed squares = distal (r = 0.67) small intestinal segment. Reproduced with permission [Yamada et al., 1981a].

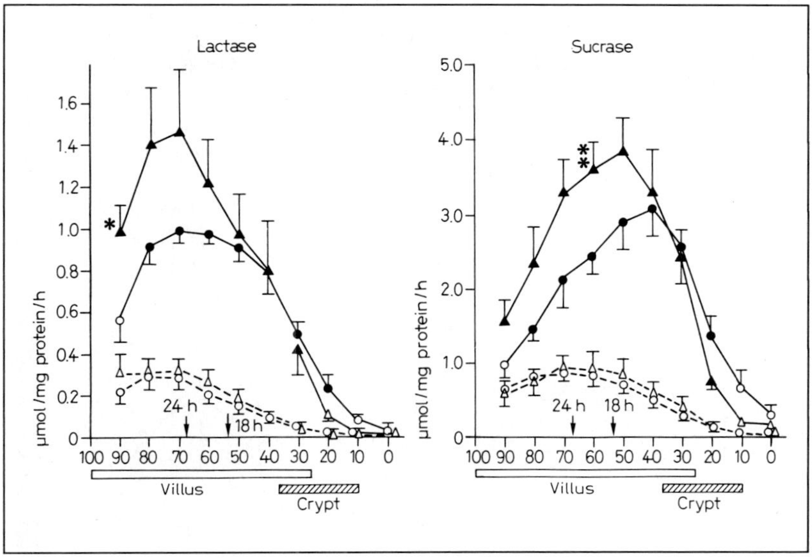

Fig. 11. Effects of high sucrose diet feeding for 18 or 24 h on jejunal lactase and sucrase specific activities along the villus-crypt columns. Abscissa depict total height of the intestinal wall with 100% representing the top portion of the villus and 0% the bottom of serosal side. Villus and crypt portions are depicted with rectangles; the overlapping area is the crypt villus transition (mix) zone. Mean and SEM are given: number of animals per group = 5–6. The dotted line represents control groups fed high fat, low starch diet (open circle = 18 h; open triangle = 24 h) and solid line represents experimental groups fed low fat, high sucrose diet (open circle = 18h; open triangle = 24 h). Full symbol depicts significantly different values from corresponding control of the same location; ** significant difference ($p < 0.02$) between the values of the group fed sucrose for 18 and 24 h; * same at $p < 0.05$ level. Arrows indicate the leading edge of thymidine-labeled cells. Reproduced with permission [Yamada et al., 1981b].

The time course of carbohydrate-induced increase of disaccharidase activities was studied at shorter time periods using force feeding techniques. Experiments with force feeding of sucrose diet revealed that the sucrose-induced increase of sucrase activity in jejunal mucosa (fig. 13) occurs within 3 h after the initial feeding of sucrose diets [Cézard et al., 1983; Goda et al., 1985a]. Cézard et al. [1983] further demonstrated that the relative rate of incorporation of ^{3}H-leucine in sucrase-isomaltase was increased by feeding a sucrose diet to rats that were previously fed carbohydrate-free high fat diets, suggesting that the rate of synthesis of sucrase-isomaltase was increased by sucrose. Sucrase activity in cytosol fraction,

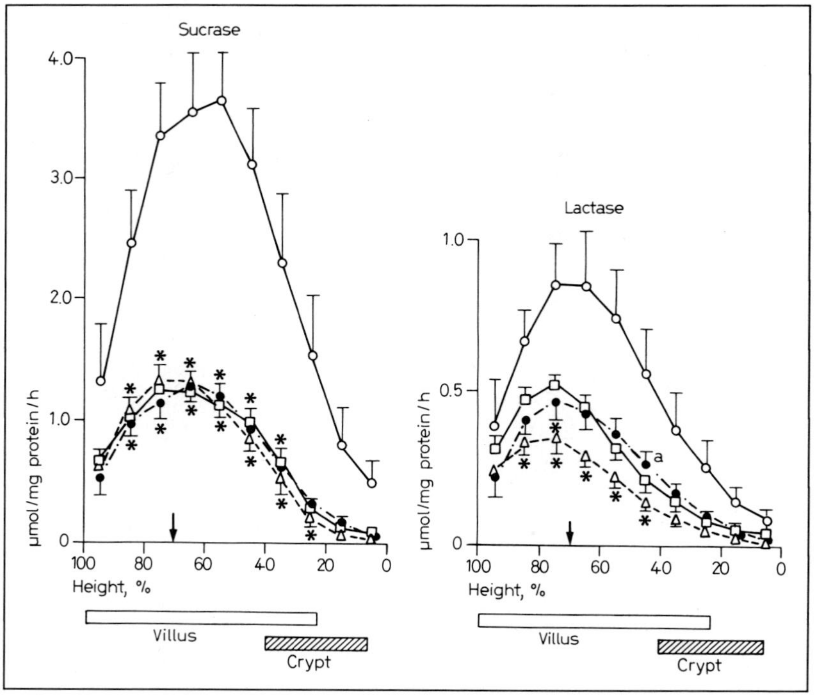

Fig. 12. Effect of feeding low starch diet on jejunal sucrase and lactase specific activity in serial sections of villus-crypt columns. Abscissa depicts total height of intestinal wall with 100% representing top part of villus and 0% bottom of serosal side. Mean and SE are given (n/group = 5). Villus and crypt portions are depicted with rectangles; overlapping area is crypt-villus transition (mix) zone. Arrow on abscissa indicates leading edge of (^{3}H)thymidine-labeled cells determined 24 h after labeled thymidine administration. Open circles = day 0 (fed high starch diet); open squares = 1 day feeding of low starch diet; open triangles = 2 day feeding of low starch diet; closed circles = 3 day feeding of low starch diet. * Significantly different values from day 0 groups at same location ($p < 0.05$). * Significantly different value from group of 2 day low starch diet feeding at same location ($p < 0.05$). Reproduced with permission [Goda et al., 1983].

presumably derived from newly synthesized sucrase-isomaltase [Cézard et al., 1979] was increased as early as 1 h after the initial feeding of the sucrose diet [Cézard et al., 1983]. Thus, the stimulation of sucrase activity in these rats (previously fed low carbohydrate diets) occurs rapidly. This rapid increase of sucrase activity was accompanied by an increase in the immunoreactive amount of sucrase-isomaltase [Cézard et al., 1983; Goda et al., 1985a]. During the short-term stimulation of sucrase activity,

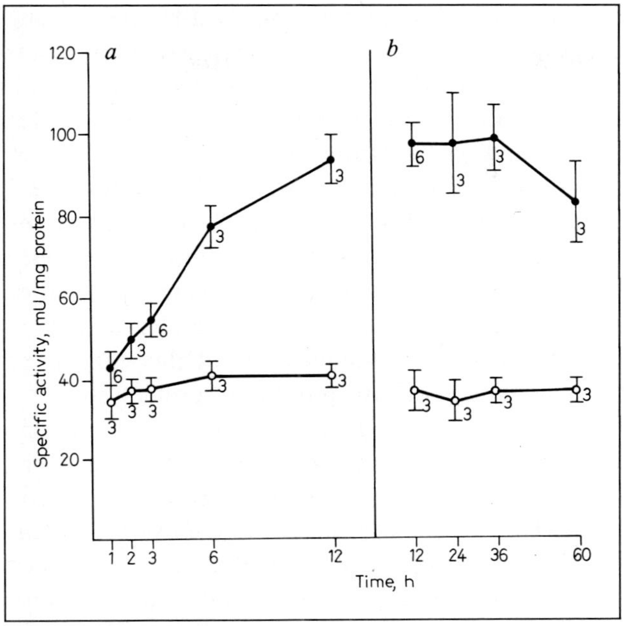

Fig. 13. Effect of sucrose diet on sucrase enzyme specific activity in mucosa homogenates. *a* Animals were fed cellulose diet for 3 days before the experiment and then force fed for the time periods noted on the abscissa with the cellulose diet (open circles) or sucrose diet (closed circles). *b* Animals were fed cellulose diet for 3 days before the experiment and then fed ad libitum (from 7:00 p.m. to 7:00 a.m.) sucrose diet (closed circles) or cellulose diet (open circles) for the time periods noted on the abscissa. The bracket represents the standard error of the mean. The numbers indicate the number of rats studied at each time point. Reproduced with permission [Cézard et al., 1983].

sucrase catalytic activity per unit of immunoreactive sucrase-isomaltase is constant [Goda et al., 1985a] or slightly increased [Cézard et al., 1983]. This discrepancy is possibly due to the method of assay of immunoreactive sucrase-isomaltase. Goda et al. [1985a] determined the amount of sucrase-isomaltase complex with electroimmunoassay (rocket technique) which quantifies only one form of antigen, e.g. either sucrase-isomaltase complex or isomaltase monomer [Goda et al., 1988a]. On the other hand, Cézard et al. [1983] measured the amount of immunoreactive sucrase-isomaltase with solid-phase radioimmunoassay which detects various forms of sucrase-isomaltase. The study of Cézard et al. [1983] suggests that some catalytically inactive sucrase is present in rats fed a low starch diet and the amount of inactive sucrase is diminished shortly after the feeding of a sucrose diet. Cézard et al. [1983] speculated that activation of inactive sucrase-isomaltase occurs shortly after the feeding of sucrose diets. In this regard, it is interesting to note that in intracellular membrane fractions obtained by precipitation with Ca^{2+} from small intestinal mucosa of pigs, catalytically inactive but immunoreactive sucrase-isomaltase was found [Sjöström et al., 1985]. Since intracellular membrane fraction contains incompletely glycosylated, high mannose glycoproteins, it is possible as the authors suggested [Sjöström et al., 1985] that complete glycosylation of a high mannose form of sucrase-isomaltase possibly results in either activation of sucrase catalytic activity or stabilization of this enzyme protein which would lead to a decrease of susceptibility to proteolysis.

Interestingly, the increase in sucrase activity per unit of immunoreactive sucrase-isomaltase is transient; after 6 h of sucrose feeding, the ratio of sucrase activity to immunoreactivity decreased again to a control level [Cézard et al., 1983]. Thus, it is likely that there are two distinct mechanisms of stimulation of activity of sucrase-isomaltase evoked by increased intake of sucrose in rats previously fed low carbohydrate diet. First, the amount of inactive sucrase-isomaltase is decreased by either activation (i.e. accelerated conversion from inactive to active enzyme) or stabilization of sucrase-isomaltase (i.e. retarded conversion from active to inactive enzyme). This rapid phase is followed by a gradual increase of enzyme protein with concomitant increase of enzyme activity; stimulation of de novo synthesis appears to occur.

Riby and Kretchmer [1984] studied the relative rates of synthesis and degradation of sucrase-isomaltase along various heights of the villus-crypt column. In rats that were fed a sucrose diet for 4 days, the rate of synthesis of sucrase-isomaltase, estimated by ^{3}H-leucine incorporation, was higher in lower villus and crypt cells than in upper villus cells (fig. 14). Maximal incorporation was observed at the villus-crypt junction. In contrast, the rate of synthesis of sucrase-isomaltase in carbohydrate-free diet fed rats was low along the entire height of the villus-crypt column [Riby and Kretchmer, 1984]. Using the double isotope method (which uses the ratio of incorporation of two isotopes as an indicator of a relative rate of degradation), Riby and Kretchmer [1984] have shown that the degradation rate of sucrase-isomaltase in rats fed a sucrose diet was lower along the entire villus height than in rats fed carbohydrate-free diet (fig. 15). Although the double isotope method does not allow quantitative comparison, the authors suggested that the modifying effect of change in degradation rate

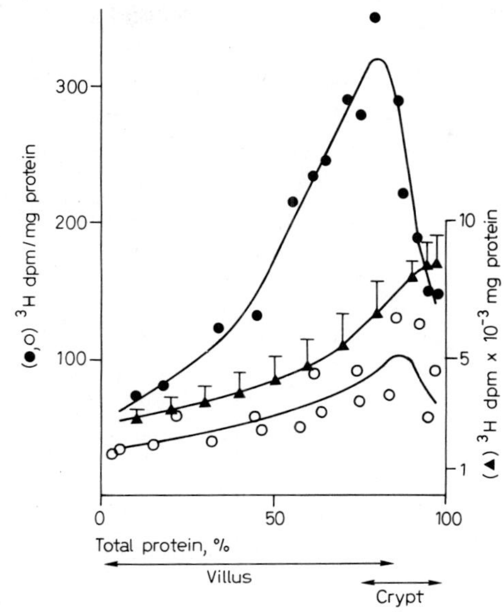

Fig. 14. Effect of dietary carbohydrate on rates of synthesis. Synthesis rate for total protein; means ± SD (n = 4) at normalized intervals of 10% of villus height (closed triangle). Synthesis rate for sucrase; individual values from 2 animals on each diet, 65% sucrose (closed circles) and carbohydrate free (open circles). Reproduced with permission [Riby and Kretchmer, 1984].

on sucrase activity might be small as compared with the change in synthesis rate [Riby and Kretchmer, 1984].

Tsuboi et al. [1985a] confirmed that the rate of synthesis of sucrase-isomaltase is stimulated in high carbohydrate (starch) diet fed rats as compared with low carbohydrate (starch) fed rats. They demonstrated that label accumulation of ^{3}H-leucine is increased not only in sucrase-isomaltase, but in glucoamylase and lactase as well. In low starch diet fed rats, a similar rate of accumulation of radioactivity was observed in sucrase-isomaltase, glycoamylase, and lactase, indicating that the basic synthesis rate of these three disaccharidases might be similar. However, the extent of stimulation of synthesis rate of these disaccharidases was different; synthesis of sucrase-isomaltase and glucoamylase was stimulated to a similar ex-

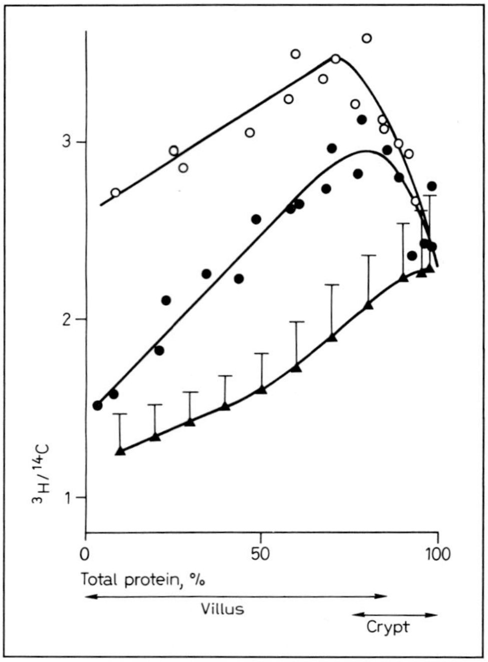

Fig. 15. Effect of dietary carbohydrate on rates of degradation. Degradation rate for total protein: means ± SD (n = 4) at normalized intervals of 10% of villus height (closed triangle). Degradation rate for sucrase: individual values from 2 animals on each diet, 65% sucrose (closed circles) and carbohydrate free (open circles). Reproduced with permission [Riby and Kretchmer, 1984].

tent (4.7–4.9 ×) whereas synthesis of lactase was stimulated to a lesser extent (2.5 ×).

The carbohydrate-mediated increase of lactase activity was studied further by force feeding sucrose and lactose diets [Goda et al., 1985a]. Within 3 h after the initial feeding of a sucrose diet, lactase activity increased as sucrase activity increased; no change thereafter was evident in lactase activity. The increase of lactase activity following the sucrose diet accompanies the increase in the immunoreactive amount of lactase protein [Goda et al., 1984a, b; 1985a]. This time course of increase in lactase activity is different from that of sucrase activity which gradually increases until reaching a constant level at 12–24 h after the initial feeding of sucrose diet [Cézard et al., 1983; Goda et al., 1985a]. The site of stimulation along the villus-crypt axis of lactase is different from that of sucrase; sucrose

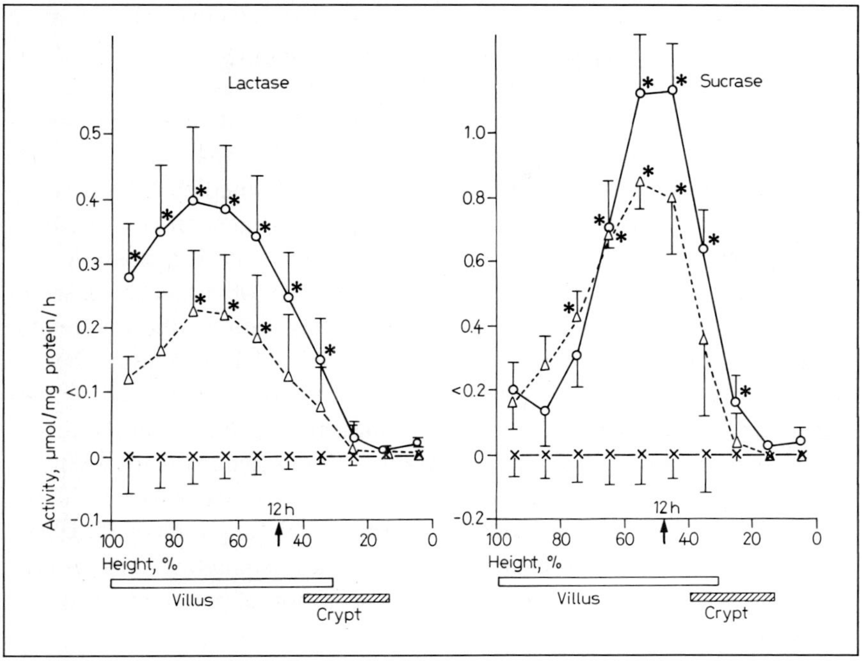

Fig. 16. The difference of lactase and sucrase activity after 12 h force feeding of sucrose and lactose (40 cal%) diet from control along the villus-crypt axis. Abscissa depicts total height of intestinal wall with 100% representing the top part of the villus and 0% the bottom of the serosal side. Means ± SEM are given. Villus and crypt portions are depicted with rectangles; overlapping area is the crypt-villus transition (mix zone). Xs = Control (fed low starch diet, n = 11); circles = sucrose diet (n = 4); triangles = lactose diet (n = 4). Reproduced with permission [Goda et al., 1985a].

stimulates sucrase activity predominantly in the lower villus, whereas lactase activity is stimulated at the broader and more apical (fig. 16) locus of villus [Goda et al., 1985a]. Feeding of lactose diet, as compared with sucrose, produces a similar stimulatory effect on sucrase and lactase activities when digestible amount of lactose (20–40 cal%) is fed. Feeding of high (70 cal%) lactose diet produces diarrhea in rats and results in a decrease in lactase activity [Goda et al., 1985a]. The similarity between the effect of sucrose and lactose suggests the importance of the common constituting monosaccharide, i.e. glucose. This is supported by the finding that force feeding of glucose diets also increases sucrase and lactase activities within 12 h in rats previously fed low starch, high fat diet [Goda et al., 1985a].

However, other monosaccharides, i.e. fructose and galactose, also increase lactase and sucrase activity. Further similar stimulatory effects are seen by feeding nonmetabolizable, but actively transported, sugars, i.e. α-methyl glucoside and 3-0-methyl glucose [Goda et al., 1985b; Goda et al., manuscript in preparation]. Therefore, some factor other than carbohydrate-derived energy might be involved in carbohydrate-mediated increase of lactase and sucrase activity. The mechanism of this general carbohydrate effect on disaccharidase activities is not clear. However, it is possible that some types of sugars affect the metabolic process of disaccharidases at more than one step. For example, sucrose affects both synthesis rate and degradation rate of sucrase [Riby and Kretchmer, 1984]. Providing there is a common regulatory step of disaccharidase metabolism affected by various sugars (including nonmetabolizable sugars), it is likely that the degradation step on brush border membrane is modified by carbohydrate. Recently, it has been shown in rats that intake of low carbohydrate diets, either with high protein [Goda et al., 1988b] or high fat [Goda et al., 1986], leads to an acceleration of degradation of sucrase-isomaltase. This is possibly due (at least partially) to a change in secretion of pancreatic proteinases [Goda et al., 1988b].

Samulitis [1986] demonstrated that the increase of disaccharidase activities induced by a sucrose diet occurred independently of diurnal variation. Thus, it appears that dietary adaptation and diurnal variation of disaccharidase activities do not share a common mechanism.

Thornburg et al. [1987] compared the responsiveness of small intestinal disaccharidases in middle-aged (12-month-old) rats with that of 3-month-old rats. Rats fed a standard laboratory diet from weaning to 3 or 12 months of age were fed a low (5 cal%) starch, high fat diet for 2 weeks and then fed a high (70 cal%) starch, low fat diet for up to 4 weeks. The initial carbohydrate-induced increases of specific activity of sucrase, maltase and lactase were identical in both age groups. Interestingly, with the exception of lactase, the middle-aged rats were unable to sustain the prolonged increases observed in younger animals.

The studies mentioned above have been conducted in rats. The dependency on carbohydrate intake of lactase activity has been reported in mice where glucose was used as carbohydrate source [Flores et al., 1987]. Therefore, the dependency on carbohydrate of lactase activity appears to be common in rats and mice, i.e. rodents. A recent study performed in young pigs [Flores et al., 1986] has shown that although sucrase activity is increased by carbohydrate (starch) intake, lactase activity is not influenced. Thus, the effect of carbohydrate intake on lactase activity in pigs is different from that in rats and mice.

In human subjects, Rosensweig and Herman [1968, 1969b, 1970] reported that diets with varying amounts of carbohydrate (glucose and sucrose) do not affect lactase activity. This conclusion was later supported by Greene et al. [1975]. However, in these studies, only subjects with high lactase activity in adulthood were used. In most mammalian species, lactase activity declines during the weanling period [Koldovsky, 1981]. Many populations of humans have a high incidence of lactose malabsorption in adulthood. Thus, lactase deficiency in adulthood is not abnormal, whereas high lactase activity in adults is considered to be more of a trait of evolution. It is possible, therefore, that lactase activity in those adults with high lactase activity is regulated by different mechanisms than those with low lactase activity. For example, starvation caused a decrease in lactase activity in subjects with high lactase activity, but it did not change lactase activity in those with low lactase activity [Knudsen et al., 1968a].

In contrast to lactase, studies in human subjects [Rosensweig and Herman, 1968, 1969b, 1970; Greene et al., 1975] have shown that activity of α-glucosidase, i.e. sucrase and maltase, is influenced by change of quality and quantity of carbohydrate in diet in a way which is similar to that discussed in rats. Both sucrose and glucose in the diets increase sucrase and maltase activities in a dose-dependent manner [Rosensweig and Herman, 1970]. Intravenous glucose administration (for a 4-day period) does not produce an increase in sucrase and maltase activities in subjects previously fed (for 5 days) a carbohydrate-free, high fat diet [Greene et al., 1975]. Following intravenous glucose administration, the feeding of a 50-cal% glucose diet led to an approximately 100% increase in sucrase and maltase activities in human subjects [Greene et al., 1975]. A diet containing sucrose elicits higher sucrase and maltase activities than a diet containing glucose [Rosensweig and Herman, 1968]. Rosensweig and Herman [1969b] studied the time required for the change in jejunal sucrase activity of human subjects; change of diets from glucose to sucrose or fructose led to an increase in sucrase activity detectable within 2–3 days and completed in about 5 days (there were no further changes 9 weeks thereafter). Since the time response for the change in sucrase activity was similar to intestinal cell turnover time, the authors proposed that the changes in sucrase activity caused by alteration of sucrose intake are mediated via the crypt cell [Rosensweig and Herman, 1969b].

The longer period required for change in sucrase activity in human subjects (than that observed in rats might partially reflect the difference of rate of migration of intestinal epithelial cells between humans and rats; the turnover rate of human intestinal cells is approximately 5 days [Shorter et al., 1964; McDonald et al., 1964], whereas that of rat intestinal cells is 2–3 days.

Long-Term Dietary Adaptation of Disaccharidases

The effect of changes in the quality of carbohydrates has been compared in long-term experiments. Many studies have been devoted to the question of inducibility of lactase in adults. Although earlier studies [Plimmer, 1906; Heilskov, 1951] utilized crude methods for lactase determination, it was clearly demonstrated that lactase activity in adult mammals (rats, rabbits, guinea pigs and pigs) is not induced to the level observed in suckling periods by the feeding of milk or a diet containing lactose. This concept was confirmed by later studies. However, a relatively small but significant change of lactase activity has been demonstrated in animals fed various kinds of carbohydrates. When a portion of starch or starch/sucrose mixture in the diet is replaced with lactose (approximately 5–30% in post weanling rats), increased lactase activity either in specific activity [Girardet et al., 1964; Cain et al., 1969; Bolin et al., 1969, 1971] or in total activity [Fischer, 1957] was demonstrated in rat jejunum after 5–8 weeks; an increase in sucrase and maltase activity was also reported [Bolin et al., 1971].

The addition of 8% lactose to a standard laboratory diet, as compared with an addition of 8% glucose, does not affect lactase or sucrase activity during 16 weeks of post weanling period in rats [Sriratanaban et al., 1971]. However, the addition of 30% lactose to the diet increased specific activity of jejunal lactase in adult rats after 12 weeks when compared with rats fed a 30% glucose diet or a standard laboratory diet. The activity of lactase in rats fed a 30% glucose diet was twice as high as that in rats fed a standard laboratory diet [Bolin et al., 1969]. When the effect of lactose (30%) in diet was compared with that of glucose/galactose mixture (30%), no difference in lactase, sucrase or maltase activity was observed during 11 weeks after birth [Leichter, 1973].

Jones et al. [1972] compared the effect of lactose, sucrose and glucose in adult rats. In this experiment, 68% carbohydrate diets containing only one type of carbohydrate (lactose, sucrose or glucose) was fed for 1–12 weeks. After 2 weeks of feeding the lactose diet, lactase-specific activity was twice as high as that of animals fed glucose or sucrose diets. Interestingly, sucrase specific activity was also higher in animals fed a lactose diet. In contrast, Reddy et al. [1968] have reported in weanling rats that feeding of liquid diets containing 47–71% (solid weight) of either lactose, sucrose, maltose or glucose produced a differential effect on lactase, sucrase, maltase and trehalase activity, respectively. The rats fed a diet containing lactose, as compared with those fed a glucose diet, exhibited a 36% higher activity of lactase at the age of 30 days; this difference was no longer present at the age of 60 days. At 60 days of age, sucrase activity in rats fed a sucrose diet was higher than rats fed glucose or lactase, whereas maltase and trehalase activities were high in rats fed a maltose diet as compared with those of rats fed glucose, sucrose or lactose. Similar effects were seen in germ-free rats [Reddy et al., 1968].

The studies mentioned above, except for those of Reddy et al. [1968], suggested that lactase activity may be modified by the nature of carbohydrate in the diet in rats, but the effect is not specific to lactase, i.e. activity of α-glucosidases is also affected. It should be noted that weaning to a lactose-containing diet in rats led to a high level of sucrase activity as compared with rats weaned to a sucrose diet at 28 days of age [Henning and Guerin, 1981]. Although a decline of lactase activity during the weaning period in rats cannot be prevented, it was suggested that the decrease of lactase activity could be delayed by dietary manipulation in rats [Reddy et al., 1968]. Lebenthal et al. [1973] examined daily changes of lactase activity in two groups of rats between days 18 and 26 postnatally. One group had access to a solid diet in addition to mothers' milk, the other had access only to mothers' milk (i.e. prolonged nursing). The latter of the two groups exhibited the higher specific lactase activity during the period studied (fig. 17).

The inevitability of the decrease of lactase activity during weaning is suggestive of genetic 'programming'. In this aspect, important results of two different experimental arrangements have to be considered: those of Reddy et al. [1968] demonstrating that postnatal consumption of lactose is not necessary for the existence of lactase activity, as well as those of Ferguson et al. [1973] and Kendall et al. [1979] reporting the presence of lactase activity in fetal intestinal isografts which had never had direct contact with lactose. The mechanism of this maturational decline of lactase activity is not clear at present. Tsuboi et al. [1981, 1985a] proposed (using rats as experimental models) that reductions in enterocyte life span (from 7–10 days to 2–3 days), and not suppressed synthesis, could possibly serve as the causal basis of lactase decline in the postweaned mammal.

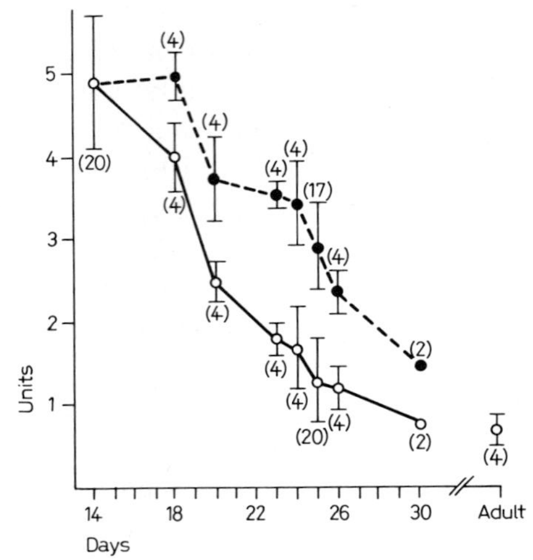

Fig. 17. Developmental pattern of lactase activity in rat jejunum. Activity is expressed as μmole of lactase hydrolyzed/mg of protein/h. Numbers in parentheses indicate number of animals studied in each age group. Each value represents mean ± SD. Prolonged nursing (closed circles); controls (open circles). Reproduced with permission [Lebenthal et al., 1973].

The mechanism whereby lactose affects lactase activity in weaning rats will be discussed herein. Lebenthal et al. [1973] demonstrated that in vitro incubation of small intestinal explants obtained from 10-day-old rats with medium containing lactose prevented the decrease of lactase activity as compared with media containing saline, glucose or sucrose. The authors suggested that lactose might protect lactase from degradation. Further, Jonas et al. [1987] demonstrated with small intestinal explants from 6-day-old rabbits that supplementation of aqueous phase of human breast milk doubled specific activities of lactase and maltase within 7 h. The active substance was identified as being lactose. Since the rate of overall protein synthesis was not increased in explants in the supplemented culture medium, the authors speculated that lactose might affect degradation rate rather than synthesis rate of these disaccharidases.

As described above, many studies exploring the effects of lactose on lactase activity were conducted using rats as the animal model. A few reports dealth with the same question in other animal species. Calves fed whole milk with supplemented 5 or 15% lactose from 3 to 77 days of age exhibited a dose-dependent increase of jejunal lactase activity [Huber et al., 1964]. Ekstrom et al. [1976] found no effect of diet containing 40% dried whey (approximately 30% lactose) on activity of mucosal lactase in pigs after 21-day feeding trials.

Studies in Monkeys. Wen et al. [1973] reported by using the lactose tolerance test that three species of adult monkeys (squirrel, rhesus and galago) were intolerant to an oral load of lactose whereas adult cebus monkeys were tolerant. The lactose intolerant adult galago monkeys were fed either a diet containing 20% lactose and 22% dextrin or a diet containing 42% dextrin. After 4 months, the lactose-fed animals exhibited a higher lactase activity in the jejunum and ileum. It is noteworthy in the light of the data reviewed from similar experiments in rats (see above), that sucrase, maltase and palatinase activities were practically the same in both groups.

Studies in Human Subjects. The question of substrate specific effects on small intestinal disaccharidase activities has been explored in humans. Rosensweig and Herman [1968] reported that a liquid diet containing sucrose elicited higher sucrase and maltase activities than a diet containing glucose at 1–4 weeks after the start of experiments; lactase activity was not modified by sucrose feeding as compared to glucose feeding. The effect of fructose was similar to that of sucrose. However, lactose, galactose or maltose (examined in one subject) did not increase sucrase and maltase activity as compared to glucose. These results suggest that the substrate of sucrase, i.e. sucrose, can alter specific activity of sucrase in human small intestine in a specific manner. The hypothesis that fructose (produced by hydrolysis of sucrose) might be the principal modulator of sucrase activity was supported by the study of Schmitz et al. [1972]. They demonstrated that in fructose intolerant children who had consumed a fructose-free diet for more than 14 months, specific activity of jejunal sucrase and isomaltase was half that of normal children. It is interesting to note that activities of lactase and heat resistant maltase (presumably originating from glucoamylase-maltase complex) were unaffected.

In contrast to the effect of dietary sucrose on sucrase activity, lactase activity in human small intestine does not seem to be dependent on dietary lactose. Complete lactose deprivation in normal caucasian adult subjects for 6 weeks resulted in no change of lactase activity [Knudsen et al., 1968b]. Adult subjects with low lactase activity given large amounts of milk (at least 0.5 l/day) or lactose (at least 50 g/day) daily for several months remained with low lactase activity and/or lactose intolerant [Cuatrecasas et al., 1965; Keusch et al., 1969b; Kretchmer, 1971; Gilat, 1971; Gilat et al., 1972]. Further, galactosemic patients (7–17 years of age) maintained on a lactose-free diet since early infancy showed no evidence of lactase 'deficiency' as measured by the lactose tolerance test [Kogut et al., 1967].

In populations with predominant lactase deficiency in adulthood, consumption of milk is low in general. Postweaning decline of lactase activity in these populations is not prevented by daily consumption of milk [Keusch et al., 1969a; Bolin et al., 1970]. Thus, postweaning decline of lactase activity is rather genetically determined and is not a result of adaptational change. A selective adult type lactase deficiency seems to be inherited by a single autosomal recessive gene [Sahi and Launiala, 1977]. Although postweaning decline of lactase activity is not prevented, there is a possibility that this decline may be modified by milk consumption. In a retrospective study, Bolin et al. [1970] found that lactose intolerance appeared at an earlier age in children who consumed less than 20 g lactose per day after the age of 9 months.

From the studies discussed above, it can be concluded that lactose intake does not exert a profound effect on lactase activity in adulthood. Lactase in human small intestine is not an adaptive enzyme in the sense that lactase is not induced by its substrate, i.e. lactose. However, it is still an open question whether lactase activity in human small intestine is modified by any dietary challenge.

Functional Significance of Dietary Mediated Change of Disaccharidase Activities

Digestion of oligo- and disaccharides and absorption of constituting monosaccharides occur sequentially in the brush border membranes of small intestinal epithelial cells. The question has been raised: Which step is the rate-limiting step? If the rate of monosaccharide absorption is relatively slow compared with rate of hydrolysis of disaccharide (i.e. monosaccharide absorption is rate-limiting), accumulated monosaccharide would inhibit hydrolysis of the disaccharide [Alpers and Cote, 1971], and the level of disaccharidase activity might not be directly related to the rate of overall digestion-absorption process of a disaccharide. Therefore, there should be a certain level of disaccharidase activity (relative to the capacity of monosaccharide absorption) below which the change in disaccharidase activity is directly reflected (by a change) in the rate of absorption of the disaccharide. To answer the question whether disaccharidase activities is the rate-limiting step and whether dietary change in disaccharidase activity is functionally significant in the overall disaccharide digestion/absorption process, several studies compared the absorption rate of disaccharides and the corresponding disaccharidase activities.

Deren et al. [1967] showed by using an intestinal perfusion technique that sucrose hydrolysis in vivo increased twofold and fructose absorption increased fourfold in rats fed sucrose diet for 34 h after 3 days fasting when compared to either fasted or casein-fed rats. Yamada et al. [1986] evaluated absorption of sucrose, maltose and glucose in everted jejunal segments of rats by measuring the change in transmural potential differences evoked by sucrose, maltose and glucose, respectively (fig. 18). After 3–5 days of fasting, decreases in specific and total activity of sucrase and maltase was accompanied by decreases in sucrose and maltose absorption. However, glucose absorption was also decreased in starved rats. The decrease in absorption of glucose, sucrose and maltose was observed within 24 h after the start of starvation when sucrase and maltase activities were similar to those in nonstarved rats. Refeeding of laboratory standard diet in starved rats exhibited a parallel increase of enzyme activities of sucrase and maltase and absorption of glucose, sucrose and maltose [Yamada et al., 1986]. Therefore, the changes of maltose and sucrose absorption appeared to be directly related to changes in glucose absorption and not to change of sucrase and maltase activity; thus, sucrase and maltase activity does not appear to be the rate-limiting step in starved and refed rats. A similar conclusion was obtained in a recent study by Leichter et al. [1987] whereas no correlation between sucrase activity and sucrose absorption in vitro was observed in rats starved 16 and 72 h. Shinohara et al. [1986] reported that the increase of sucrase and maltase activity induced by increased intake of starch was accompanied by an increase of sucrose and maltose absorption in everted jejunal segments of rats (evaluated by transmural difference). In this study, glucose absorption was also increased by a greater starch intake. Since absorption of trehalose was increased in rats fed a high starch diet whereas trehalase activity was not modified, it was apparent that change in glucose absorption produced a profound effect on disaccharide absorption. Therefore, it is not clear from these studies at which (low) level of sucrase and maltase activity the hydrolysis of sucrose

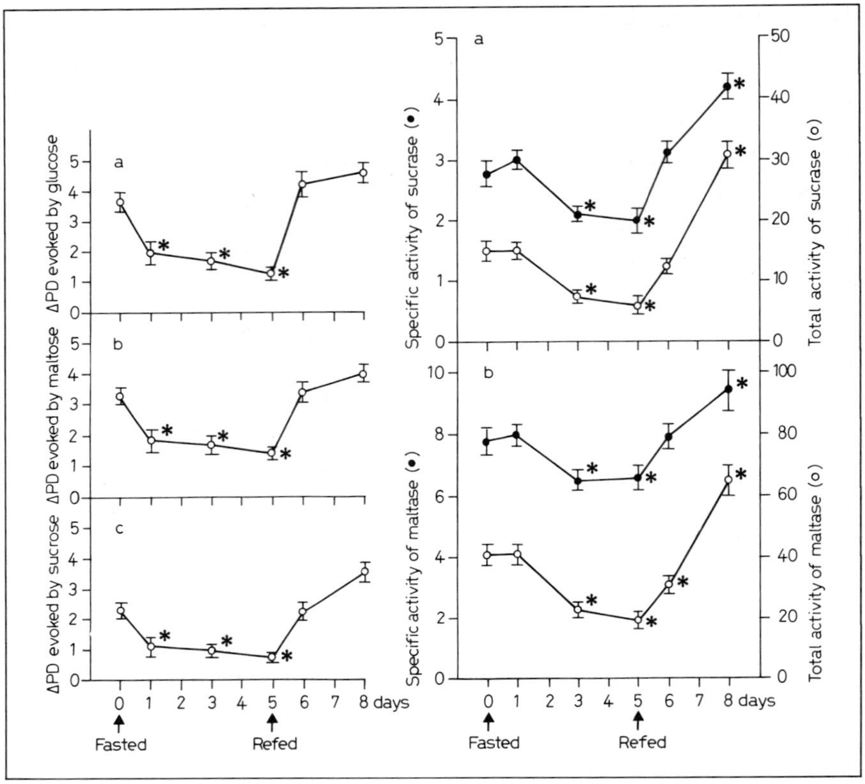

Fig. 18. Left Panel: Transmural potential difference (ΔPD) evoked by glucose, maltose or sucrose in the rat jejunum during fasting and refeeding. Results are expressed as means ± SE of 7–15 animals. ΔPD was measured at the concentration of 20 m*M* glucose (*a*), 10 m*M* maltose (*b*) or 40 m*M* sucrose (*c*) in the standard solution containing 50 m*M* Na_2SO_4 (pH 7.4). *Significantly different from control at $p < 0.05$. Right Panel: Sucrase and maltase activities in the rat jejunum during fasting and refeeding. Results are expressed as means ± SE of 7–15 animals. Enzyme activities were measured in the homogenate of jejunal mucosa after the measurement of ΔPD. Substrate concentration was 40 m*M* sucrose (*a*) or 10 m*M* maltose (*b*) in the standard solution (pH 7.4). *Significantly different from control at $p < 0.05$. Specific activity, μmol substrate/mg protein/h. Total activity, μmol substrate/cm gut/h. Reproduced with permission [Yamada et al., 1986].

and maltose becomes the rate-limiting step. It appears that at present the increase in sucrase activity over the level seen in normal rats fed standard laboratory diet (2–3 μmol/mg protein/h) would not be functionally significant as suggested by Bury [1972]. In order to determine the level of sucrase activity below which sucrose hydrolysis is rate-limiting in sucrose absorption, an experimental condition which affects only the hydrolysis step (but not glucose transport) is required. An inhibitor of α-glucosidases, such as acarbose [Schmidt et al., 1977; Puls et al., 1977], might be useful for this purpose. Acarbose is a potent competitive type of inhibitor of small intestinal sucrase [Caspary and Graf, 1979; Hanozet et al., 1981; Goda et al., 1981] and glucoamylase [Goda et al., 1981; Moriuchi et al., 1982] that does not affect glucose transport [Hanozet et al., 1981]. Recently, Madariaga et al. [1987] reported that dose-dependent decrease of sucrase activity in the presence of acarbose was reflected in a parallel decrease of blood glucose in portal vein after administration of sucrose solution into isolated jejunal loops of rats. This study suggests that in a decreased level of sucrase activity, sucrase hydrolysis might be a rate-limiting step in the overall digestion/absorption process of sucrose.

In contrast to α-glucosidases (i.e. sucrase-isomaltase, glucoamylase and trehalase), the activity of lactase is low in adulthood in most mammalian species. The few exceptions have been reported in some populations of primates [Wen et al., 1973] and in humans. In adult rats, lactase activity in the jejunum is approximately one third of that of sucrase activity (when a standard laboratory diet is fed). Leichter et al. [1984] studied the relationship between dietary induced increase of lactase activity and lactose absorption in adult rats. In animals fed a high starch diet, lactase specific activity was higher than that in the low starch group. The higher lactase activity in animals fed high starch diet was reflected by higher lactose absorption, determined in vivo (fig. 19) or in everted sac in vitro (fig. 20). In both experiments, significant linear regression was observed between lactase activity and lactose absorption (fig. 21). Further, Leichter et al. [1987] demonstrated recently that by using the everted sac technique, the short-term (3 days) starvation induced increase in lactase activity in rats was reflected in enhanced absorption of lactose. These studies suggest that the increase in lactase activity in adult rats induced by either increased capacity to hydrolyze lactose and absorb the constituting monosaccharides. It should be noted that the range of lactase activity modified in these studies was 0.5–1.0 μmol/mg protein/h. This level of lactase activity is comparable to or even higher than that of jejunal biopsies obtained from human subjects with 'lactase deficiency' [Lebenthal et al., 1975; Welsh et al., 1978]. Therefore, it is possible that a change in lactase activity in human subjects with 'lactase deficiency' could be functionally significant whereas a change in lactase activity in human subjects without 'lactase deficiency' might not.

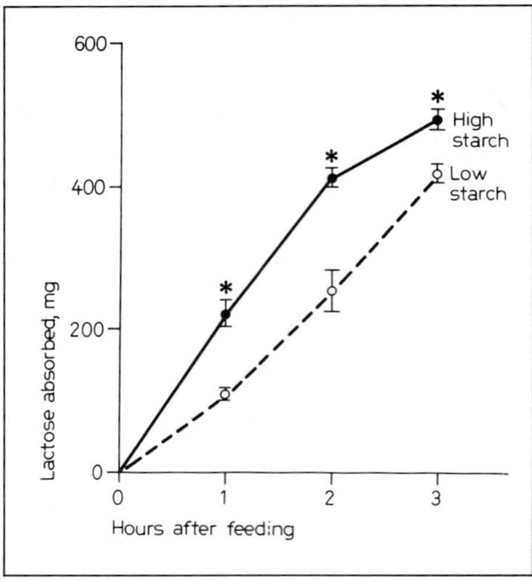

19

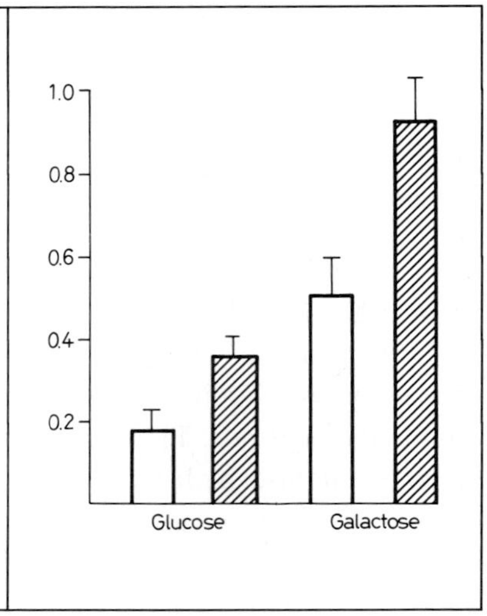

20

Fig. 19. Effect of feeding low starch and high starch diets for 7 days on intestinal lactose absorption. Rats were given 600 mg of lactose orally at time 0. Amount of lactose absorbed was calculated from amount of lactose and galactose remaining in gastrointestinal tract. Mean ± 2 SE are given. Number of animals = 4–5/group. *Significantly different from low starch groups at $p < 0.01$. Reproduced with permission [Leichter et al., 1984].

Fig. 20. Serosal appearance of monosaccharides in everted small intestinal sacs from rats fed low and high starch diets. Results are expressed as means ± SE for 11 animals per group. Absorption of galactose and glucose from lactose by everted sac was significantly different ($p < 0.01$) between animals on low and high starch diets. Open bars = low starch diet; hatched bars = high starch diet. Ordinate: glucose in μmoles/100 mg intestine. Reproduced with permission [Leichter et al., 1984].

Concluding Remarks

A considerable amount of information has been accumulated regarding the adaptive response of small intestinal disaccharidases. Sucrase and maltase activities are closely dependent on the quantity and nature of dietary carbohydrate. Dietary regulation of lactase may be variable among species. Little is known about the regulation of trehalase activity. Most of the studies have described only the changes in enzyme activities, the mechanisms of which are still unclear. The molecular and cellular basis of dietary related change of disaccharidases needs to be elucidated. For discussion on the molecular basis, the absolute amount, i.e. immunoreactive amount,

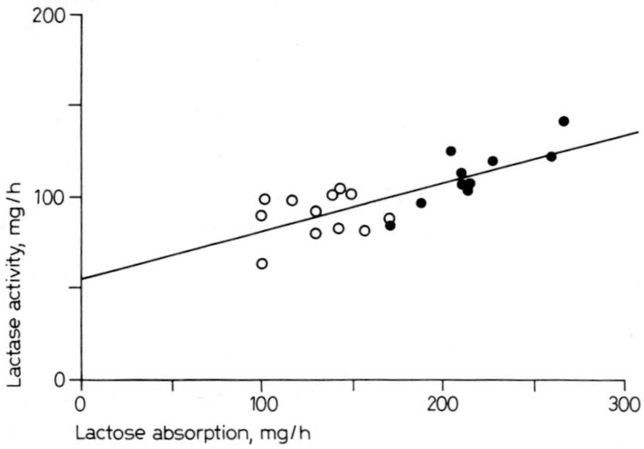

Fig. 21. Linear regression between lactose absorption in vivo and lactase activity in small intestine of rats fed high starch diet (closed circle) and low starch diet (open circle). Lactase activity was expressed as total activity in upper two thirds of small intestine (mg lactose hydrolyzed/h/segment), $n = 22$, $r = 0.77$, $p < 0.001$. Lactase activity $= 0.267 \times$ lactose absorption $+ 54.2$. Reproduced with permission [Leichter et al., 1984].

rather than enzyme activity of disaccharidases is required. This line of studies involves determination of rates of metabolite processes of disaccharidases in small intestinal epithelial cells and determination of specific mRNA. Although some established adenocarcinoma cell lines express disaccharidase activities, i.e. caco cells [Pinto et al., 1983], attempts at primary culture of normal villus cells of adult animals have not succeeded [Quaroni and May, 1980]. This is one of the major obstacles in exploring the mechanisms of dietary regulation of small intestinal disaccharidases. More investigation needs to be encouraged in this area to deal with the problem.

It has been clearly established that some hormone, e.g. corticosterone in rats, rather than dietary factors plays a critical role in expression of sucrase activity during the postnatal period [Lebenthal et al., 1972; Herbst and Koldovsky, 1972; Raul et al., 1981; Goda et al., 1985c]. However, it is not clear whether dietary related change of disaccharidase activities in adult mammals involves changes in hormonal status. Adrenal hormones are the only ones that have been examined. Adrenalectomy does not prevent a carbohydrate-induced increase of activity of sucrase [Deren et al., 1967; Goda et al., 1984a] and lactase [Goda et al., 1984b] in rat jejunum. The possible involvement of other hormones, especially gastrointestinal hormones, should be explored in future studies.

The other line of studies should explore the functional significance of dietary related change of disaccharidase activity. The exact relation between digestive process of carbohydrate and absorptive process of constituting monosaccharidase is not clear. Both of these processes might be regulated by the concentration of substrate available in the microenvironment on the brush border membrane. The microenvironment present in vivo may not be reproduced in vitro. Further, starch digestion process is probably more complicated in the actual situation than is expected. Although change in sucrase activity over a certain level does not seem to be functionally significant for digestion and absorption of sucrose, this does not necessarily indicate that change in sucrase activity (and the amount of sucrase-isomaltase) is not functionally significant for digestion and absorption of *all* carbohydrates.

References

Alpers, D.H.; Cote, M.N.: Inhibition of lactose hydrolysis by dietary sugars. Am. J. Physiol. *221:* 865–868 (1971).

Alpers, D.H.; Tedesco, F.J.: The possible role of pancreatic proteases in the turnover of intestinal brush border proteins. Biochim. biophys. Acta *401:* 28–40 (1975).

Altmann, G.G.: Morphological effects of a large single dose of cycloheximide on the intestinal epithelium of the rat. Am. J. Anat. *143:* 219–240 (1975).

Beam, H.E.; Henning, S.J.: Development of the circadian rhythm of jejunal sucrase activity in the weanling rat. Am. J. Physiol. *235:* E437–E442 (1978).

Bernard, A.; Carlier, H.: Inhibition of protein synthesis and intestinal absorptive cell ultrastructure in cycloheximide or puromycin-treated rats. Repro. Nutr. Develop. *25:* 451–464 (1985).

Blair, D.G.R.; Yakimets, W.; Tuba, J.: Rat intestinal sucrase. II. The effects of rat age and sex and of diet on sucrase activity. Can. J. Biochem. Physiol. *41:* 917–929 (1963).

Bolin, T.D.; Davis, A.E.; Seah, C.S.; Chua, K.L.; Yong, V.; Kho, K.M.; Siak, C.L.; Jacob, E.: Lactose intolerance in Singapore. Gastroenterology *59:* 76–84 (1970).

Bolin, T.D.; McKern, A.; Davis, A.E.: The effect of diet on lactase activity in the rat. Gastroenterology *60:* 432–437 (1971).

Bolin, T.D.; Pirola, R.C.; Davis, A.E.: Adaptation of intestinal lactase in the rat. Gastroenterology *57:* 406–409 (1969).

Bolles, R.C.; Stokes, L.W.: Rat's anticipation of diurnal and a-diurnal feeding. J. comp. physiol. Psychol. *60:* 290–294 (1965).

Boyle, J.T.; Celano, P.; Koldovský, O.: Demonstration of a difference in expression of

maximal lactase and sucrase activity along the villus in the adult rat jejunum. Gastroenterology *70:* 503–507 (1980).
Boyle, J.T.; Kelly, K.; Krulich, L.; Koldovský, O.: Site of thyroxine-evoked decrease of jejunal lactase in the rats. Am. J. Physiol. *243:* G359–G364 (1982).
Bury, K.D.: Carbohydrate digestion and absorption after massive resection of the small intestine. Surgery Gynec. Obstet. *135:* 177–187 (1972).
Bustamante, S.; Gasparo, M.; Kendall, K.; Coates, P.; Brown, S.; Sonawane, B.; Koldovský, O.: Increased activity of rat intestinal lactase due to increased intake of α-saccharides (starch, sucrose) in isocaloric diets. J. Nutr. *111:* 943–953 (1981).
Bustamante, S.; Goda, T.; Koldovský, O.: Dietary regulation of intestinal glucohydrolases in adult rats: comparison of the effect of solid and liquid diets containing glucose polymers, starch or sucrose. Am. J. clin. Nutr. *43:* 891–897 (1986).
Cain, G.D.; Moore, P., Jr.; Patterson, M.; McElveen, M.A.: The stimulation of lactase by feeding lactose. Scand. J. Gastroent. *4:* 545–550 (1969).
Caspary, W.F.; Graf, S.; Inhibition of human intestinal α-glucoside-hydrolases by a new complex oligosaccharide. Res. exp. Med. *175:* 1–6 (1979).
Celano, P.; Jumawan, J.; Koldovský, O.: Thyroxine-evoked decrease of jejunal lactase activity in adult rats. Gastroenterology *73:* 425–428 (1977).
Cézard, J.-P.; Broyart, J.P.; Cuisinier-Gleizes, P.; Mathieu, H.: Sucrase-isomaltase regulation by dietary sucrose in the rat. Gastroenterology *84:* 18–25 (1983).
Cézard, J.-P.; Conklin, K.A.; Das, B.C.; Gray, G.M.: Incomplete intracellular forms of intestinal surface membrane sucrase-isomaltase. J. biol. Chem. *254:* 8969–8975 (1979).
Cuatrecasas, P.; Lockwood, D.H.; Caldwell, J.R.: Lactose deficiency in the adult. A common occurrence. Lancet *i:* 14–18 (1965).
Danielsen, E.M.; Skovbjerg, H.; Noŕen, O.; Sjöström, H.: Biosynthesis of microvillar proteins. Nature of precursor forms of microvillar enzymes from Ca^{2+}-precipitated enterocyte membranes. FEBS Lett. *132:* 197–200 (1981).
Danielsen, E.M.; Skovbjerg, H.; Noŕen, O.; Sjöström, H.: Biosynthesis of intestinal microvillar protein. Intracellular processing of lactase-phlorizin hydrolase. Biochem. biophys. Res. Commun. *122:* 82–90 (1984).
Deren, J.J.; Broitman, S.A.; Zamcheck, N.: Effect of diet upon intestinal disaccharidases and disaccharide absorption. J. clin. Invest. *46:* 186–195 (1967).
Ecknauer, R.: Starvation and sucrase activity in small intestinal mucosa. An evaluation of different tissue preparations and reference systems. Biomedicine *29:* 129–133 (1978).
Ekstrom, K.E.; Grummer, R.H.; Benevenga, N.J.: Effects of a diet containing 40% dried whey on the performance and lactase activities in the small intestine and cecum of hampshire and chester white pigs. J. Ani. Sci. *42:* 106–113 (1976).
Ferguson, A.; Gerskowitch, V.P.; Russell, R.I.: Pre- and postweaning disaccharidase patterns in isografts of fetal mouse intestine. Gastroenterology *64:* 292–297 (1973).
Fischer, J.E.: Effects of feeding a diet containing lactose upon β-*D*-galactosidase activity and organ development in the rat digestive tract. Am. J. Physiol. *188:* 49–53 (1957).
Flores, C.; Bezerra, J.; Goda, T.; Bustamante, S.; MacDonald, M.P.; Kaplan, M.; Koldovský, O.: Effect of a high dextrose diet on sucrase and lactase activity in jejunum of obese mice (C57 BL/6J obob). J. Am. Coll. Nutr. *5:* 565–575 (1987).

Flores, C.; Bezerra, J.; Goda, T.; Bustamante, S.; Pongratz, G.; Koldovský, O.: Effect of diet on intestinal sucrase, lactase, and maltase activity in pigs. Am. J. clin. Nutr. *43:* abstr. No. 124 (1986).

Furuya, S.; Sitren, H.S.; Zeigen, S.; Offord, C.E.; Stevenson, N.R.: Alterations in the circadian rhythmicity of rat small intestinal functions. J. Nutr. *109:* 1962–1973 (1979).

Galand, G.: Purification and characterization of kidney and intestinal brush border membrane trehalases from the rabbit. Biochim. biophys. Acta *789:* 10–19 (1984).

George, D.E.; Lebenthal, E.; Landis, M.; Lee, P.C.: Circadian rhythm of the pancreatic enzymes in rats: its relation to small intestinal disaccharidase. Nutr. Res. *5:* 651–662 (1985).

Gilat, T.: Lactase – an adaptive enzyme? Gastroenterology *60:* 346–347 (1971).

Gilat, T.; Russo, S.; Gelman-Malachi, E.; Aldor, T.A.M.: Lactase in man: nonadaptable enzyme. Gastroenterology *62:* 1125–1127 (1972).

Girard-Globa, A.; Bourdel, G.; Lardeux, B.: Regulation of protein synthesis and enzyme accumulation in the rat pancreas by amount and timing of dietary protein. J. Nutr. *110:* 1380–1390 (1980).

Girardet, P.P.; Richterich, R.; Antener, I.: Adaptation de la lactase intestinale à l'administration de lactose chez le rat adulte. Helv. physiol. Acta *22:* 7–14 (1964).

Goda, T.; Bustamante, S.; Grimes, J.; Koldovský, O.: Dietary induced increase of lactase activity in adult rats is independent of adrenals. Experientia *40:* 1287–1288 (1984a).

Goda, T.; Bustamante, S.; Koldovský, O.: Dietary regulation of intestinal lactase and sucrase in adult rats: quantitative comparison of effect of lactose and sucrose. J. pediat. Gastroenterol. Nutr. *4:* 998–1008 (1985a).

Goda, T.; Bustamante, S.; Koldovský, O.: Effect of feeding various monosaccharides on the activity and the immunoreactive amount of lactase and sucrase in adult rat jejunum. Pediat. Res. *19:* 219A (1985b).

Goda, T.; Bustamante, S.; Thornburg, W.; Koldovský, O.: Dietary-induced increase of lactase activity and in immunoreactive lactase in adult rat jejunum. Biochem. J. *221:* 261–263 (1984b).

Goda, T.; Koldovský, O.: Evidence of degradation process of sucrase-isomaltase in jejunum of adult rats. Biochem. J. *229:* 751–758 (1985).

Goda, T.; Koldovský, O.: Role of pancreatic proteases in degradation of lactase and sucrase-isomaltase in rat jejunum. Am. J. clin. Nutr. *43:* abstr. No. 48 (1986).

Goda, T.; Quaroni, A.; Koldovský, O.: Characterization of degradation process of sucrase-isomaltase in rat jejunum with monoclonal antibody-based enzyme-linked immunosorbent assay (ELISA). Biochem. J. *250:* 41–46 (1988a).

Goda, T.; Raul, F.; Gossé, F.; Koldovský, O.: Short-term effects of a high protein-low carbohydrate diet on the degradation of sucrase-isomaltase in adult rat jejunoileum. Am. J. Physiol., in press (1988b).

Goda, T.; Samulitis, B.K.; Koldovský, O.: Effect of starch intake on degradation process of sucrase-isomaltase in jejunum of rats. Fed. Proc. *45:* 539 (1986).

Goda, T.; Yamada, K.; Bustamante, S.; Edmond, J.; Grimes, J.; Koldovský, O.: Precocious increase of sucrase activity by carbohydrates in the small intestine of suckling rats. I. Significance of the stress effect of sugar-induced diarrhea. J. pediat. Gastroenterol. Nutr. *4:* 468–475 (1985c).

Goda, T.; Yamada, K.; Bustamante, S.; Koldovský, O.: Dietary-induced rapid decrease of microvillar carbohydrase activity in rat jejunoileum. Am. J. Physiol. *245:* G418–G423 (1983).

Goda, T.; Yamada, K.; Hosoya, N.; Moriuchi, S.: Effect of α-glucosidase inhibitor BAY g 5421 on rat intestinal disaccharidases. Food Nutr. (in Japanese) *34:* 139–144 (1981).

Gorostiza, E.; Marche, C.; Broyart, J.P.; Balmain, N.; Cézard, J.P.: Influence of starvation on sucrase regulation by dietary sucrose in the rat. Am. J. clin. Nutr. *40:* 1017–1022 (1984).

Grand, R.J.; Chong, D.A.; Isselbacher, K.J.: Intracellular processing of disaccharidases: the effect of actinomycin D. Biochim. biophys. Acta *261:* 341–352 (1972).

Grand, R.J.; Jaksina, S.: Additional studies on the regulation of carbohydrate-dependent enzymes in the jejunum: changes in amino acid pools, protein synthesis, and the effect of actinomycin-D. Gastroenterology *64:* 429–437 (1973).

Gray, G.M.; Lally, B.C.; Conklin, K.A.: Action of intestinal sucrase-isomaltase and its free monomers on an α-limit dextrin. J. biol. Chem. *254:* 6038–6043 (1979).

Greene, H.L.; Stifel, F.B.; Hagler, L.; Herman, R.H.: Comparison of the adaptive changes in disaccharidase, glycolytic enzyme and fructose diphosphatase activities after intravenous and oral glucose in normal men. Am. J. clin. Nutr. *28:* 1122–1125 (1975).

Hanozet, G.; Pircher, H.-P.; Vanni, P.; Oesch, B.; Semenza, G.: An example of enzyme hysteresis. The slow and tight interaction of some fully competitive inhibitors with small intestinal sucrase. J. biol. Chem. *256:* 3703–3711 (1981).

Hauri, H.-P.: Use of monoclonal antibodies to investigate the intracellular transport and biogenesis of intestinal brush-border proteins. Biochem. Soc. Transact. *14:* 161–163 (1986).

Heilskov, N.S.C.: Studies on animal lactase. II. Distribution in some of the glands of the digestive tract. Acta physiol. scand. *24:* 84–89 (1951).

Henning, S.J.; Guerin, D.M.: Role of diet in the determination of jejunal sucrase activity in the weanling rats. Pediat. Res. *15:* 1068–1072 (1981).

Herbst, J.; Koldovský, O.: Cell migration and cortisone induction of sucrase activity in jejunum and ileum. Biochem. J. *127:* 795–800 (1972).

Huber, J.T.; Rifkin, R.J.; Keith, J.M.: Effect of level of lactose upon lactase concentrations in the small intestines of young calves. J. Dairy Sci. *97:* 789–792 (1964).

Hunziker, W.; Spiess, M.; Semenza, G.; Lodish, H.F.: The sucrase-isomaltase complex: primary structure, membrane-orientation, and evolution of a stalked, intrinsic brush border protein. Cell *46:* 227–234 (1986).

James, W.P.T.; Alpers, D.H.; Gerber, J.E.; Isselbacher, K.J.: The turnover of disaccharidases and brush border proteins in rat intestine. Biochim. biophys. Acta *230:* 194–203 (1971).

Jonas, A.; Oren, M.; Diver-Haber, A.; Kaplan, B.; Passwell, J.: Effects of the components of breast milk on mucosal enzyme activity of the newborn small intestine. Pediat. Res. *21:* 126–130 (1987).

Jones, D.P.; Sosa, F.R.; Skromak, E.: Effects of glucose, sucrose, and lactose on intestinal disaccharidases in the rat. J. Lab. clin. Med. *79:* 19–30 (1972).

Kaufman, M.A.; Korsmo, H.A.; Olsen, W.A.: Circadian rhythm of intestinal sucrase activity in rats. J. clin. Invest. *65:* 1174–1181 (1980).

Kelly, J.J.; Alpers, D.H.: Properties of human intestinal glucoamylase. Biochim. biophys. Acta *315:* 113–120 (1973).

Kendall, K.; Jumawan, J.; Koldovský, O.: Development of jejunoileal differences of activity of lactase, sucrase and acid β-galactosidase in isografts of fetal rat intestine. Biol. Neonate *36:* 206–214 (1979).

Kerzner, B.; Kelly, M.H.; Gall, D.G.; Butler, D.G.; Hamilton, J.R.: Transmissible gastroenteritis: sodium transport and the intestinal epithelium during the course of viral enteritis. Gastroenterology *72:* 457–461 (1979).

Keusch, G.T.; Troncale, F.J.; Miller, L.H.; Promadhat, V.; Anderson, P.R.: Acquired lactose malabsorption in Thai children. Pediatrics *43:* 540–545 (1969a).

Keusch, G.T.; Troncale, F.J.; Thavaramara, B.; Prinyanont, P.; Anderson, P.R.; Bhamarapravathi, N.: Lactase deficiency in Thailand: Effect of prolonged lactose feeding. Am. J. clin. Nutr. *22:* 638–641 (1969b).

Kim, Y.S.; McCarthy, D.M.; Lane, W.; Fong, W.: Alterations in the levels of peptide hydrolases and other enzymes in brush-border and soluble fractions of rat small intestinal mucosa during starvation and refeeding. Biochim. biophys. Acta *321:* 262–273 (1973).

Kimura, T.; Seto, A.; Yoshida, A.: Effect of diets on intestinal disaccharidase and leucineaminopeptidase activities in refed rats. J. Nutr. *108:* 1087–1097 (1978).

Knudsen, K.B.; Bradley, E.M.; Lecocq, F.R.; Colonel, L.; Bellamy, H.M.; Welsh, J.D.: Effect of fasting and refeeding on the histology and disaccharidase activity of the human intestine. Gastroenterology *55:* 46–51 (1968a).

Knudsen, K.B.; Welsh, J.D.; Kronenberg, R.S.; Vanderveen, J.E.; Heidelbaugh, N.D.: Effect of a nonlactose diet on human intestinal disaccharidase activity. Am. J. dig. Dis. *13:* 593–597 (1968b).

Kogut, M.D.; Donnell, G.N.; Shaw, K.N.F.: Studies of lactose absorption in patients with galactosemia. J. Pediat. *71:* 75–81 (1967).

Koldovský, O.: Developmental, dietary and hormonal control of intestinal disaccharidases in mammals (including man); in Randle, Steiner, Whelan, Carbohydrate metabolism and its disorders, vol. 3, pp. 482–522 (Academic Press, London 1981).

Koldovský, O.; Sunshine, P.; Kretchmer, N.: Cellular migration of intestinal epithelia in suckling and weaned rats. Nature *212:* 1389–1390 (1966).

Kretchmer, N.: Memorial lecture: lactose and lactase – a historical perspective. Gastroenterology *61:* 805–813 (1971).

Lebenthal, E.; Antonowicz, I.; Shwachman, H.: Correlation of lactase activity, lactose tolerance test and milk consumption in different age groups. Am. J. clin. Nutr. *28:* 595–600 (1975).

Lebenthal, E.; Sunshine, P.; Kretchmer, N.: Effect of carbohydrate and corticosteroids on activity of α-glucosidases in intestine of the infant rat. J. clin. Invest. *51:* 1244–1250 (1972).

Lebenthal, E.; Sunshine, P.; Kretchmer, N.: Effect of prolonged nursing on the activity of intestinal lactase in rats. Gastroenterology *64:* 1136–1141 (1973).

Leblond, C.P.; Stevens, C.E.: The constant renewal of the intestinal epithelium of the albino rat. Anat. Rec. *100:* 357–378 (1948).

Leese, H.J.; Semenza, G.: On the identity between the small intestinal enzymes phlorizin hydrolase and glycosylceramidase. J. biol. Chem. *248:* 8170–8173 (1973).

Leichter, J.: Effect of dietary lactose on intestinal lactase activity in young rats. J. Nutr. *103:* 392–396 (1973).

Leichter, J.; Goda, T.; Bhandari, S.D.; Bustamante, S.; Koldovský, O.: Relation between dietary-induced increase of intestinal lactase activity and lactose digestion and absorption in adult rats. Am. J. Physiol. *247:* G729–G735 (1984).

Leichter, J.; Goda, T.; Koldovský, O.: Dependency of lactase absorption on lactase activity in starved rats. Can. J. Physiol. Pharmacol. *65:* 2287–2290 (1987).

Loran, M.R.; Althausen, T.L.: Cellular proliferation of intestinal epithelia in the rat two months after partial resection of the ileum. J. biophys. biochem. Cytol. *7:* 667–672 (1960).

MacDonald, W.C.; Trier, J.S.; Everett, N.B.: Cell proliferation and migration in stomach, duodenum and rectum of man: radioautographic studies. Gastroenterology *46:* 405–417 (1964).

Madariaga, H.; Lee, P.C.; Heitlinger, L.; Lebenthal, E.: Carbohydrate (C) hydrolysis as the determining step in the uptake of disaccharides (DS) absorption in normal rat intestine (Abstract). Mead Johnson Nutritional Division of Research for Pediatric Gastroenterology, Annual Pediatric Gastroenterology Research Forum for Pediatric Gastroenterologists (Mead Johnson, Phoenix 1987).

Markiewicz, A.; Kaminski, M.; Chocilowski, W.; Gomoluch, T.; Boldys, H.; Skrzypek, B.: Circadian rhythms of four marker enzymes activity of the jejunal villi in man. Histochem. Acta *72:* 91–99 (1983).

McCarthy, D.M.; Nicholson, J.A.; Kim, Y.S.: Intestinal enzyme adaptation to normal diets of different composition. Am. J. Physiol. *239:* G445–G451 (1980).

McNeill, L.K.; Hamilton, J.R.: The effect of fasting on disaccharidase activity in the rat small intestine. Pediatrics *47:* 65–72 (1971).

Moriuchi, S.; Bunya, Y.; Endo, S.; Kamai, K.; Yoshizawa, S.; Goda, T.; Hosoya, N.: The effect of α-glucosidase inhibitor (acarbose) feeding on rat intestinal disaccharidases. J. Jap. Soc. Nutr. Food Sci. *35:* 351–356 (1982).

Nakano, M.; Sumi, Y.; Miyakawa, M.: Purification and properties of trehalase from rat intestinal mucosal cells. J. Biochem. *81:* 1041–1049 (1977).

Nishida, T.; Saito, M.; Suda, M.: Parallel between circadian rhythms of intestinal disaccharidases and food intake of rats under constant lighting conditions. Gastroenterology *74:* 224–227 (1978).

Nördström, C.; Dahlqvist, A.: Qualitative distribution of some enzymes along the villi and crypts of human small intestine. Scand. J. Gastroent. *8:* 407–416 (1973).

Nördström, C.; Dahlqvist, A.; Josefsson, L.: Quantitative determination of enzymes in different parts of the villi and crypts of rat small intestine. Comparison of alkaline phosphatase, disaccharidases and dipeptidases. J. Histochem. Cytochem. *15:* 713–721 (1967).

Nördström, C.; Koldovský, O.; Dahlqvist, O.: Localization of β-galactosidases and acid phosphatase in the small intestinal wall: comparison of adult and suckling rat. J. Histochem. Cytochem. *17:* 341–347 (1969).

Nsi-Emvo, E.; Launay, J.-F.; Raul, F.: Modulation by thyroxine of the amount of lactase protein in the jejunum of adult rats. Enzyme *36:* 216–220 (1986).

Nsi-Emvo, E.; Raul, F.: Stimulation of lactase synthesis induced by starvation in the jejunum of adult rat. Enzyme *31:* 45–49 (1984).

Pinto, M.; Robine-Leon, S.; Appay, M.-D.; Kedinger, M.; Triadou, N.; Dussaulx, E.;

Lacroix, B.; Simon-Assmann, P.; Haffen, K.; Fogh, J.; Zweibaum, A.: Enterocyte-like differentiation and polarization of the human colon carcinoma cell line Caco-2 in culture. Biol. Cell *47:* 323–330 (1983).

Plimmer, R.H.A.: On the presence of lactase in the intestines of animals and on the adaptation of the intestine to lactose. J. Physiol., Lond. *35:* 20–31 (1906).

Powell, G.K.; McElveen, M.A.: Effect of prolonged fasting on fatty acid and re-esterification in rat intestinal mucosa. Biochim. biophys. Acta *369:* 8–15 (1974).

Puls, W.; Keup, U.; Krause, H.P.; Thomas, G.; Hoffmeister, F.: Glucosidase inhibition. A new approach to the treatment of diabetes, obesity, and hyperlipoproteinaemia. Naturwissenschaften *64:* S536 (1977).

Quaroni, A.; May, R.J.: Establishment and characterization of intestinal epithelial cell cultures. Methods Cell Biol. *21B:* 403–427 (1980).

Raul, F.; Decken, A. von der: Modulation of RNA polymerase activities in the intestine of adult rats by dietary sucrose. J. Nutr. *113:* 2134–2140 (1983).

Raul, F.; Decken, A. von der: Dietary sugar promotes gene activation in intestinal cell chromatin of adult rats. Experientia *40:* 364–365 (1984).

Raul, F.; Decken, A. von der: Changes in chromatin structure and transcription activity by starvation and dietary sucrose in mature and immature intestinal epithelial cells of the rat. Cell. mol. Biol. *31:* 299–304 (1985).

Raul, F.; Kedinger, M.; Simon, P.M.; Grenier, J.-F.; Haffen, K.: Comparative in vivo and in vitro effect of mono- and disaccharides on intestinal brush border enzyme activities in suckling rats. Biol. Neonate *39:* 200–207 (1981).

Raul, F.; Launay, J.-F.: Stimulation of intestinal chromatin template activity by dietary carbohydrates in adult rats. Experientia *39:* 166–167 (1983).

Raul, F.; Noriega, R.; Doffoel, M.; Grenier, J.-F.; Haffen, K.: Modifications of brush border enzyme activities during starvation in the jejunum and ileum of adult rats. Enzyme *28:* 328–335 (1982a).

Raul, F.; Noriega, R.; Nsi-Emvo, E.; Doffoel, M.; Grenier, J.-F.: Lactase activity is under hormonal control in the intestine of adult rat. Gut *24:* 648–652 (1983).

Raul, F.; Pousse, A.; Grenier, J.-F.; Haffen, K.: La stimulation de l'activité de la saccharase par le saccharose est-elle sous la dépendance d'une synthèse d'acides ribonucléiques dans l'intestin de rat adulte? Gastroentérol. clin. biol. *6:* 424–429 (1982b).

Raul, F.; Simon, P.M.; Kedinger, M.; Grenier, J.-F.; Haffen, K.: Effect of sucrose refeeding on disaccharidase and aminopeptidase activities of intestinal villus and crypt cells in adult rats. Evidence for a sucrose-dependent induction of sucrase in the crypt cells. Biochim. biophys. Acta *630:* 1–9 (1980).

Reddy, B.S.; Pleasants, J.R.; Wostmann, R.S.: Effect of dietary carbohydrates on intestinal disaccharidases in germ free and conventional rats. J. Nutr. *95:* 413–419 (1968).

Riby, J.; Galand, G.: Rat intestinal brush border membrane trehalase: some properties of the purified enzyme. Compar. Biochem. Physiol. *82B:* 821–827 (1985).

Riby, J.E.; Kretchmer, N.: Effect of dietary sucrose on synthesis and degradation of intestinal sucrase. Am. J. Physiol. *246:* G757–G763 (1984).

Riby, J.E.; Kretchmer, N.: Participation of pancreatic enzymes in the degradation of intestinal sucrase-isomaltase. J. Ped. Gastroenterol. Nutr. *4:* 971–979 (1985).

Rosensweig, N.S.; Herman, R.H.: Control of jejunal sucrase and maltase activity by dietary sucrose or fructose in man. A model for the study of enzyme regulation in man. J. clin. Invest. *47:* 2253–2262 (1968).

Rosensweig, N.S.; Herman, R.H.: Diet and disaccharidases. Am. J. clin. Nutr. *22:* 99–102 (1969a).
Rosensweig, N.S.; Herman, R.H.: Time response of jejunal sucrase and maltase activity to a high sucrose diet in normal man. Gastroenterology *56:* 500–505 (1969b).
Rosensweig, N.S.; Herman, R.H.: Dose response of jejunal sucrase and maltase activities to isocaloric high and low carbohydrate diets in man. Am. J. clin. Nutr. *23:* 1373–1377 (1970).
Sahi, T.; Launiala, K.: More evidence for the recessive inheritance of selective adult type lactose malabsorption. Gastroenterology *73:* 231–232 (1977).
Saito, M.: Daily rhythmic changes in brush border enzymes of the small intestine and kidney in rat. Biochim. biophys. Acta *286:* 212–215 (1972).
Saito, M.; Kato, H.; Suda, M.: Circadian rhythm of intestinal disaccharidases of rats fed with adiurnal periodicity. Am. J. Physiol. *238:* G97–G101 (1980).
Saito, M.; Murakami, E.; Nishida, T.; Fujisawa, Y.; Suda, M.: Circadian rhythms in digestive enzymes in the small intestine of rats. I. Patterns of the rhythms in various regions of the small intestine. J. Biochem. *78:* 475–480 (1975).
Saito, M.; Murakami, E.; Nishida, T.; Fujisawa, Y.; Suda, M.: Circadian rhythms of digestive enzymes in the small intestine of the rat. II. Effects of fasting and refeeding. J. Biochem. *80:* 563–568 (1976a).
Saito, M.; Murakami, E.; Suda, M.: Circadian rhythms in disaccharidases of rat small intestine and its relation to food intake. Biochim. biophys. Acta *421:* 177–179 (1976b).
Saito, M.; Sato, Y.; Suda, M.: Circadian rhythm and dietary response of disaccharidase activities in isolated rat jejunum. Gastroenterology *75:* 828–831 (1978a).
Saito, M.; Suda, M.: Effect of diet on enzymes of the brush border of the small intestine and kidney of rats. J. Nutr. Sci. Vitaminol. *21:* 207–215 (1975).
Saito, M.; Suda, M.: Disaccharidase rhythm in rat small intestine; no relationship with mitosis rhythm. Experientia *34:* 700–701 (1978).
Saito, M.; Suda, M.; Matzuda, H.: Postnatal development of circadian rhythms in disaccharidase activities in rat small intestine. Am. J. Physiol. *234:* E500–E503 (1978b).
Samulitis, B.: Effect of carbohydrate intake on rat small intestinal disaccharidase activities, with special respect to diurnal rhythm; master's thesis, University of Arizona, Tucson (1986).
Sasajima, K.; Kawachi, T.; Sato, S.; Sugimura, T.: Purification and properties of α′-trehalase from the mucosa of rat small intestine. Biochim. biophys. Acta *403:* 139–146 (1975).
Sasaki, M.; Yamada, K.; Goda, T.; Moriuchi, S.; Hosoya, N.: The diurnal rhythm of intestinal digestive enzymes in diabetic rats. J. Jap. Soc. Nutr. Food Sci. *33:* 185–189 (1980).
Schmidt, D.D.; Frommer, W.; Junge, B.; Müller, L.; Wingender, W.; Truscheit, E.: α-Glucosidase inhibitors. New complex oligosaccharides of microbial origin. Naturwissenschaften *64:* 3535 (1977).
Schmitz, J.; Odièvre, M.; Rey, J.: Specificity of the effects of a fructose-free diet on the activity of intestinal α-glucosidases in man. A study in hereditary fructose intolerance. Gastroenterology *62:* 389–392 (1972).
Semenza, G.: Intestinal oligo- and disaccharidases; in Randle, Steiner, Whelan, Carbohy-

drate metabolism and its disorders, vol. 3, pp. 425–479 (Academic Press, London 1981).

Semenza, G.: Anchoring and biosynthesis of stalked brush border membrane proteins; glycosidases and peptidases of enterocytes and of renal tubuli. Annu. Rev. Cell. Biol. *2:* 255–313 (1986).

Shinohara, H.; Tsuji, Y.; Yamada, K.; Hosoya, N.: Effects of carbohydrate intake on disaccharidase activity and disaccharide-evoked transmural potential difference in rat small intestine. J. Jap. Soc. Nutr. Food Sci. *39:* 35–41 (1986).

Shorter, E.G.; Moertel, C.G.; Titus, J.L.; Reitemeier, R.J.: Cell kinetics in the jejunum and rectum of man. Am. J. dig. Dis. *9:* 760–763 (1964).

Siegel, P.S.: Food intake in the rat in relation to the dark-light cycle. J. comp. physiol. Psychol. *54:* 294–301 (1961).

Sjöström, H.; Norén, O.; Christiansen, L.; Wacker, H.; Semenza, G.: A fully active, two active site, single-chain-sucrase-isomaltase from pig small intestine. J. biol. Chem. *255:* 11332–11338 (1980).

Sjöström, H.; Norén, O.; Danielsen, E.M.: Enzymatic activity of 'high-mannose' glycosylated forms of intestinal microvillar hydrolases. J. Ped. Gastroenterol. Nutr. *4:* 980–983 (1985).

Soares, F.C.; Collares, E.F.; Rosario, M.D.; Brasil, L.: Invertase no jejuno do rato: tipos de resposta ao estìmulo com sacarose. Arq. Gastroent. *13:* 89–96 (1976).

Sriratanaban, A.; Symynkywicz, L.A.; Thayer, W.R., Jr.: Effect of physiologic concentration of lactose on prevention of postweaning decline of intestinal lactase. Dig. Dis. *16:* 839–844 (1971).

Stevenson, N.R.; Day, S.E.; Sitren, H.: Circadian rhythmicity in rat intestinal villus length and cell number. Int. J. Chronobiol. *6:* 1–12 (1979).

Stevenson, N.R.; Ferrigni, F.; Parnicky, K.; Day, S.; Fierstein, J.S.: Effect of changes in feeding schedule on the diurnal rhythms and daily activity levels of intestinal brush border enzymes and transport systems. Biochim. biophys. Acta *406:* 131–145 (1975).

Stevenson, N.R.; Fierstein, J.S.: Circadian rhythms of intestinal sucrase and glucose transport: cued by time of feeding. Am. J. Physiol. *230:* 731–735 (1976).

Stevenson, N.R.; Sitren, H.S.; Furuya, S.: Circadian rhythmicity in several small intestinal functions is independent of use of the intestine. Am. J. Physiol. *238:* G203–G207 (1980).

Thornburg, W.; Grimes, J.; Goda, T.; Bustamante, S.; Pollack, P.; Koldovský, O.: The response of activity of jejunal disaccharidases and pancreatic amylase in young and middle aged rats to a high carbohydrate diet. J. Nutr. *117:* 63–69 (1987).

Tsuboi, K.K.; Kwong, L.K.; D'Harlingue, A.E.; Stevenson, D.K.; Kerner, J.A., Jr.; Sunshine, P.: The nature of maturational decline of intestinal lactase activity. Biochim. biophys. Acta *840:* 69–78 (1985a).

Tsuboi, K.K.; Kwong, L.K.; Neu, J.; Sunshine, P.: A proposed mechanism of normal intestinal lactase decline in the postweaned mammal. Biochem. biophys. Res. Commun. *101:* 645–652 (1981).

Tsuboi, K.K.; Kwong, L.K.; Yamada, K.; Sunshine, P.; Koldovský, O.: Nature of elevated rat intestinal carbohydrase activities after high-carbohydrate diet feeding. Am. J. Physiol. *249:* G510–G518 (1985b).

Ulshen, M.H.; Grand, R.J.: Site of substrate stimulation of jejunal sucrase in the rat. J. clin. Invest. *64:* 1097–1102 (1979).

Welsh, J.D.; Poley, J.R.; Bhatia, M.; Stevenson, D.E.: Intestinal disaccharidase activities in relation to age, race, and mucosal damage. Gastroenterology *75:* 847–855 (1978).

Wen, C.-P.; Antonowicz, I.; Tovar, E.; McGandy, R.B.; Gershoff, S.N.: Lactose feeding in lactose-intolerant monkeys. Am. J. clin. Nutr. *26:* 1224–1228 (1973).

Yamada, K.; Abe, M.; Hosoya, N.: Diurnal rhythm of rat intestinal disaccharidase activities along the villus-crypt axis. J. Jap. Soc. Nutr. Food Sci. *38:* 51–56 (1985).

Yamada, K.; Bustamante, S.; Koldovský, O.: Time- and dose-dependency of intestinal lactase activity in adult rat on starch intake. Biochim. biophys. Acta *676:* 108–112 (1981a).

Yamada, K.; Bustamante, S.; Koldovský, O.: Dietary-induced rapid increase of rat jejunal sucrase and lactase activity in all regions of the villus. FEBS Lett. *129:* 89–92 (1981b).

Yamada, K.; Goda, T.; Bustamante, S.; Koldovský, O.: Different effect of starvation on activity of sucrase and lactase in rat jejunoileum. Am. J. Physiol. *244:* G449–G455 (1983).

Yamada, K.; Shinohara, H.; Hyodo, R.; Soneda, F.; Sugiyama, M.; Moriuchi, S.; Yamada, N.; Osumi, M.; Hosoya, N.: Adaptive changes of sugar absorption in rat small intestine during fasting and refeeding. J. clin. Biochem. Nutr. *1:* 39–51 (1986).

Yatvin, M.B.: Action of actinomycin D on the GI tract: Implications for enzyme induction studies. Proc. Soc. exp. Biol. Med. *136:* 1010–1013 (1971).

Zucker, I.: Light-dark rhythms in rat eating and drinking behavior. Physiol. Behav. *6:* 115–126 (1971).

Otakar Koldovský, MD, PhD, Department of Pediatrics,
Arizona Health Sciences Center, Tucson, AZ 85724 (USA)

Subject Index